Advances in Gastroenterology

Editor

FRÉDÉRIC P. GASCHEN

VETERINARY CLINICS OF NORTH AMERICA: SMALL ANIMAL PRACTICE

www.vetsmall.theclinics.com

January 2021 • Volume 51 • Number 1

ELSEVIER

1600 John F. Kennedy Boulevard • Suite 1800 • Philadelphia, Pennsylvania, 19103-2899
http://www.vetsmall.theclinics.com

**VETERINARY CLINICS OF NORTH AMERICA: SMALL ANIMAL PRACTICE Volume 51, Number 1
January 2021 ISSN 0195-5616, ISBN-13: 978-0-323-76187-1**

Editor: Stacy Eastman
Developmental Editor: Nicole Congleton

Veterinary Clinics of North America: Small Animal Practice (ISSN 0195-5616) is published bimonthly by Elsevier Inc., 360 Park Avenue South, New York, NY 10010-1710. Months of issue are January, March, May, July, September, and November. Business and Editorial Offices: 1600 John F. Kennedy Blvd., Ste. 1800, Philadelphia, PA 19103-2899. Customer Service Office: 3251 Riverport Lane, Maryland Heights, MO 63043. Periodicals postage paid at New York, NY and additional mailing offices. Subscription prices are $358.00 per year (domestic individuals), $933.00 per year (domestic institutions), $100.00 per year (domestic students/residents), $451.00 per year (Canadian individuals), $998.00 per year (Canadian institutions), $488.00 per year (international individuals), $998.00 per year (international institutions), $100.00 per year (Canadian students/residents), and $220.00 per year (international students/residents). To receive student/resident rate, orders must be accompanied by name of affiliated institution, date of term, and the *signature* of program/residency coordinator on institution letterhead. Orders will be billed at individual rate until proof of status is received. Foreign air speed delivery is included in all *Clinics* subscription prices. All prices are subject to change without notice. **POSTMASTER:** Send address changes to *Veterinary Clinics of North America: Small Animal Practice*, Elsevier Health Sciences Division, Subscription Customer Service, 3251 Riverport Lane, Maryland Heights, MO 63043. Customer Service (orders, claims, online, change of address): Elsevier Periodicals Customer Service, Elsevier Health Sciences Division Subscription **Customer Service 3251 Riverport Lane Maryland Heights, MO 63043. Tel: 1-800-654-2452 (U.S. and Canada); 314-447-8871 (outside U.S. and Canada). Fax: 314-447-8029. E-mail: journalscustomerservice-usa@elsevier.com (for print support); journalsonlinesupport-usa@elsevier.com (for online support).**

Reprints. For copies of 100 or more of articles in this publication, please contact the Commercial Reprints Department, Elsevier Inc., 360 Park Avenue South, New York, NY 10010-1710. Tel.: 212-633-3874; Fax: 212-633-3820; E-mail: reprints@elsevier.com.

Veterinary Clinics of North America: Small Animal Practice is also published in Japanese by Inter Zoo Publishing Co., Ltd., Aoyama Crystal-Bldg 5F, 3-5-12 Kitaaoyama, Minato-ku, Tokyo 107-0061, Japan.

Veterinary Clinics of North America: Small Animal Practice is covered in *Current Contents/Agriculture, Biology and Environmental Sciences, Science Citation Index, ASCA, MEDLINE/PubMed (Index Medicus), Excerpta Medica,* and *BIOSIS.*

Contributors

EDITOR

FRÉDÉRIC P. GASCHEN, Dr med vet, Dr habil
Diplomate, American College of Veterinary Internal Medicine (Small Animal Internal Medicine); Diplomate, European College of Veterinary Internal Medicine-Companion Animals (Internal Medicine); Professor, Department of Veterinary Clinical Sciences, School of Veterinary Medicine, Louisiana State University, Baton Rouge, Louisiana, USA

AUTHORS

KARIN ALLENSPACH, Dr med vet, PhD, FVH, FHEA, AGAF
Diplomate, European College of Veterinary Internal Medicine (Companion Animals); Professor of Translational Health and Internal Medicine, College of Veterinary Medicine, Iowa State Unversity, Ames, Iowa, USA

KATHRIN BUSCH, DVM, Dr medvet
Diplomate, European College of Veterinary Internal Medicine (Companion Animals); Clinic of Small Animal Medicine, Centre for Clinical Veterinary Medicine, Ludwig-Maximilians-University, München, Germany

JENNIFER CHAITMAN, VMD
Diplomate, American College of Veterinary Internal Medicine (Small Animal Internal Medicine); Veterinary Internal Medicine and Allergy Specialists, New York, New York, USA

JULIEN RODOLPHE SAMUEL DANDRIEUX, BSc, Dr med vet, PhD
Diplomate, American College of Veterinary Internal Medicine (Small Animal Internal Medicine); Lecturer, Department of Veterinary Clinical Sciences, Melbourne Veterinary Schoo, Faculty of Veterinary and Agricultural Sciences, University of Melbourne, Werribee, Victoria, Australia

VALÉRIE FREICHE, DVM, PhD
DESV-MI, Unité de Médecine Interne, CHUVA, Ecole Nationale Vétérinaire d'Alfort, Maisons-Alfort Cedex, France

FRÉDÉRIC P. GASCHEN, Dr med vet, Dr habil
Diplomate, American College of Veterinary Internal Medicine (Small Animal Internal Medicine); Diplomate, European College of Veterinary Internal Medicine-Companion Animals (Internal Medicine); Professor, Department of Veterinary Clinical Sciences, School of Veterinary Medicine, Louisiana State University, Baton Rouge, Louisiana, USA

ALEXANDER J. GERMAN, BVSc, PhD, CertSAM, SFHEA, FRCVS
Diplomate, European College of Veterinary Internal Medicine (Companion Animals); Institute of Life Course and Medical Sciences, University of Liverpool, Neston, Merseyside, United Kingdom

MEGAN GROBMAN, DVM, MS, PhD
Diplomate, American College of Veterinary Internal Medicine (Small Animal Internal Medicine); Assistant Professor, Auburn University, Department of Clinical Sciences, Auburn, Alabama, USA

JUAN HERNANDEZ, Dr med vet, PhD
Diplomate, American College of Veterinary Internal Medicine (Small Animal Internal Medicine); Diplomate, European College of Veterinary Internal Medicine; Associate Professor, Department of Clinical Sciences, Nantes-Atlantic College of Veterinary Medicine and Food Sciences (Oniris), University of Nantes, Nantes, France; Institut Micalis, INRAE, AgroParisTech, Université Paris-Saclay, Jouy-en-Josas, France

ROMAN HUSNIK, MVDr, PhD
Department of Veterinary Clinical Sciences, College of Veterinary Medicine, Purdue University, West Lafayette, Indiana, USA

CHELSEA IENNARELLA-SERVANTEZ, BS, MS
College of Veterinary Medicine, Iowa State University, Ames, Iowa, USA

AARTI KATHRANI, BVetMed (Hons), PhD, FHEA, MRCVS
Diplomate, American College of Veterinary Internal Medicine; Diplomate, American College of Veterinary Nutrition; Royal Veterinary College, Hatfield, Hertfordshire, United Kingdom

PETER HENDRIK KOOK, PD, Dr med. vet
Diplomate, American College of Veterinary Internal Medicine; Diplomate, European College of Veterinary Internal Medicine (Companion Animals); Faculty Member, Department of Small Animals, Clinic for Small Animal Internal Medicine, Vetsuisse Faculty, University of Zurich, Zurich, Switzerland

SINA MARSILIO, Dr med vet, PhD
Diplomate, American College of Veterinary Internal Medicine (Small Animal Internal Medicine); Diplomate, European College of Veterinary Internal Medicine (Companion Animals); Department of Veterinary Medicine and Epidemiology, UC Davis School of Veterinary Medicine, Davis, California, USA

SILKE SALAVATI SCHMITZ, Dr med vet, PhD, FHEA, MRCVS
Diplomate, European College of Veterinary Internal Medicine (Companion Animals); Senior Lecturer in Small Animal Internal Medicine, Hospital for Small Animals, Royal (Dick) School of Veterinary Studies, The Roslin Institute, College of Medicine and Veterinary Medicine, University of Edinburgh, Easter Bush, Midlothian, United Kingdom

JAN S. SUCHODOLSKI, Dr med vet, PhD, AGAF
Diplomate, American College of Veterinary Microbiologists; Gastrointestinal Laboratory, College of Veterinary Medicine, Texas A&M University, College Station, Texas, USA

M. KATHERINE TOLBERT, DVM, PhD
Diplomate, American College of Veterinary Internal Medicine; Clinical Associate Professor, Texas A&M University, Gastrointestinal Laboratory, College Station, Texas, USA

STEFAN UNTERER, DVM, Dr med vet, Dr habil
Diplomate, European College of Veterinary Internal Medicine (Companion Animals); Clinic of Small Animal Medicine, Centre for Clinical Veterinary Medicine, Ludwig-Maximilians-University, München, Germany

ANNA-LENA ZIESE, Dr med vet
Clinic of Small Animal Medicine, Ludwig Maximilian University of Munich, Munich, Germany

Contents

 Video content accompanies this article at http://www.vetsmall.
theclinics.com.

Esophagitis in cats and dogs is a consequence of increased exposure of the esophageal mucosa to gastroduodenal reflux. Causes can include anesthesia-related reflux, frequent vomiting, or lodged foreign bodies. An exception is eosinophilic esophagitis, an emerging primary inflammatory disease of the esophagus with a presumed allergic etiology. Reflux esophagitis owing to lower esophageal sphincter incompetence is often suspected; a tentative diagnosis can be made by endoscopic assessment, wireless esophageal pH-monitoring, or histologic examination. Because it can be difficult to distinguish diet-responsive upper gastrointestinal disease from esophagitis, response to treatment with gastric acid suppressants is needed to confirm the tentative diagnosis.

 Video content accompanies this article at http://www.vetsmall.
theclinics.com.

Aerodigestive disorders (AeroDs) in people encompass a wide range of clinical syndromes, reflecting the complex relationship between the respiratory and digestive tracts. In veterinary medicine, aspiration is used interchangeably with aspiration pneumonia. Although aspiration pneumonia is a common disorder in dogs, it does not reflect the breadth of AeroDs. Unfortunately, AeroDs rarely are investigated in veterinary medicine because of lack of clinical recognition, limitations in available diagnostics, and the fact that AeroDs may be caused by occult digestive disease. Recognizing patients with AerodD represents an area of significant clinical importance that may provide additional areas of clinical intervention.

A range of gastroprotective drugs are available for the treatment of esophagitis and gastroduodenal mucosal injury including acid suppressants (ie, histamine-2 receptor antagonists, proton pump inhibitors), coating agents, prostaglandin analogs, and antacids. Of these, the proton pump inhibitors are the most effective drugs for the medical treatment of upper gastrointestinal injury. However, proton pump inhibitors are not effective for all causes of upper gastrointestinal injury. The choice of gastroprotective drug should be guided by the cause and location of gastrointestinal injury and the potential for adverse effects.

Gastric motility disorders present both diagnostic and therapeutic challenges and likely are under-recognized in small animal practice. This review includes a comparative overview of etiopathogenesis and clinical presentation of gastric motility disorders, suggests a practical approach to the diagnosis of these conditions, and provides an update on methods to evaluate gastric motor function. Furthermore, management of gastric dysmotility is discussed, including a review of the documented effect of gastric prokinetics.

In addition to presenting with respiratory signs, many dogs with brachycephalic airway obstructive syndrome show digestive tract signs related to the same conformational abnormalities. A detailed diagnostic investigation is usually required, including clinicopathologic analyses, thoracic radiographs, fluoroscopic studies, abdominal ultrasound examinations and both upper airway and gastrointestinal tract endoscopy. In most cases, medical therapies are successful in managing clinical signs, but surgery can occasionally be required to resolve hiatal hernia or pyloric stenosis. In determining prognosis, the features of each individual case should be considered, with the overall prognosis depending on the severity and extent of all the identified lesions.

Acute hemorrhagic diarrhea syndrome is defined as sudden onset of severe bloody diarrhea frequently associated with vomiting, which results in severe, sometimes life-threatening dehydration. Although there is strong evidence that clostridial overgrowth and toxin release is responsible for the pathogenesis of the disease, the diagnosis is still based on exclusion of other causes for acute hemorrhagic diarrhea. With early and appropriate treatment, mainly based on fluid therapy, the prognosis is good and complications such as sepsis or severe hypoalbuminemia rarely occur.

Differentiation of feline inflammatory bowel disease and intestinal small cell lymphoma can be challenging, and some clinicians argue that it is unnecessary because prognosis and treatment are similar. Differentiation of feline inflammatory bowel disease and intestinal small cell lymphoma can be challenging and some clinicians argue that it is unnecessary since prognosis and treatment are similar. Altough the body of research on this topic has increased over time, we still know little about etiopathogenesis, progression, alternative treatment modalities and prognosis of the different forms of FCE. While differentiating IBD from SCL might not alter a single patients' disease course, further research efforts are required to alter the disease course for our feline patient population as a whole.

Canine protein–losing enteropathies occur commonly in small animal practice, and their management is often challenging with a long-term survival rate of only about 50%. Recent studies have investigated prognostic factors that may determine outcome in individual cases. In particular, systemic complications such as hypercoagulability, vitamin D3 deficiency, and tryptophan deficiency may play an important role and should be investigated in severely affected cases in order to maximize outcome.

Nutrition can influence those functions of the gastrointestinal tract that can be adversely affected in chronic enteropathy, such as microbiota, mucosal immune system, intestinal permeability, and motility. Diet serves as a possible risk factor in disease pathogenesis and as a target for treatment in chronic enteropathy. Malnutrition is prevalent in people with inflammatory bowel disease and negatively affects outcome. Approximately two-thirds of dogs with protein-losing enteropathy due to chronic enteropathy or lymphangiectasia are underweight. Commercial diets and home-prepared diets have been used successfully in the management of chronic enteropathy. Fat restriction is the main dietary strategy for intestinal lymphangiectasia.

In this article, we review different tests that have been researched in dogs with chronic enteropathy. The usefulness of these tests either to assess etiology, to differentiate between treatment response, or to monitor treatment response is discussed. The tests are divided in those that are commercially available and those that hold promises for further development.

The intestinal microbiome is an important immune and metabolic organ in health and disease. Recent molecular and metabolomic approaches have provided a better characterization of different types of dysbiosis, including mucosa-adherent bacteria and functional changes in the microbiome. This article summarizes recent advances in assessment of dysbiosis, the importance of the bile acid–converting Clostridium hiranonis as an important beneficial bacterium in the canine gut, and different therapeutic approaches to dysbiosis.

Silke Salavati Schmitz

Probiotics/or synbiotics products for small animals do not fulfill the criteria required to qualify as a probiotic. Studies explaining modes of action are lacking. Outcome measures are inconsistent, with some trials assessing only nonspecific routine diagnostic parameters or fecal scores. Preliminary evidence shows that specific preparations are beneficial in parvovirus infections and acute hemorrhagic diarrhea syndrome in dogs and in Tritrichomonas fetus infection in cats. In dogs, inflammatory bowel disease specific probiotics can decrease clinical severity. More studies focusing on functional outcomes in dogs and cats with well-defined diseases to allow evidence-based clinical use of probiotics and synbiotics are needed.

Jennifer Chaitman and Frédéric Gaschen

In people, fecal microbiota transplantation is recognized as the best treatment modality for recurrent Clostridioides difficile infection, and its value is currently investigated in the treatment of other diseases associated with an abnormal gut microbiome. In dogs, intestinal dysbiosis has been documented in many acute and chronic digestive diseases as well as in diseases of other organ systems. There are only few published studies evaluating the benefits of fecal microbiota transplantation (FMT) in canine gastrointestinal disorders. They provide evidence that FMT may be beneficial in the treatment of acute intestinal diseases and hope that the technique might also be useful for the management of chronic enteropathies.

VETERINARY CLINICS OF NORTH AMERICA: SMALL ANIMAL PRACTICE

FORTHCOMING ISSUES

March 2021
Forelimb Lameness
Kevin P. Benjamino and Kenneth A.
Bruecker, *Editors*

May 2021
Small Animal Nutrition
Dottie Laflamme, *Editor*

July 2021
Working Dogs: An Update for Veterinarians
Maureen McMichael and Melissa
Singletary, *Editors*

RECENT ISSUES

November 2020
Emergency and Critical Care of Small Animals
Elisa M. Mazzaferro, *Editor*

September 2020
Feline Practice: Integrating Medicine and Well-Being (Part II)
Margie Scherk, *Editor*

July 2020
Feline Practice: Integrating Medicine and Well-Being (Part I)
Margie Scherk, *Editor*

SERIES OF RELATED INTEREST

Veterinary Clinics of North America: Exotic Animal Practice
https://www.vetexotic.theclinics.com/

VETERINARY CLINICS OF NORTH AMERICA: SMALL ANIMAL PRACTICE

FORTHCOMING ISSUES

March 2021
Forelimb Lameness
Kevin S. Benjamino and Kenneth A.
Bruecker, Editors

May 2021
Small Animal Nutrition
Dottie Laflamme, Editor

July 2021
Working Dogs: An Update for Veterinarians
Maureen McMichael and Melissa
Singletary, Editors

RECENT ISSUES

November 2020
Emergency and Critical Care of Small
Animals
Elisa M. Mazzaferro, Editor

September 2020
Feline Practice: Integrating Medicine and
Well-Being (Part III)
Margie Scherk, Editor

July 2020
Feline Practice: Integrating Medicine and
Well-being (Part I)
Margie Scherk, Editor

SERIES OF RELATED INTEREST

Veterinary Clinics of No rth America: Exotic Animal Practice
https://www.vetexotic.theclinics.com

THE CLINICS ARE NOW AVAILABLE ONLINE!
Access your subscription at:
www.theclinics.com

Preface

A Much-Needed Update on Digestive Diseases of Cats and Dogs

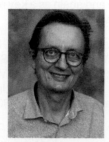

Frédéric P. Gaschen, Dr med vet, Dr habil
Editor

It has been 10 years already since an issue of *Veterinary Clinics of North America: Small Animal Practice* was entirely devoted to gastroenterology. Needless to say, the current issue is long overdue. We have learned a lot since 2011 thanks to research performed both in the laboratory setting and on the clinic floor. For instance, our understanding of the gastrointestinal (GI) microbiome in health and disease has greatly expanded. Also, new technologies, such as pH capsules, have been useful to generate relevant clinical data. Finally, numerous clinical and benchtop studies have been published, for instance, about acute and chronic enteropathies and other common conditions. These advances should help guide our decisions in our daily practice of canine and feline medicine. Therefore, the goal of this issue is to provide the busy clinician with a quick but complete reference on the current knowledge about diagnostic approach and management of a selection of common digestive diseases of cats and dogs.

Numerous authors from around the world have agreed to share their expertise and wisdom in this issue. They have invested a significant amount of time to provide concise state-of-the-art reviews in their fields of research. And they did it while COVID-19 was forcing everyone to do whatever they do very differently or to stop doing it altogether. I am very grateful to them all for their extraordinary commitment under these exceptional circumstances. Thank you also to Nicole Congleton and the staff at Elsevier for their support and for making sure this project would be completed on time.

The contents of this issue will appeal to clinicians dealing with cats and dogs with digestive disorders. The reader will find reviews describing clinical presentation, pathogenesis, diagnostic approach, and management for diseases affecting the esophagus, stomach, and small and large intestine. While some articles summarize the current understanding of conditions, such as esophagitis, acute hemorrhagic diarrhea

Vet Clin Small Anim 51 (2021) xiii–xiv
https://doi.org/10.1016/j.cvsm.2020.09.013
0195-5616/21/© 2020 Published by Elsevier Inc.

vetsmall.theclinics.com

syndrome, and protein-losing enteropathy, other articles explore the relationship be-tween airway and digestive diseases, or the approach and management of GI motility disorders. The optimal use of various ancillary tests in the approach of our GI patients is also discussed. The importance of the GI microbiota in digestive diseases is high-lighted in an eye-opening review. The difficulty in differentiating inflammatory from neoplastic infiltration of the feline gut is addressed in another article. Finally, a group of articles focuses on various key aspects in the management of GI patients, such as protection of the gastric mucosa, benefits of diet and nutrition in chronic intestinal dis-eases, and use of probiotics and fecal microbiota transplantation.

I hope that the reader will use this newest GI issue again and again as a key resource to guide their decisions for their own patients. Happy reading!

Frédéric P. Gaschen, Dr med vet, Dr habil
Department of Veterinary Clinical Sciences
School of Veterinary Medicine
Louisiana State University
Baton Rouge, LA 70803, USA

E-mail address:
fgaschen@lsu.edu

Esophagitis in Cats and Dogs

Peter Hendrik Kook, PD, Dr. med. vet

KEYWORDS

- Esophagitis • Gastroesophageal • Reflux • Esophageal • Biopsy • Dog • Cat

KEY POINTS

- Esophagitis is mostly a consequence of increased exposure to gastroduodenal reflux owing to various primary causes.
- An exception is eosinophilic esophagitis, an emerging primary inflammatory disease of the esophagus with a presumed allergic etiology.
- Clinical signs can vary and it can be difficult to differentiate esophagitis from other upper (mostly food-responsive) gastrointestinal diseases.
- When no extraesophageal disease can explain clinical signs, gastroesophageal reflux disease owing to an incompetent lower esophageal sphincter, similar to the well-known condition in people, is suspected.
- Esophagitis owing to gastroesophageal reflux can be confirmed with wireless esophageal pH-monitoring (Bravo capsule), endoscopy, or esophageal endoscopic biopsies and histology.

 Video content accompanies this article at http://www.vetsmall.theclinics.com.

INTRODUCTION

Esophagitis denotes a localized or diffuse inflammation of the esophageal mucosa. It is generally thought to result from a caustic or chemical (ie, gastric acid, bile acids) injury. In humans, the most frequent mechanism causing esophagitis is gastroesophageal reflux (GER) leading to GER disease (GERD). GERD is thought to result from lower esophageal sphincter (LES) incompetence.[1] In small animal medicine, GERD secondary to a primary functional LES abnormality is poorly understood, most probably because diagnosing GERD based on a detailed questionnaire on perceived symptoms, as it is done in human medicine, is not applicable. The situation becomes even more complicated when considering that the nonerosive form of GERD (ie, absence of visible lesions on esophagoscopy and the presence of reflux-associated symptoms) comprises the majority of patients in human medicine.[1]

Department of Small Animals, Clinic for Small Animal Internal Medicine, Vetsuisse Faculty, University of Zurich, Winterthurerstrasse 260, Zurich 8057, Switzerland
E-mail address: pkook@vetclinics.uzh.ch

Vet Clin Small Anim 51 (2021) 1–15
https://doi.org/10.1016/j.cvsm.2020.08.003
0195-5616/21/© 2020 The Author(s). Published by Elsevier Inc. This is an open access article under the CC BY-NC-ND license (http://creativecommons.org/licenses/by-nc-nd/4.0/).

vetsmall.theclinics.com

It should also be noted in this context that, independent of the cause of esophagitis, esophageal inflammation in itself can cause esophageal hypomotility and thus gastro-esophageal sphincter weakness by impairing the excitatory cholinergic pathways to the gastroesophageal sphincter. In cats, induction of experimental esophagitis has been shown to attenuate the release of acetylcholine and lowered gastroesophageal pressures. These changes were reversible on healing of the esophagus.[2,3]

CONDITIONS ASSOCIATED WITH ESOPHAGITIS

Esophagitis is for the most part not an independent disease in cats and dogs, but develops secondary to gastro(duodenal) reflux, which in turn can have various causes. The most common scenario for esophagitis in cats and dogs is perianesthetic reflux. Clinical signs usually begin a couple of days after anesthesia, and the diagnosis is usually based on a combination of medical history and ensuing clinical signs. It has been reported that intraabdominal procedures have a higher risk for GER, also the duration of preoperative fasting and choice of preanesthetic drugs influence the incidence of GER during anesthesia.[4-7] In extreme cases, lethal esophageal rupture secondary to perianesthetic acid reflux is possible[8]; however no information exists on associations between magnitude of intraoperative esophageal acid exposure and the risk of subsequent esophageal inflammation. Further causes are medication-induced cases of esophagitis. Cats seem to be particularly susceptible to pill-induced esophagitis when receiving peroral medication, and antibiotics such as clindamycin and doxycycline (doxycycline hyclate is known to cause a strong acidic solution [pH 2–3] compared with doxycycline monohydrate) have been frequently implicated.[9,10] Thus, the routine administration of a small water bolus to facilitate esophageal clearance is recommended in this species.[11] Further causes are lodged foreign bodies, frequent vomiting, malpositioned esophageal feeding tubes, and distal esophageal neoplasia (often leiomyoma),[12,13] all of which permit increased exposure of the esophageal mucosa to gastro(duodenal) reflux. Primary gastric hyperacidity conditions such as Zollinger–Ellison syndrome[14,15] or delayed gastric emptying owing to acute pancreatitis or pyloric outflow obstructions can also lead to esophagitis when refluxing gastric contents injure the esophageal mucosa. Hiatal hernias also predispose to esophagitis in dogs and cats because of the altered functional anatomy of the gastroesophageal pressure barrier (loss of the intrinsic support of the crural diaphragm) and impaired esophageal acid (Video 1).[16-18] Hiatal hernias and associated GER resulting from upper airway obstruction are common problems in brachycephalic dog breeds.[19-21] Less commonly, non–breed-specific upper airway obstruction may also cause reflux esophagitis.[22,23] The supposed pathomechanism is the negative intrathoracic pressure generated by increased inspiratory effort. Yeast esophagitis (Candida spp) can rarely develop as a secondary complication in cases of idiopathic megaesophagus owing to the chronic effects of lodging food.

Probably the only primary inflammatory esophageal disease without an underlying condition predisposing to GER is eosinophilic esophagitis (EE). This entity is a recently recognized inflammatory disorder of the esophagus in dogs and cats suspected to be a hypersensitivity disorder that results in marked accumulation of eosinophils within the esophageal tissue.[24,25] Eosinophil presence and activity then results in tissue damage, edema, inflammation, and fibrosis. Only case reports have been reported up to now and it is currently unclear whether EE is underdiagnosed in cats and dogs.

Reflux esophagitis owing to a LES incompetence similar to GERD in humans is also frequently suspected in dogs and cats based on a variety of clinical signs assumed to reflect esophageal pain. Specific diagnostic criteria for GERD are lacking and a tentative diagnosis is made based on clinical and endoscopic findings, exclusion of other esophageal and extraesophageal diseases, and an adequate response to treatment.[18,26-29] The crux is that diagnosing GERD in people is largely based on symptom perception, and ideally a close correlation between reflux and symptom during ambulatory esophageal pH-metry.[1] However, although symptoms are by definition inherently subjective experiences and communicated to the health care professional by the human patient, cats and dogs naturally exhibit clinical signs that can or cannot reflect sensations associated with esophagitis. This is why GERD is mostly a diagnosis of exclusion in our patients and ideally based on a clear response to treatment. Recently, the 3-year incidence of suspected canine GERD presented to a specialty practice was estimated at 0.9%, diagnoses have been based on a combination of historical and clinical signs, as well as radiographic, endoscopic, or histopathologic findings without actual demonstration of increased esophageal reflux events.[29] It is still controversial if GERD is truly an independent disease in cats and dogs, because inflammatory small bowel disease can present with similar clinical signs.[28,30] In the authors' experience, many patients with clinical signs originally attributed to reflux esophagitis have chronic inflammatory enteropathies and can in fact be successfully managed in the long term with dietary changes, high-dose multistrain probiotics or budesonide.

Cats with chronic gingivostomatitis have recently been shown to have a high incidence of concurrent esophagitis based on endoscopy and histology.[31] It remains difficult to determine to what extent esophageal inflammation causes clinical signs in these patients as clinical features are limited and cannot distinguish with certainty stomatitis from esophagitis. Dogs with idiopathic laryngeal paralysis can also have increased acidic reflux events compared with clinically normal dogs with refluxes even reaching the most proximal part of the esophagus.[32] However, these findings were not accompanied by endoscopic evidence of esophagitis and esophageal biopsies were not collected in that study.

CLINICAL SIGNS

Esophagitis may lead to immediate signs caused by inflammation or delayed signs caused by stricture formation. Animals with mild esophagitis may show no clinical signs, whereas animals with more severe esophagitis can show decreased appetite, anorexia, odynophagia or dysphagia, ptyalism, increased empty swallowing motions, extension of head and neck while swallowing, retching, vomiting, regurgitation, sudden unexplained discomfort, belching, drooling, excessive grass eating, or surface licking. Brachycephalic breeds (especially French Bulldogs) usually show a mixture of regurgitation and retching of frothy material mostly during increased activity or excitement.

Clinical signs reported in the literature include retching, gagging, repeated swallowing motions, smacking, discomfort at night, sudden nervousness, restlessness or discomfort, and refusal to eat despite apparent interest in food.[18,24-26,28,29]

Pruritus and other manifestations of allergic skin disease may be seen in cases of EE. Concurrent borborygmi may indicate that it is a small bowel disease after all, even in the absence of diarrhea. Although it would seem to be plausible that the severity of clinical signs depends on the extent and depth of esophageal lesions, they do not always correlate and may vary greatly. Hoarseness, stridor, and cough could reflect injury to the epiglottis, larynx, and upper airway.[30] The onset of anesthesia-associated reflux esophagitis varies from 1 to 3 days to 2 weeks after a causative anesthetic event.[33,34] On physical examination, patients may have evidence of halitosis and laryngeal signs with redness, hyperemia, and edema of the vocal folds and arytenoids. However, the majority of patients have normal physical examinations. Clinical signs of strictures depend on the degree of obstruction; the narrower the stricture the more pronounced is the regurgitation; however, regurgitation also could be caused by painful swallowing. Strictures closer to the pharynx may cause more immediate regurgitation. Mild to moderate strictures may cause no clinical signs until the patient swallows a large food bolus or firm food (**Fig. 1**A, B). Sometimes there is gradual progression in severity as the stricture continues to contract, causing greater luminal narrowing.

Care should be taken to evaluate the respiratory system as, analogous to humans, it is surmised that esophagitis can also cause inflammatory airway disease. Pulmonary manifestations of esophagitis may include aspiration pneumonia, chronic bronchitis, and potentially interstitial pulmonary fibrosis. Concerning this aspect, it is of particular interest to note that idiopathic pulmonary fibrosis is seen nearly exclusively in older West Highland White Terriers, a breed that is at the same time notoriously famous for lodged esophageal foreign bodies.[35–37] Chronic intermittent microaspiration of gastric acid secondary to an esophageal dysmotility may be a contributing causative event in this breed. A recent study found that, although gastric juice microaspirations occurred in various canine respiratory diseases, bile acids measured in bronchoalveolar lavage fluid as a surrogate marker for microaspirations of gastroduodenal content were detected only in healthy West Highland White Terriers.[38]

DIAGNOSIS
Diagnostic Imaging

Although historical and clinical findings may be suggestive of esophagitis, the results of routine laboratory testing are usually normal. Radiography is of limited use for the detection of esophagitis; compatible findings may be mild esophageal dilations or fluid

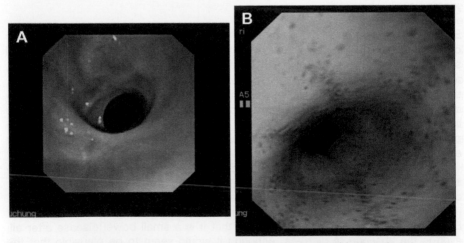

Fig. 1. (*A*) Partial midthoracic esophageal stricture in an 8-year-old King Charles Cavalier Spaniel with esophagitis secondary to a lodged foreign body (chewing bone) that had been sitting in the esophagus for 2 days. The dog started to regurgitate again 5 days after removal of the foreign body when fed a regular amount. Small portion were well-tolerated. (*B*) Distal esophagus of the same dog with multiple brownish dots representing a proliferative response of submucosal glands to increased acidic reflux.

accumulation in the distal esophagus. However, foreign bodies, hiatal hernias, esophageal dilation, ring anomalies, or masses could be detected and a pathologic lung pattern may reflect aspiration injury to the lungs. Mediastinal or pleural air or liquid accumulation may indicate esophageal perforation. If a perforation is considered likely, an iodinated contrast medium should be used instead of barium. Although contrast esophagrams are inexpensive, readily available, and noninvasive tests, they are only useful in demonstrating stenotic narrowing or intramural masses of the esophagus. The sensitivity of barium esophagram to detect esophagitis is low. Mucosal irregularities and a prolonged retention of the contrast medium can be seen with moderate to severe inflammation, whereas milder forms of esophagitis will be missed.[4] Fluoroscopic swallow studies have the benefit to assess esophageal motility during the whole swallow with less of a chance to miss the moment, when the contrast medium passes a narrow point, as could be the case with static images. It is of importance to do wet swallows with liquid contrast medium and dry swallows with a barium–food mixed bolus, because liquids can sometimes pass a partial stricture, whereas a food bolus may be retained. Although swallow studies can assess causes (reflux episodes, hiatal hernia [see Video 1], mural masses) as well as consequences (dysmotility, strictures, reflux episodes) of esophagitis, it is not a useful modality to diagnose esophagitis.

ENDOSCOPY

Endoscopic examination is the most sensitive method to diagnose esophagitis, although reliable endoscopic criteria for diagnosis of esophagitis as well as grading of severity of esophagitis have not been established in small animals. Of note, no descriptive endoscopic work larger than case reports has been published on canine or feline esophagitis, and it is likely that subtle lesions go undetected. Only 1 in 22 dogs presenting with clinical signs attributed to esophagitis also had endoscopic evidence of esophagitis in a recent study.[28] Early signs of esophagitis are erythema and edema usually above the LES (**Fig. 2**), but these findings depend on the quality of endoscopic equipment. Other signs include increased vascularity, because enlarged capillaries develop in response to acid near the mucosal surface (**Fig. 3**A, B). Prolonged acidic injury leads to proliferation of submucosal esophageal glands in dogs,[39] and their excretory ducts can readily be seen as round dots (**Fig. 4**). Another common sign is increased granularity; the mucosal surface seems to be rough and puckered (**Fig. 5**). Findings compatible with severe esophagitis are areas of exudative pseudomembranes and ulcerative mucosa. The esophageal mucosa of published cases of EE of cats and dogs seems to be clearly abnormal with marked proliferative mucosal lesions similar to a cobblestone appearance, friable and hyperemic mucosa with exudative and ulcerated mucosa, and the presence of benign structure formation.[24,25] Typical gross endoscopic findings in humans with EE comprise concentric rings, furrows, exudate, and strictures. However, a normal endoscopic examination has been reported in up to 40% of cases and EE can be missed without biopsies.[40] This author has been actively looking for EE in esophageal biopsies from patients with compatible clinical signs and unremarkable esophageal linings, but has not found a case as of yet. Although typical for reflux esophagitis, circular inflammation just above the LES should not be confused with the squamocolumnar junction (the demarcation line between the squamous esophageal lining and the columnar gastric lining, the so-called z-line), that may seem to be sharply delineated in cats and dogs with erythematous and reddened gastric mucosa. This is especially the case with esophageal overinsufflation. Strictures are usually obvious at endoscopy; exceptions could

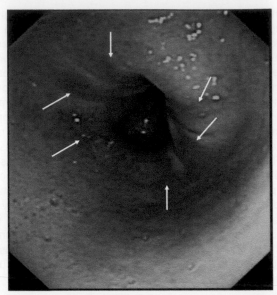

Fig. 2. Distal esophagitis in a 1-year-old male French Bulldog presenting for daily regurgitation. Streaky erosions can be seen just above the LES (*arrows*). Final diagnosis was reflux owing to brachycephalic obstructive airway syndrome.

be large breeds with esophageal diameters much bigger than the scope where strictures could be missed. In these cases, generous air insufflation will usually help to demonstrate the focally reduced esophageal diameter. The endoscopic examination should always include a full gastric inspection with special attention to the cardia and pylorus to exclude underlying abnormality, such as obstructive leiomyoma or radiolucent foreign bodies, to confirm that the esophagitis is the primary problem. Concurrent duodenoscopy and biopsies seems reasonable given the unspecific clinical signs that could also reflect the presence of small bowel disease.

Narrow band imaging uses only blue and green light that is absorbed by vessels but reflected by mucosa, and can better capture the microstructures of the superficial mucosa and reveal subtle changes of patients with esophagitis in human medicine.[41] The value of narrow band imaging has still to be determined in canine and feline esophagitis (**Fig. 6**).

ESOPHAGEAL HISTOLOGY

It could be argued that esophagoscopy without biopsy is insufficient to rule out esophagitis, because cases with grossly normal appearing mucosa on endoscopy and necropsy, but histopathologic evidence of esophagitis, have been reported in cats and dogs.[12,26,31,42,43] This finding is in accordance with findings in humans, where endoscopic findings in patients with GERD vary from no visible mucosal damage (termed nonerosive esophageal reflux disease) to esophagitis, peptic strictures, or Barrett's esophagus.[1] Unfortunately, it can be difficult to obtain adequate esophageal biopsies, except in the more severe cases of esophagitis, because the esophagus is lined with a robust stratified squamous epithelium, and even repeated biopsies with serrated forceps from the same location may yield only epithelial bits. Münster and colleagues[44,45] advocate taking biopsies from the gastroesophageal junction using standard forceps

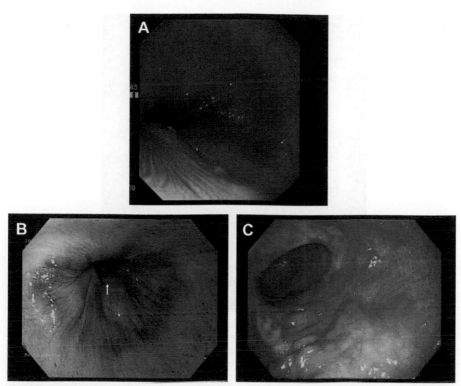

Fig. 3. (*A*) Distal esophagitis just above the LES in a 6-year-old female spayed Bernese Mountaindog presented for inappetence. No cause could be identified. (*B*) Esophagoscopy of a 9-year-old Labrador Retriever presented for increased lip smacking and empty swallowing. There is circumferential increased vascularity around the LES beginning at the Z-line (*white arrow*). Gastroscopy (*C*) of the dog under 3B revealed increased granularity, erythema, and protruding bulges. Histopathology revealed severe lymphocytic gastritis with fibrosis, a differential diagnosis was small cell lymphoma.

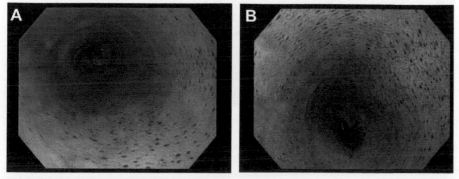

Fig. 4. (*A*) Same dog as in **Fig. 3**B and C. Prolonged acidic injury leads to proliferation of submucosal esophageal glands and their excretory ducts can be seen as round brown spots. (*B*) Narrow band imaging.

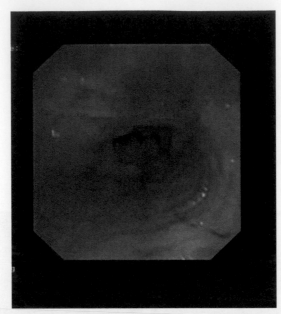

Fig. 5. Distal esophagus of an 18-month-old male neutered Maine Coon cat 14 months after surgical correction (Y-U cardioplasty) and subsequent ballooning of a congenital esophageal stenosis. The cat could eat again and thrived to a normal sized clinically healthy Maine Coon cat. A side effect of the surgery was incomplete closure of the LES, and twice daily omeprazole was prescribed. The esophageal mucosa seems to be edematous, with patchy erythema and increased granularity, the typical ringed structure of the feline esophagus is only partially visible.

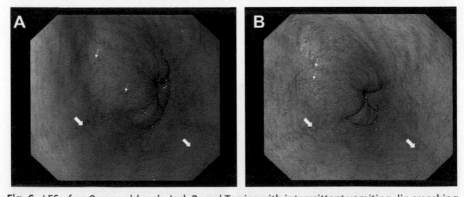

Fig. 6. LES of an 8-year-old male Jack Russel Terrier with intermittent vomiting, lip smacking, and refusal to eat. White light endoscopy (*A*) shows mild mucosal vein dilation (*thin arrows*) and discrete longitudinal stripes (*thick arrows*) reflecting activated excretory ducts of submucosal glands. (*B*) Narrow band imaging (*blue green* endoscopy) accentuates these findings. Wireless esophageal pH-monitoring revealed a fractional time pH less than 4 of 1% (0%–3.1%). Histopathology revealed moderate gastric and duodenal lymphoplasmacytic inflammation. No improvement was seen with gastric acid suppression, and clinical signs finally disappeared with a novel protein diet and budesonide.

for single use with open elliptical branches, and a lancet. Structural microscopic abnormalities such as fibrosis, inflammation, elongation of the stromal papillae, and increased thickness of the basal cell layers can be found in biopsies comprising only the squamous epithelium and the lamina propria mucosae.[27,29] Before the advent of esophageal pH-metry, esophageal histology was used in the research on GERD in people, and hyperplastic thickening of the basal cell layer and abnormal elongation of stromal papillae of the lamina propria were found to reflect excessive regeneration and thus were considered pathognomonic for GERD in humans.[46,47] Histologic evidence of hyper-regeneratory changes in esophageal biopsies was recently also reported in 20 dogs presenting with clinical signs suggestive of reflux esophagitis (**Fig. 7**).[29] So far, the sensitivity of these histologic lesions for the diagnosis reflux esophagitis has not been evaluated against a quantifiable gold standard, such as intraesophageal pH-metry, but the predominant clinical signs regurgitation and ptyalism improved in 8 of 11 dogs with hyper-regeneratory esophagopathy after treatment with proton pump inhibitors.[29] The specificity of esophageal histologic lesions has not been assessed so far, and this endeavor seems to be challenging because clinically silent reflux esophagitis cannot be ruled out with certainty. But still, hyper-regeneratory esophageal lesions were significantly less common in age-matched control dogs (n = 19) undergoing endoscopy for clinical signs unrelated to the esophagus (eg, chronic diarrhea).[29] Clearly, further work is necessary to clarify the prevalence and thus significance of esophageal histologic lesions of cats and dogs. Endoscopic findings of severe chronic acid exposure such as Barrett's esophagus (replacement of the normal squamous epithelium of the distal esophagus with metaplastic columnar epithelium) are exceedingly rare in cats and dogs, further illustrating that GERD might not be as common as in humans.[18,48]

In contrast, the histologic findings of EE seem to be straightforward; eosinophils are not found in the healthy esophagus, making the presence of these cells indicative of disease. Guidelines in humans recommend that a diagnosis of EE is made when a patient presents with symptoms of esophageal dysfunction and esophageal biopsies demonstrate 15 or more eosinophils in a high power field in the absence of competing

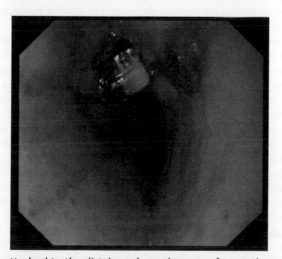

Fig. 7. pH capsule attached to the distal esophageal mucosa for continuous esophageal pH monitoring in a dog with suspicion of reflux esophagitis.

causes such as GERD.[49] Reported eosinophil counts in mucosal biopsies of cats and dogs with EE ranged from 20 to 40 eosinophils per high power field.[24,25]

ESOPHAGEAL pH-METRY

All these procedures may aid in the diagnosis of esophagitis, but still fail to detect and quantify reflux when GERD is suspected. In humans, catheter-free esophageal pH monitoring has become the gold standard in diagnosing GERD. This technique not only provides information on esophageal acid exposure, but is also able to assess symptoms associated with acid reflux episodes. A widely used system in humans is the Bravo system. It includes a small capsule (26.0 mm × 5.5 mm × 6.5 mm) containing an antimony pH electrode with internal reference, miniaturized electronics with radiofrequency transmitter and battery, and a capsule delivery system, as well as an external receiver to monitor intraesophageal pH. This wireless pH monitoring system was found to be a useful tool for extended (generally 4 days; some capsules adhere up to 7 days to the mucosa and esophageal pH measurement can be extended accordingly) ambulatory catheterless esophageal pH monitoring in dogs.[28] Endoscopic capsule placement was quick and easy, and adverse clinical signs have not been observed.[28] Current disadvantages of the system are the high cost of the pH capsule, receiver, and software, as well as the need for brief anesthesia for accurate placement. Our clinical experience indicates that this technique seems to be safe and patients from 6 to 55 kg body weight tolerate the measurements well. The capsule is positioned in the distal esophagus 3 to 5 cm above the LES and attached (ie, pierced) to the mucosa (see **Fig. 7**). Mucosal attachment is achieved by the use of vacuum suction and a lock and pin mechanism. Once released from the delivery system, pH data are recorded by a receiver attached to the dog's collar and owners are instructed to maintain a logbook to record all events presumed to be related to GER. The receiver has so-called symptom buttons that can be individually programmed. At discharge, owners are familiarized with the receiver and instructed to press the appropriate buttons if the dog shows the corresponding clinical signs. An association between clinical signs and reflux is considered positive if the clinical signs occurs within 1 to 2 minutes of the reflux event. In people, the so-called symptom index is defined as the percentage of symptom events that are temporally related to a reflux episode. A symptom index of 50% usually is considered positive.[50]

Our results contradicted the hypothesis that minute amounts of acid can severely damage the esophagus in dogs. In healthy dogs, the number of refluxes (defined as an esophageal pH of <4) and the duration of long refluxes (>5 minutes) varied considerably over the course of 96 hours. The median total number of refluxes was 10 (range, 1–65), the median number of refluxes lasting longer than 5 minutes was 1 (range, 0–4), the median duration of longest reflux was 8 minutes (range, 0–27). The overall fraction time of a pH of less than 4 was low and usually ranged between 0% and 3%.[28] These numbers are actually lower compared with what has been established as normal in humans (4.0%–6.7%).[51,52] Results in dogs with clinical signs commonly attributed to reflux esophagitis were insofar surprising as clinically relevant reflux episodes could not be demonstrated in 17 of 22 suspected dogs and a temporal relationship between clinical signs observed by owners and reflux episodes could also not be established. Still, dogs with clinical signs had overall higher esophageal pH parameters when compared with healthy dogs.[28] A clear limitation of the study was that esophageal pH recordings were available from only 7 healthy control dogs and therefore no robust reference range exists for comparison of esophageal pH data at this point. Another conclusion from that study was that the differential diagnosis diet-responsive enteropathy should be ruled out as best as possible before pursuing treatment for esophagitis, because both diseases can have similar clinical signs.[28] Since that study, we have used this system frequently in dogs with clinical signs suggestive of esophagitis, but could detect abnormal esophageal pH profiles in only a handful of dogs. In fact, complete resolution of clinical signs is rarely achieved with gastric acid suppression alone,[30] and most dogs ultimately respond to dietary changes, probiotics, and less commonly budesonide.

THERAPY

Treatment should ideally be directed at the underlying causes of the esophagitis and it is important to eliminate predisposing factors (eg, oral medication). In case of a chronic obstructive upper respiratory problem, corrective surgery minimizing or eliminating the obstruction may also resolve inflammatory esophageal lesions.[19] The same would apply to hiatal hernias. Because anesthesia is the most common cause of esophagitis, it would be desirable to prevent acidic reflux in patients undergoing anesthesia, especially in those that already have a history of anesthesia-related esophagitis. Pretreatment with high doses of metoclopramide yielded conflicting results and the administration of ranitidine before surgery also did not reduce the incidence of GER.[53,54] Although preanesthetic administration of cisapride and esomeprazole together decreased the number of reflux episodes in anesthetized dogs in a recent study, the administration of esomeprazole alone was felt to be less effective because it only decreased the acidity of refluxes but not the overall quantity of reflux episodes.[55] In cats, esophageal pH during anesthesia could be significantly increased when 2 oral doses of omeprazole were given 18 to 24 and 4 hours before anesthesia, and no reflux episodes (defined as a pH of <4) were recorded during anesthesia compared with placebo-treated cats.[56]

The same principle of increasing the LES pressure together with gastric acid suppression to prevent further injury and allow esophageal healing has been recommended in the treatment of suspected reflux esophagitis. In cats, experimentally induced esophagitis decreases esophageal peristalsis, decreases the LES pressure, and diminishes esophageal clearance.[3] These changes were reversible with healing of the esophagus.[3] Contradictory to common belief, orally administered metoclopramide administration did not result in significant changes in the LES pressure in dogs. Only cisapride administration significantly increased LES pressure in a placebo-controlled study.[57] A mainstay of treatment for suspected esophagitis is a combination of gastric acid suppression and sucralfate. In dogs and cats, proton pump inhibitors (ie, omeprazole) provide superior gastric acid suppression compared with H2 receptor antagonists (ranitidine, famotidine) and should therefore be considered more effective for the treatment of acid-related disorders.[58]

Twice daily dosing (1–1.5 mg/kg) is advised to maximize gastric acid suppression in canine and feline esophagitis. An exception may be esomeprazole in dogs, because once-daily oral dosing in a recent study also lead to an adequate increase of intragastric pH.[59] Sucralfate, an aluminum salt of a sulfated disaccharide, is a mucosal protectant that binds to inflamed tissue to create a protective barrier. It is supposed to block diffusion of gastric acid and pepsin across the esophageal mucosa and inhibit the erosive action of pepsin and possibly bile.[58] Although the rationale for its effectiveness is based on its protective adherence to denuded mucosal surface in an acidic environment, and the canine esophageal milieu is weakly alkaline,[28] clinically it seems to soothe the patient's discomfort when dosed multiple times daily.[58] In people, intensive high-dose sucralfate therapy (2 g of sucralfate given orally every 2 hours for the first

3 days, followed by 2 g 8 times daily for 21 days) has been shown to be beneficial in enhancing mucosal healing and preventing stricture formation in advanced-grade corrosive esophagitis.[60] EE has been successfully treated with dietary antigen elimination (ie, hydrolyzed diet) in a cat and with corticosteroids in a dog.[24,25] When present, strictures may need esophageal bougienage or balloon dilation. Budesonide orodispersible tablets have recently been shown to be a promising new option for the induction of clinical and histologic remission in a placebo-controlled trial in humans with EE.[61] Lifestyle changes are part of the initial management of reflux esophagitis in people and include losing weight if overweight, avoiding bed time snacks, and elevating the head at night. Although this therapy intuitively makes sense, no data are available on this strategy in small animals.

SUMMARY

Esophagitis in cats and dogs is largely a consequence of prolonged esophageal exposure to acid, which in turn can have various underlying causes. Analogous to GERD in humans, an incompetent LES is also often suspected to cause clinical signs, but the validity of these clinical signs remains currently unclear. The diagnosis can be confirmed endoscopically, with esophageal biopsies, with esophageal wireless pH monitoring or through a clear response to therapeutic trials with sufficiently dosed proton pump inhibitors. In unclear cases that do not respond satisfyingly to treatment, chronic enteropathy should be suspected and strict dietary trials should be tried out.

DISCLOSURE

The author has nothing to disclose.

SUPPLEMENTARY DATA

Supplementary data related to this article can be found online at https://doi.org/10.1016/j.cvsm.2020.08.003.

REFERENCES

1. Savarino E, de Bortoli N, De Cassan C, et al. The natural history of gastroesophageal reflux disease: a comprehensive review. Dis Esophagus 2017; 30(2):1–9.
2. Salapatek AMF, Diamant NE. Assessment of neural inhibition of the lower esophageal sphincter in cats with esophagitis. Gastroenterology 1993;104(3):810–8.
3. Zhang X, Geboes K, Depoortere I, et al. Effect of repeated cycles of acute esophagitis and healing on esophageal peristalsis, tone, and length. Am J Physiol Gastrointest Liver Physiol 2005;288(6):G1339–46.
4. Galatos AD, Raptopoulos D. Gastro-oesophageal reflux during anaesthesia in the dog: the effect of preoperative fasting and premedication. Vet Rec 1995;137: 479–83.
5. Galatos AD, Raptopoulos D. Gastro-oesophageal reflux during anaesthesia in the dog: the effect of age, positioning and type of surgical procedure. Vet Rec 1995; 137:513–6.
6. Wilson DV, Evans AT, Miller RA. Effects of preanesthetic administration of morphine on gastroesophageal reflux and regurgitation during anesthesia in dogs. Am J Vet Res 2004;66(3):386–90.

7. Viskjer S, Sjöström L. Effect of the duration of food withholding prior to anesthesia on gastroesophageal reflux and regurgitation in healthy dogs undergoing elective orthopedic surgery. Am J Vet Res 2017;78(2):144–50.

8. Adami C, Palma SD, Gendron K, et al. Severe esophageal injuries occurring after general anesthesia in two cats: case report and literature review. J Am Anim Hosp Assoc 2011;47(6):436–42.

9. Beatty JA, Swift N, Foster DJ, et al. Suspected clindamycin-associated oesophageal injury in cats: five cases. J Feline Med Surg 2006;8(6):412–9.

10. Schulz BS, Zauscher S, Ammer H, et al. Side effects suspected to be related to doxycycline use in cats. Vet Rec 2013;172(7):184–5.

11. Westfall DS, Twedt DC, Steyn PF, et al. Evaluation of esophageal transit of tablets and capsules in 30 cats. J Vet Intern Med 2001;15(5):467–70.

12. Kook PH, Wiederkehr D, Makara M, et al. Megaesophagus secondary to an esophageal leiomyoma and concurrent esophagitis. Schweiz Arch Tierheilkd 2009;151(10):497–501.

13. Rolfe DS, Twedt DC, Seim HB. Chronic regurgitation or vomiting caused by esophageal leiomyoma in three dogs. J Am Anim Hosp Assoc 1994;30:425–30.

14. Gal A, Ridgway MD, Frederickson RL. An unusual clinical presentation of a dog with gastrinoma. Can Vet J 2011;52(6):641–4.

15. Shaw DH. Gastrinoma (Zollinger-Ellison syndrome) in the dog and cat. Can Vet J 1988;29(5):448–52.

16. Frowde PE, Battersby IA, Whitley NT, et al. Oesophageal disease in 33 cats. J Feline Med Surg 2011;13(8):564–9.

17. Gaskell CJ, Gibbs C, Pearson H. Sliding hiatus hernia with reflux esophagitis in two dogs. J Small Anim Pract 1974;15(8):503–9.

18. Gualtieri M, Olivero D. Reflux esophagitis in three cats associated with metaplastic columnar esophageal epithelium. J Am Anim Hosp Assoc 2006;42(1): 65–70.

19. Lecoindre P, Richard S. Digestive disorders associated with the chronic obstructive respiratory syndrome of brachycephalic dogs: 30 cases (1999-2001). Revue Méd Vét 2004;155(3):141–6.

20. Poncet CM, Dupre GP, Freiche VG, et al. Prevalence of gastrointestinal tract lesions in 73 brachycephalic dogs with upper respiratory syndrome. J Small Anim Pract 2005;46(6):273–9.

21. Reeve EJ, Sutton D, Friend EJ, et al. Documenting the prevalence of hiatal hernia and oesophageal abnormalities in brachycephalic dogs using fluoroscopy. J Small Anim Pract 2017;58(12):703–8.

22. Pearson H, Darke PGG, Gibbs C, et al. Reflux esophagitis and stricture formation after anaesthesia: a review of seven cases in dogs and cats. J Small Anim Pract 1978;19(9):507–19.

23. Boesch RP, Shah P, Vaynblat M, et al. Relationship between upper airway obstruction and gastroesophageal reflux in a dog model. J Invest Surg 2005; 18(5):241–5.

24. Mazzei MJ, Bissett SA, Murphy KM, et al. Eosinophilic esophagitis in a dog. J Am Vet Med Assoc 2009;235(1):61–5.

25. Pera J, Palma D, Donovan TA. Eosinophilic esophagitis in a kitten. J Am Anim Hosp Assoc 2017;53(4):214–20.

26. Han E, Broussard J, Baer KE. Feline esophagitis secondary to gastroesophageal reflux disease: clinical signs and radiographic, endoscopic, and histopathological findings. J Am Anim Hosp Assoc 2003;39(2):161–7.

27. Münster M, Kook P, Araujo R, et al. Determination of hyperregeneratory esophagopathy in dogs with clinical signs attributable to esophageal disease. Tierarztl Prax Ausg K Kleintiere Heimtiere 2015;43(3):147–55.
28. Kook PH, Kempf J, Ruetten M, et al. Wireless ambulatory esophageal pH monitoring in dogs with clinical signs interpreted as gastroesophageal reflux. J Vet Intern Med 2014;28(6):1716–23.
29. Muenster M, Hoerauf A, Vieth M. Gastro-oesophageal reflux disease in 20 dogs (2012 to 2014). J Small Anim Pract 2017;58(5):276–83.
30. Lux CN, Archer TN, Lunsford KV. Gastroesophageal reflux and laryngeal dysfunction in a dog. J Am Vet Med Assoc 2012;240(9):1100–3.
31. Kouki MI, Papadimitriou SA, Psalla D, et al. Chronic gingivostomatitis with esophagitis in cats. J Vet Intern Med 2017;31(6):1673–9.
32. Tarvin KM, Twedt DC, Monnet E. Prospective controlled study of gastroesophageal reflux in dogs with naturally occurring laryngeal paralysis. Vet Surg 2016; 45(7):916–21.
33. Sellon RK, Willard MD. Esophagitis and esophageal strictures. Vet Clin North Am Small Anim Pract 2003;33(5):945–67.
34. Wilson DV, Walshaw R. Postanesthetic esophageal dysfunction in 13 dogs. J Am Anim Hosp Assoc 2004;40(6):455–60.
35. Gianella P, Pfammatter NS, Burgener IA. Oesophageal and gastric endoscopic foreign body removal: complications and follow-up of 102 dogs. J Small Anim Pract 2009;50(12):649–54.
36. Juvet F, Pinilla M, Shiel RE, et al. Oesophageal foreign bodies in dogs: factors affecting success of endoscopic retrieval. Ir Vet J 2010;63(3):163–8.
37. Jankowski M, Spuzak J, Kubiak K, et al. Oesophageal foreign bodies in dogs. Pol J Vet Sci 2013;16(3):571–2.
38. Määttä OLM, Laurila HP, Holopainen S, et al. Reflux aspiration in lungs of dogs with respiratory disease and in healthy West Highland White Terriers. J Vet Intern Med 2018;32(6):2074–81.
39. Van Nieuenhove Y, Willems G. Gastroesophageal reflux triggers proliferative activity of the submucosal glands in the canine esophagus. Dis Esophagus 1998; 11(2):89–93.
40. Mackenzie SH, Go M, Chadwick B. Eosinophilic esophagitis in patients presenting with dysphagia – a prospective analysis. Aliment Pharmacol Ther 2008;28(9): 1140–6.
41. LV J, Liu D, Ma S, et al. Investigation of relationships among gastroesophageal reflux disease subtypes using narrow band imaging magnifying endoscopy. World J Gastroenterol 2013;19(45):8391–7.
42. Dodds WJ, Goldberg HI, Montgomery C, et al. Sequential gross, microscopic, and roentgenographic features of acute feline esophagitis. Invest Radiol 1970; 5:209–19.
43. Lobetti R, Leisewitz A. Gastroesophageal reflux in two cats. Feline Pract 1996; 24(1):5–9.
44. Münster M, Bilzer T, Dettmann K, et al. Assessment of the histological quality of endoscopic biopsies obtained from the canine gastro-esophageal junction. Tierarztl Prax Ausg K Kleintiere Heimtiere 2012;40(5):318–24.
45. Münster M, Vieth M, Hörauf A. Evaluation of the quality of endoscopically obtained esophageal biopsies in the dog. Tierarztl Prax Ausg K Kleintiere Heimtiere 2013;41(6):375–82.
46. Ismail-Beigi F, Horton PF, Pope CE. Histological consequences of gastroesophageal reflux in man. Gastroenterology 1970;58(2):163–74.

47. Elster K. Morphology of esophagitis. Leber Magen Darm 1972;2(2):44–7.
48. Gualtieri M, Cocci A, Olivero D et al. Esophageal and gastric intestinal metaplasia in the dog and the cat: a retrospective study of 41 cases (2003-2007). Proceedings 18th ECVIM-CA Congress. Ghent, 2008, p. 217.
49. Furuta GT, Liacouras CA, Collins MH, et al. Eosinophilic esophagitis in children and adults: A systematic review and consensus recommendations for diagnosis and treatment. Gastroenterology 2007;133:1342–63.
50. Richter JE, Pandolfino JE, Vela MF, et al. Utilization of wireless pH monitoring technologies: a summary of the proceedings from the Esophageal Diagnostic Working Group. Dis Esophagus 2013;26:755–65.
51. Shay SS, Tutuian R, Sifrim D, et al. Twenty-four hour ambulatory simultaneous impedance and pH monitoring: a multicenter report of normal values from 60 healthy volunteers. Am J Gastroenterol 2004;99(6):1037–43.
52. Zerbib F, des Varannes SB, Roman S, et al. Normal values and day-to-day variability of 24-h ambulatory oesophageal impedance-pH monitoring in a Belgian-French cohort of healthy subjects. Aliment Pharmacol Ther 2005;22(10):1011–21.
53. Wilson DV, Evans AT, Mauer WA. Influence of metoclopramide on gastroesophageal reflux in anesthetized dogs. Am J Vet Res 2006;67(1):26–31.
54. Favarato ES, Souza MV, Costa PR, et al. Evaluation of metoclopramide and ranitidine on the prevention of gastroesophageal reflux episodes in anesthetized dogs. Res Vet Sci 2012;93(1):466–7.
55. Zacuto AC, Marks SL, Osborn J, et al. The influence of esomeprazole and cisapride on gastroesophageal reflux during anesthesia in dogs. J Vet Intern Med 2012; 26(3):518–25.
56. Garcia RS, Belafsky PC, Della Maggiore A, et al. Prevalence of gastroesophageal reflux in cats during anesthesia and effect of omeprazole on gastric pH. J Vet Intern Med 2017;31(3):734–42.
57. Kempf J, Fraser L, Reusch CE, et al. High-resolution manometric evaluation of the effects of cisapride and metoclopramide hydrochloride administered orally on lower esophageal sphincter pressure in awake dogs. Am J Vet Res 2014;75(4): 361–6.
58. Marks SL, Kook PH, Papich MG, et al. ACVIM consensus statement: support for rational administration of gastrointestinal protectants to dogs and cats. J Vet Intern Med 2018;32(6):1823–40.
59. Hwang JH, Jeong JW, Song GH, et al. Pharmacokinetics and acid suppressant efficacy of esomeprazole after intravenous, oral, and subcutaneous administration to healthy Beagle dogs. J Vet Intern Med 2017;31(3):743–50.
60. Gümürdülü Y, Karakoç E, Kara B, et al. The efficiency of sucralfate in corrosive esophagitis: a randomized, prospective study. Turk J Gastroenterol 2010; 21(1):7–11.
61. Lucendo AJ, Miehlke S, Schlag C, et al. Efficacy of budesonide orodispersible tablets as induction therapy for eosinophilic esophagitis in a randomized placebo-controlled trial. Gastroenterology 2019;157(1):74–86e.

Aerodigestive Disease in Dogs

Megan Grobman, DVM, MS, PhD

KEYWORDS

- Aspiration • Dysphagia • Motility • Pneumonia • Reflux • Megaesophagus
- Respiratory

KEY POINTS

- Aerodigestive disorders span a wide range of important clinical syndromes affecting the upper and lower airways, bronchioles, and pulmonary parenchyma (ie, alveoli and interstitium).
- Aerodigestive diseases frequently reflect defects in swallowing and/or airway protection.
- Aerodigestive diseases can occur in the absence of digestive signs and in the face of normal radiographs.
- The role of bacterial infection in cases of aspiration pneumonia is unclear.
- Videofluoroscopic swallow studies represent the criterion standard for diagnosis of dysphagia in veterinary medicine.

 Video content accompanies this article at http://www.vetsmall.theclinics.com.

INTRODUCTION

Although aspiration pneumonia is the most well-recognized aerodigestive disorder (AeroD) in veterinary clinical practice, AeroDs span a range of common and clinically important conditions (**Table 1**). AeroDs reflect failures in airway protection, abnormal swallowing, or a combination of these that result in, or contribute to, respiratory disease. In people, AeroDs have been implicated in the pathogenesis and progression of several acute and chronic respiratory diseases. Reflux, for example, has been implicated in chronic cough, asthma, pulmonary fibrosis, and chronic obstructive pulmonary disease.[1,2] Importantly, treatment of reflux was found to reduce the frequency of disease exacerbations and slow the rate of decline in lung function.[3]

A similar association has been documented in dogs. A study evaluating dogs presenting exclusively for cough, in the absence of clinical signs of digestive disease, found swallowing abnormalities in 80.6%, including 9/11 dogs with normal thoracic radiographs.[4] Furthermore, there is a demonstrated correlation between gastrointestinal (GI) signs and the severity of respiratory disease in brachycephalic dogs, with 88% of

Auburn University, Department of Clinical Sciences, 1220 Wire Road, Auburn, AL 36849, USA
E-mail address: Meg0098@auburn.edu

Vet Clin Small Anim 51 (2021) 17–32
https://doi.org/10.1016/j.cvsm.2020.09.003
0195-5616/21/© 2020 Elsevier Inc. All rights reserved.

vetsmall.theclinics.com

Table 1	
Aerodigestive syndromes reported in the veterinary literature by anatomic location	
Condition	
Upper airway	Laryngitis,[35,74] laryngeal paralysis/ dysfunction,[19,33,35,74] larygopharyngeal reflux,[4] nasopharyngeal reflux,[4] otitis,[21] upper airway obstruction,[23] rhinitis,[4] sleep disordered breathing (apnea)[23]
Bronchi, bronchioles, and pulmonary parenchyma	Acute respiratory distress syndrome,[35] aspiration pneumonia/pneumonitis,[35] bronchiectasis,[65] bronchomalacia,[4] diffuse aspiration bronchiolitis,[35] exogenous lipid pneumonia,[75] interstitial lung disease,[35,43] large airway obstruction[76]
Oral preparatory defects	Cranial nerve defects,[53] periodontal disease,[4] myopathy/neuropathy[53,77]
Pharyngeal swallow defects	Cricopharyngeal achalasia,[56] cricopharyngeal dyssynchrony,[56] myopathy/neuropathy,[53] pharyngeal hypomotility,[4] pharyngeal spasticity,[4] pharyngeal mucocele,[78] reflux (laryngopharyngeal)[4]
Esophageal swallow defects	Esophageal hypomotility,[4] LES-AS,[4] megaesophagus,[4] myopathy/neuropathy[53] hiatal hernia,[4,79] reflux (gastroesophageal)[4]
Gastric	Vomiting (acute or chronic)[53]

Otitis is included the upper airway disorders due to the connection of the Eustachian tube to the nasopharynx. This list is not exhaustive but is intended to reflect the more common diseases encountered in clinical veterinary practice.
Data from Refs. [4,19,21,23,33,35,43,53,56,65,74,76–79]

brachycephalic dogs treated medically for GI disease demonstrating clear and sustained improvement after brachycephalic airway surgery.[5] Additionally, investigators found a decreased complication rate and improved prognosis in brachycephalic dogs treated for reflux prior to brachycephalic airway surgery.[5] This suggests that a subpopulation dogs with respiratory signs have AeroDs and, like humans, may respond to treatment targeting the digestive tract. Unfortunately, AeroDs may present with occult digestive signs, representing a significant clinical challenge for the practitioner.

PHYSIOLOGY OF SWALLOWING

Swallowing is a complex act involving several muscles of the upper respiratory and digestive tracts and can be considered both a feeding and an airway protective behavior. The cooperation between swallowing and breathing is not limited to the removal of oral and respiratory secretions and prevention of aspiration during swallowing. Safe swallowing also requires centrally mediated coordination to ensure breathing and swallowing do not occur at the same time, that there is time to clear secretions after coughing to prevent reaspiration, and to reset the respiratory cycle to ensure a fairly consistent respiratory rate and rhythm.[6]

The act of swallowing can be separated into voluntary and involuntary phases. The voluntary phase involves the prehension and mastication of food and propulsion to the oropharynx. This phase in entirely voluntary and absent in reflexive swallows, such as may be seen when swallowing accumulated oral secretions[7–10]

The presence of a bolus in the rostral oropharynx initiates the pharyngeal phase of the swallow. This and all subsequent phases are involuntary. The pharyngeal phase is mediated by sensory afferents of cranial nerves IX and X and involves passage of the bolus through the upper esophageal sphincter into the esophagus.[6,11] This phase of swallowing also is characterized by the initiation of airway protective behaviors, including the blockage of the nasopharynx and larynx, which are absent during the oral preparatory and esophageal phases.[12,13]

Passage of the bolus into the esophagus marks the beginning of the esophageal phase of swallowing. Contraction of the upper esophageal sphincter and accompanying peristaltic contraction is the primary wave. Luminal distention triggers progressive contractions (secondary waves). The esophageal phase ends with the opening of the lower esophageal sphincter (LES) to allow the passage of food into the stomach and closure to prevent reflux.[14]

DYSPHAGIA, REGURGITATION, AND VOMITING

The term, *dysphagia*, can be used to describe a defect in any of the phases of swallowing. Dysphagia may be classified based on location/phase (oral preparatory, pharyngeal, or esophageal) and/or mechanism (mechanical vs functional). Dysphagia may be secondary to functional defects in swallowing (eg, myasthenia gravis, pharyngeal hypomotility, and cricopharyngeal achalasia) or secondary to structural abnormalities (eg, severe dental disease, trauma, foreign bodies, strictures, and neoplasia). Key clinical features associated with dysphagia include difficulty with prehension, gagging, repetitive swallowing while eating, and regurgitation. Additional clinical features of aerodigestive disease are listed in **Table 2**. Although these features may help a practitioner localize the problem to a specific location/swallowing phase, treatment depends on the specific underlying etiology. Although some conditions can be managed medically (esophagitis and myasthenia gravis), disorders of motility (cricopharyngeal achalasia and LES–achalasia-line syndrome [AS]) require targeted intervention. Incorrect localization may lead to significant worsening of clinical signs, making correct identification critically important.[14–16]

The clinical feature most commonly associated with defects in the esophageal phase of swallowing is regurgitation. Regurgitation refers to the retrograde passive expulsion of esophageal contents. Importantly, in regurgitation the airway protective behaviors that occur during vomiting (ie, laryngeal adduction and soft palate elevation) are absent. Obstructive disorders causing regurgitation include but are not limited to esophageal foreign bodies, vascular ring anomalies, strictures, and esophageal/paraesophageal tumors. Functional disorders include defects of the LES (eg, LES-AS), muscle (eg, esophageal hypomotility), inflammatory disease (eg, esophagitis), neuromuscular dysfunction (eg, botulism, myasthenia gravis, and polyneuropathy/polymyopathy), and toxins (eg, lead, thallium, and organophosphates).[15–17]

In contrast to regurgitation, vomiting is a centrally mediated process, resulting in the active expulsion of GI contents from the stomach and proximal duodenum. Vomiting also involves coordinated efforts to protect the airways. Despite this, vomiting, like regurgitation, is considered a major risk factor for respiratory disease by overwhelming these protective mechanisms.[15–18]

REFLUX AND REFLUX DISEASE

A less well-known, but important, link between respiratory and digestive disease is gastroesophageal reflux (GER). GER refers to the back flow of stomach contents into the esophagus. An extraesophageal manifestation of GER is extraesophageal

Table 2
Aerodigestive signs and related clinical mechanisms in dogs

Aerodigestive Signs	Related Clinical Mechanism
Cough	Airway protective mechanism, nonspecific marker of respiratory disease. The severity of cough does not reflect disease severity because chronic aspiration may diminish the cough reflex.[80]
Dysphonia	Laryngeal dysfunction
Gagging while eating	Pharyngeal swallow dysfunction
Increased effort while swallowing	Pharyngeal swallow dysfunction
Lip licking	Reflux
Neck extension	Esophageal pain, reflux, pharyngeal swallow dysfunction (when observed while eating)
Night restlessness, flank biting, prayer position	Epigastric pain frequently encountered with reflux and sliding hiatal hernia
Regurgitation	Reflux, esophageal dysphagia, esophagitis
Repetitive dry swallowing (not while eating)	Reflux
Repetitive swallowing attempts per bolus (while eating)	Pharyngeal swallow dysfunction
Respiratory distress	Acute upper airway obstruction, severe aspiration event
Reverse sneezing	Nasopharyngeal reflux, pharyngeal collapse, pharyngitis
Stridor	Laryngeal dysfunction
Stertor	Nasal or pharyngeal disease
Throat clear	Airway protective mechanism suggestive of poor pharyngeal clearance, nasopharyngeal reflux, postnasal drip

reflux (EER). The broader category of EER includes laryngopharyngeal reflux, where the refluxate contacts the larynx, and pharynx and nasopharyngeal reflux, where the refluxate extends into the nasopharynx. Reflux often is an occult process in veterinary species, but it has been implicated in laryngeal dysfunction, increased mortality after brachycephalic airway surgery, otitis media via the eustachian tube, and chronic rhinitis.[5,19–22] In pediatric animals, reflux can cause apnea, bradycardia, laryngeal closure, and pediatric death.[23] GER occurs commonly in healthy, asymptomatic humans and has been documented in up to 41% of asymptomatic dogs.[24] Pathologic and physiologic reflux differ, however, in terms of volume, timing, and location within the esophagus. Discrimination is possible by several imaging modalities, including videofluoroscopic swallow studies (VFSSs). Reflux often remains occult until patients develop complications: esophagitis, laryngeal dysfunction, regurgitation, and a wide spectrum of respiratory diseases.

The combinations of GER, clinical signs, and gross pathology (dependent on site) are termed, *GER disease (GERD), EER disease (EERD), laryngopharyngeal reflux disease*, and *nasopharyngeal reflux disease*. Clinical signs are dependent on frequency, volume, and duration of contact between the refluxate and the esophagus, larynx, and pharynx. Causes of reflux include spontaneous transient relaxations of the LES (most common), diminished basal LES pressure, straining (coughing, vomiting, or increased intra-abdominal pressure), and hiatal hernia.[1,2,5,19,20,25] Pathology associated with

GERD can occur by direct contact of low pH refluxate and digestive enzymes, leading to tissue damage and stimulation of regional nerve terminals, and by macroaspiration/microaspiration. The pathophysiology of tissue damage secondary to reflux and aspiration is discussed in more detail later. VFSS clips depicting EER and pathologic GER with a sliding hiatal hernia are provided in the supplemental materials.

AERODIGESTIVE DISORDERS

Because AeroDs can reflect dysfunction in any phase of swallowing as well as failures in airway protection, the number of potential conditions is substantial. Failures in airway protection include both mechanical and functional defects (eg, laryngeal mass and laryngeal paralysis, respectively) as well as clinical scenarios where the normal airway protective mechanisms are overwhelmed (eg, vomiting and regurgitation).

Additional complications are multifocal disease and comorbid conditions contributing to clinical signs. A study using VFSSs to evaluate patients for occult AeroDs identified 72% of dogs with swallowing abnormalities had defects in more than one location.[4] Additionally 55% of those with swallow abnormalities had respiratory disease contributing to their clinical signs. This relationship is well established in people where the act of coughing induces reflux events in patients with known reflux induced chronic cough.[26] Similarly, in dogs with reflux and laryngeal paralysis, the degree of negative pressure associated with upper airway obstruction is sufficient to induce additional reflux events.[27] These studies suggest that in many patients both digestive and respiratory disease contribute to disease progression, likely in a self-perpetuating cycle. In such cases, case management is dependent on identifying and addressing both the digestive and respiratory components of disease.

Aspiration-related respiratory disorders reflect a subpopulation of AeroDs where gastric and/or oropharyngeal contents are aspirated into the respiratory tract. Detection of aspiration events presents an additional challenge because both macroaspiration and microaspiration events (ie, aspiration of microscopic particulates) can cause respiratory disease.[28] The ultimate prevalence of aspiration syndromes in dogs currently is unknown; however, they represent a significant source of morbidity and mortality in human patients and are associated with disease progression, exacerbations of clinical signs, and treatment costs.[29] Numerous conditions recognized in people also have been reported in dogs through individual case reports and case series.[19,30–33] A review of aspiration-related respiratory disorders in dogs has been published previously[30] and aspiration-associated respiratory syndromes reported in dogs are listed in **Table 1**.

Tissue Damage Secondary to Reflux and Aspiration

Reflux of GI secretions has been linked to diseases of the larynx, pharynx, and middle ear (via the eustachian tube) through the action of acid, digestive enzymes (ie, pepsin), and bile acids.[34,35] Although each substance is capable of causing damage independently, increased tissue damage is documented when they occur in combination, suggesting that management should address both the acidic and nonacidic components of reflux.[19,27,34]

Damage to the airways, and pulmonary parenchyma occurs through the aspiration of acid, digestive enzymes, and foreign material.[17,30,36–38] Aspiration events may be oropharyngeal or gastroesophageal in origin and may or may not be clinically observed.[39] Because 50% of healthy people aspirate during sleep without apparent clinical significance,[40] it is likely that the development of respiratory disease depends on the composition and volume of the aspirated material, and the presence of functional airway protective mechanisms (ie, mucociliary clearance, and innate immunity).[41]

Inflammation in acidic aspiration is characterized by a biphasic response.[42] After aspiration, direct damage to the respiratory epithelium occurs immediately, followed hours later by neutrophilic inflammation. As in the upper airway, digestive enzymes also play a role in inflammation. Pepsin is directly cytotoxic, and bile acids have been documented in bronchoalveolar lavage fluid in human patients with reflux-associated respiratory disease and in dogs with pulmonary fibrosis.[43–47] In addition to acid and digestive enzymes, the aspiration of small particles also contributes to respiratory inflammation. In small animal models, tracheal instillation of small (<10 um) particles leads to neutrophilic inflammation.[48] Importantly, the combination of acidic aspiration and particulate aspiration appears to have a synergistic effect, where the combination results in more severe inflammation than either alone.[39,48]

Aspiration and Antibiotics

In people, the inhalation of low pH gastric fluid, digestive enzymes, and/or particulate material frequently leads to sterile inflammation (ie, aspiration pneumonitis).[49] This may or may not lead to a secondary bacterial complication (ie, aspiration pneumonia).[39,50] The distinction between aspiration pneumonitis and aspiration pneumonia is important, because treatment differs between these 2 conditions.[51] Aspiration pneumonitis is treated supportively, whereas aspiration pneumonia is treated with antimicrobials.[49,51] This distinction rarely is made in veterinary medicine and antibiotics frequently are initiated without objective evidence of bacterial infection. In dogs, the prevalence of secondary bacterial infection in aspiration pneumonia is unknown. Although prospective studies are needed, it is possible that antimicrobials are not always necessary and, as in people, inappropriate antibiotic use in dogs with aspiration pneumonitis may contribute to the development of resistant bacterial pathogens.[51]

Risk Factors

Increased risk for AeroDs have been reported for human patients with decreased consciousness, deficits in airway protection, dysphagia, and conditions where barriers to aspiration are overwhelmed (eg, vomiting and regurgitation).[48] Similar risk factors are seen in dogs. Diminished consciousness, body position during anesthetic recovery, duration of anesthesia, vomiting and regurgitation, seizures, cranial nerve deficits, and the presence of megaesophagus are independent risk factors for aspiration.[52,53] More than 1 risk factor may be present: 32% of dogs with aspiration pneumonia had greater than or equal to 2 risk factors.[53]

Common disorders associated with aspiration are esophageal disease (39.8%), vomiting (38.6%), neurologic disease (27.3%), laryngeal disease (18.2%), and anesthesia (13.6%).[53] Of those with esophageal disease, megaesophagus was identified in 71.4% of dogs. The remaining dogs were diagnosed with non-ME esophageal dysmotility, hiatal hernia, and an unknown disorder in 17.1%, 2.8%, and 8.6%, of dogs respectively.[53] Although focusing specifically on aspiration pneumonia, these studies highlight the role of digestive disease, in particular esophageal dysfunction, in the development of respiratory disease.

CLINICAL APPROACH

The range of conditions contributing to aerodigestive disease is broad and may be present in the absence of digestive signs. As such, conscious clinical recognition of these syndromes on the part of the veterinary practitioner is required.

Signalment can be used to help identify specific disease states. For example, congenital abnormalities usually are diagnosed at a young age and include persistent right aortic arch, cleft palate, and cricopharyngeal achalasia. Likewise, certain breeds are associated with a high incidence of dysphagia, including German shepherd dogs (vascular ring anomaly),[54] large breed dogs (masticatory muscle disorders),[55] golden retrievers (cricopharyngeal achalasia), and French bulldogs with sliding hiatal hernia.[56,57] Ultimately, however, AeroDs can occur in any breed regardless of age. Evaluation for AeroDs requires a thorough history. Identification may be aided by specific lines of questioning. These include identifying patients with recurrent disease (eg, recurrent aspiration pneumonia), identification and localization of dysphagia (ie, oral preparatory, pharyngeal, or esophageal), and inciting events (ie, eating and drinking or time of day) as well as historical vomiting/regurgitation events or recent anesthesia.[4] A thorough physical examination, including evaluation for comorbidities, and observation of swallowing are critically important components of evaluation for AeroDs. Specific clinical features suggestive of AeroDs are provided in **Table 2** and supplemental Video 1.

Initial Evaluation

Observation
Clinical episodes may be observed either at home or in the clinic. Observing a patient during feeding may allow a clinician to identify and localize dysphagia. Recording episodes is extremely helpful in patients with intermittent clinical signs (eg, reflux, sliding hiatal hernia).

Oral examination
A through oral examination is recommended in patients with evidence of AeroDs (**Fig. 1**). For example, patients with EER frequently have evidence of significant pharyngeal erythema. This may be performed in combination with a laryngeal function examination.

Minimum database
A minimum database may include, complete blood count, serum biochemical profile, and urinalysis. Unfortunately, findings may be non-specific. Changes in CBC, chemistry panel and urinalysis may be nonspecific.

Thoracic radiographs
Thoracic radiographs (minumum 3 views) are recommended. At least 1 lateral view should include the cervical trachea. Radiographs provide critical information on both primary diseases and comorbid conditions (eg, megaesophagus and/or aspiration pneumonia). When investigating reflux, fluid in the distal esophagus on thoracic radiographs occasionally may be observed in normal patients. Clinical significance is difficult to determine based on this finding alone. Unfortunately, radiographs lack the sensitivity to detect dynamic functional disorders or subtle pulmonary pathology. Furthermore, patients with AeroDs may present with normal thoracic radiographs.[4] AeroDs cannot be ruled out in patients with normal radiographs in the presence of supporting clinical signs.

Abdominal imaging
Abdominal imaging (radiographs/abdominal ultrasound) may be considered in patients with clinical signs suggestive of abdominal disorders (eg, vomiting and abdominal pain).

Treatment trials with client reporting
Treatment trials with client reporting are best used where reflux is suspected. Treatment trials are used in people with suspected reflux disease due to their simplicity,

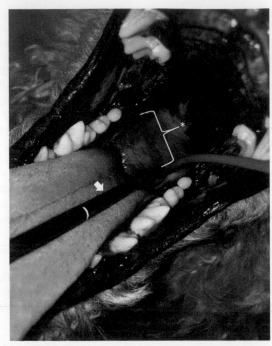

Fig. 1. A 13-year-old female spayed standard poodle was presented for aspiration pneumonia, a 4-week history of repetitive swallowing while eating, and increased upper respiratory noise (stertor). Oral examination prior to bronchoscopy (*white arrow*) revealed a large pharyngeal mucocele (*white brackets* and *asterisk*). Red rubber catheter is used to provide supplemental oxygen (*black arrow*).

noninvasiveness, and availability.[58] Although classically performed with proton pump inhibitors (eg, omeprazole, 1 mg/kg orally, every 12 hours, 30 minutes before feeding), a treatment trial also may include prokinetics (eg, metoclopramide, erythromycin or cisapride), especially where delayed gastric emptying is suspected. In human medicine, it is recommended that treatment trials for suspected reflux be performed for at least 8 weeks to 12 weeks in order to allow adequate time for a treatment response.[58]

Unfortunately, treatment trials are dependent on client reporting. Client reporting is inherently prone to bias due to variable client vigilance and a failure to recognize episodic, subtle clinical signs. Pretreatment and post-treatment surveys and visual analog scale (VAS) scores can help mitigate bias in client reporting.[59] Those patients who fail to respond to treatment trials should have such treatments discontinued appropriately to reduce risk of complications.[60] Additional diagnostics then are needed.

Advanced Testing

Laryngeal function examination

Laryngeal function examination is an important part of evaluation in patients with AeroDs. This is true particularly for patients with pharyngeal or esophageal dysphagia due to shared innervation between the pharynx, larynx, and the proximal esophagus.[4,33] Laryngeal dysfunction has been documented in dogs with reflux and in dogs lacking overt evidence of laryngeal disease (eg, stridor).[4,19] Because of this relationship, swallow evaluation may be indicated prior to surgical correction of laryn-geal paralysis to identify occult swallow dysfunction that may further increase the risk of aspiration events.[61] Laryngeal function examination may be performed in general practice but requires careful attention to technique.[61]

Videofluoroscopic swallow study

VFSSs have the benefit of allowing real time imaging (**Fig. 2**). They are considered the criterion standard for the evaluation of dysphagia in dogs.[24] Historically, these have been performed with dogs held in lateral recumbency and force-fed. This has limited use of VFFS in several disorders due to unacceptable risks of aspiration. Recent

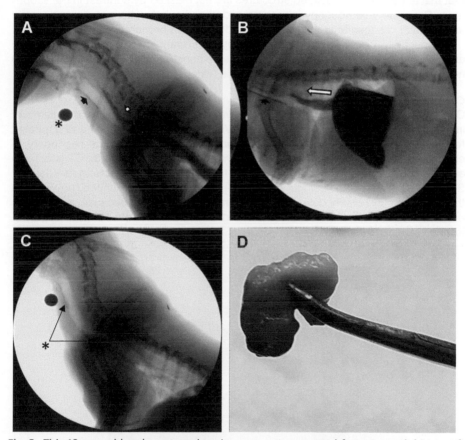

Fig. 2. This 12-year-old male castrated terrier cross was presented for a 4-month history of coughing while eating and drinking and nighttime restlessness. (*A, B, C*) Still images from a VFSS. (*A*) The dog was consuming a meal of liquid consistency. Liquid bolus is denoted by the white arrow. The degree of liquid accumulation in the esophagus was considered a normal variant due to multiple rapid swallow inhibition. Aspirated material is denoted by the black arrow; 1-cm size marker is denoted by the asterisk. (*B*) Aspirated contrast material is visible distal to the thoracic inlet (*black arrow*). Spontaneous reflux is denoted by the white arrow. (*C*) The arrows denote residual contrast material in the proximal and distal esophagus. Attempts at clearing this material (ie, cough) was conspicuously absent during image collection; 1-cm size marker is denoted by the asterisk. (*D*) On oral examination, a mass was found to obstruct normal adduction of the arytenoids. This was identified as an inflammatory polyp on histopathology.

studies have advocated an alternative which, by allowing free feeding, reduces risk of aspiration to what would be expected from feeding at home. Natural feeding position and bolus sizes further increase the physiologic relevance of VFSSs in dogs.[24,62] Objective swallowing metrics established using standardized recipes with rheological properties objectively consistent with commercially available products have been recently published.[24] Numerous swallowing abnormalities, including esophageal hypomotility, LES-AS, moderate–large volume reflux and macroaspiration, are detectable using this method. To date, LES-AS has been detected only by VFSSs.[63,64]

Respiratory fluoroscopy may be performed alone or in combination with VFSSs. If combined, it is recommended that respiratory fluoroscopy be performed first so that that airways and associated structures are not masked by contrast in the esophagus. Respiratory fluoroscopy is recommended particularly where static or dynamic architectural changes to larynx, trachea, and mainstem bronchi are suspected.

Unfortunately, the availability of fluoroscopy is currently limited to specialty practice and veterinary teaching hospitals. VFSS clips demonstrating EER and a sliding hiatal hernia are available in supplemental materials (Video 2 and Video 3, respectively).

Computed tomography

Computed tomography (CT) is useful for evaluating thoracic masses, extraluminal/intraluminal esophageal lesions, pharyngeal/retropharyngeal masses, and aspirated foreign material and for thorough evaluation of pulmonary diseases secondary to chronic aspiration (aspiration bronchiolitis and bronchiectasis) (**Fig. 3**). CT is considered the most sensitive diagnostic modality for the identification of bronchiectasis.[65] Survey radiography and a single breathing phase CT are both limited, however, in that they can only reliably detect static abnormalities changes. Because swallow disorders are dynamic, a more sensitive imaging modality is one that can evaluate swallowing in real time (ie, VFSSs).

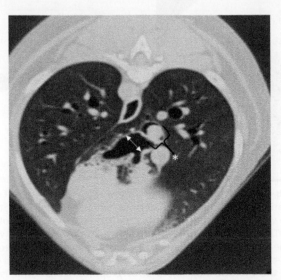

Fig. 3. This 8-year-old female spayed cocker spaniel was presented for a 9-month history of cough. Transverse CT image showed marked bronchiectasis of the accessory lobar bronchus (*double-headed arrow*) with soft tissue attenuating foreign material in the bronchial lumen of the accessory lung lobe (*brackets* and *asterisk*). Subsequent bronchoscopy identified complete occlusion of the accessory lobar bronchus with secretions and kibble foreign material.

Endoscopy

Endoscopy (**Fig. 4**) is routinely available in most specialty practices. Esophageal mucosal lesions may strongly support reflux esophagitis in dogs.[66] In human studies, however, endoscopy identified abnormalities in less than 50% of patients with known GERD.[67] A study in dogs demonstrated similar results, and supports this interpretation that esophagoscopy is a specific but poorly sensitive test for reflux disease in dogs.[66] Endoscopic evaluation of the nasopharynx and bronchoscopy with bronchoalveolar lavage fluid analysis (cytology and culture) remain an important mainstay for evaluation of airway and pulmonary parenchymal disease in dogs.

pH monitoring

Tests evaluating esophageal and gastric pH are rare outside of tertiary care centers or veterinary teaching hospitals. pH monitoring has proved invaluable in optimizing antacid therapy in dogs.[60,68] Diagnostic tests relying on esophageal or pharyngeal pH, however, fail to recognize reflux in human patients treated with proton pump inhibitors or those with nonacidic reflux (ie, secondary to digestive enzymes), which is increasingly implicated in disease representing up to 90% cases in some human studies.[47,69–71] The importance of nonacidic reflux in dogs currently is unknown.

Manometry

High-resolution manometry is considered a mainstay in evaluation of dysphagia in people. In veterinary medicine, however, it is significantly limited by availability, cost, and the need for substantial operator training.[72,73]

MANAGEMENT

Management is dependent on the underlying etiology. The key to management is appropriate patient identification and disease localization.

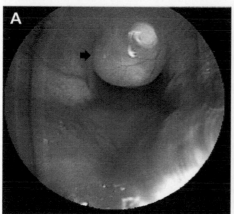 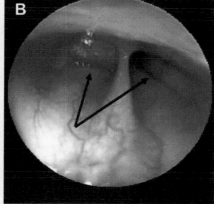

Fig. 4. This 9-year-old male castrated shih tzu was presented for a chronic history of cough, nasal discharge, suspected obstructive sleep apnea, and otitis media. Body condition score was 9/9. (*A*) Retroflexed choanal examination showed an obstructive fluctuant cyst (*arrow*) as well as diffuse nasopharyngeal erythema. (*B*) Rostral to the cyst, obstructive edematous nasopharyngeal turbinates (*arrows*) were noted. In addition, bilateral laryngeal paresis was noted on laryngeal function examination. A treatment-trial for EER was initiated. Weight loss also was recommended. Treatment response was noted after 4 weeks with decreased nasal discharge, nocturnal apneic episodes, and cough.

SUMMARY

The understanding of AeroDs in veterinary medicine is still in its infancy. Current evidence suggests, however, that dogs with AeroDs may represent a large and underrecognized patient population. Identification requires conscious awareness of the relationship between the respiratory and digestive tracts and AeroDs should be considered even in the absence of clinical signs of digestive disease and in dogs with normal thoracic radiographs.

DISCLOSURE

The author does not have any financial or personal relationships that could inappropriately influence or bias the content of this article. United States Patent No. 9,107,385 for the free-feeding kennels is held by the Curators of the University of Missouri, listing as inventors: Teresa Lever, Joan Coates, Mitchell Allen, and Laila Al-Khashti.

SUPPLEMENTARY DATA

Supplementary data to this article can be found online at https://doi.org/10.1016/j.cvsm.2020.09.003.

REFERENCES

1. Groome M, Cotton JP, Borland M, et al. Prevalence of laryngopharyngeal reflux in a population with gastroesophageal reflux. Laryngoscope 2007;117(8):1424–8.
2. Koufman JA. Laryngopharyngeal reflux is different from classic gastroesophageal reflux disease. Ear Nose Throat J 2002;81(9 Suppl 2):7–9.
3. Celli BR, Thomas NE, Anderson JA, et al. Effect of pharmacotherapy on rate of decline of lung function in chronic obstructive pulmonary disease: results from the TORCH study. Am J Respir Crit Care Med 2008;178(4):332–8.
4. Grobman ME, Masseau I, Reinero CR. Aerodigestive disorders in dogs evaluated for cough using respiratory fluoroscopy and videofluoroscopic swallow studies. Vet J 2019;251:105344.
5. Poncet CM, Dupre GP, Freiche VG, et al. Long-term results of upper respiratory syndrome surgery and gastrointestinal tract medical treatment in 51 brachycephalic dogs. J Small Anim Pract 2006;47(3):137–42.
6. Logemann J. Swallowing physiology and pathophysiology. Otolaryngol Clin North Am 1988;21(4):613–23.
7. Nishino T. Swallowing as a protective reflex for the upper respiratory tract. Anesthesiology 1993;79(3):588–601.
8. Paterson WG, Hynna-Liepert TT, Selucky M. Comparison of primary and secondary esophageal peristalsis in humans: effect of atropine. Am J Physiol 1991;260(1 Pt 1):G52–7.
9. Matsuo K, Palmer JB. Anatomy and physiology of feeding and swallowing: normal and abnormal. Phys Med Rehabil Clin N Am 2008;19(4):691–707,vii.
10. Bautista TG, Sun Q-J, Pilowsky PM. The generation of pharyngeal phase of swallow and its coordination with breathing: interaction between the swallow and respiratory central pattern generators. Progress in brain research, vol. 212. Elsevier; 2014. p. 253–75.
11. Hollshwandner CH, Brenman HS, Friedman MH. Role of afferent sensors in the initiation of swallowing in man. J Dent Res 1975;54(1):83–8.
12. Shaker R, Dodds WJ, Ren J, et al. Esophagoglottal closure reflex: a mechanism of airway protection. Gastroenterology 1992;102(3):857–61.

13. Shaker R, Ren J, Medda B, et al. Identification and characterization of the esophagoglottal closure reflex in a feline model. Am J Physiol 1994;266(1 Pt 1): G147–53.
14. Pollard RE. Imaging evaluation of dogs and cats with dysphagia. ISRN Vet Sci 2012;2012:238505.
15. Ettinger SJ, Feldman EC. Textbook of veterinary internal medicine: diseases of the dog and the cat, vol. 7. St. Louis (MO): Elsevier Saunders; 2010.
16. Smith JA, Houghton LA. The oesophagus and cough: laryngo-pharyngeal reflux, microaspiration and vagal reflexes. Cough 2013;9:12.
17. Houghton LA, Lee AS, Badri H, et al. Respiratory disease and the oesophagus: reflux, reflexes and microaspiration. Nat Rev Gastroenterol Hepatol 2016;13: 445–60.
18. Praud JP. Upper airway reflexes in response to gastric reflux. Paediatr Respir Rev 2010;11(4):208–12.
19. Lux CN, Archer TM, Lunsford KV. Gastroesophageal reflux and laryngeal dysfunction in a dog. J Am Vet Med Assoc 2012;240(9):1100–3.
20. Lecoindre P, Richard S. Digestive disorders associated with the chronic obstructive respiratory syndrome of brachycephalic dogs: 30 cases (1999-2001). Rev Med Vet (Toulouse) 2004;155(3):141–6.
21. Salguero R, Herrtage M, Holmes M, et al. Comparison between computed tomographic characteristics of the middle ear in nonbrachycephalic and brachycephalic dogs with obstructive airway syndrome. Vet Radiol Ultrasound 2016; 57(2):137–43.
22. Flouraki E, Kazakos G, Savvas I, et al. Rhinitis following intraoperative gastro-oesophageal reflux in a dog. Vet Rec Case Rep 2019;7(2):e000792.
23. Boesch RP, Shah P, Vaynblat M, et al. Relationship between upper airway obstruction and gastroesophageal reflux in a dog model. J Invest Surg 2005; 18(5):241–5.
24. Harris R, Grobman M, Allen M, et al. Standardization of a videofluoroscopic swallow study protocol to investigate dysphagia in dogs. J Vet Intern Med 2017;31(2): 383–93.
25. Gaude GS. Pulmonary manifestations of gastroesophageal reflux disease. Ann Thorac Med 2009;4(3):115–23.
26. Kahrilas PJ, Smith JA, Dicpinigaitis PV. A causal relationship between cough and gastroesophageal reflux disease (GERD) has been established: a pro/con debate. Lung 2014;192(1):39–46.
27. Tarvin KM, Twedt DC, Monnet E. Prospective controlled study of gastroesophageal reflux in dogs with naturally occurring laryngeal paralysis. Vet Surg 2016; 45(7):916–21.
28. Cardasis JJ, MacMahon H, Husain AN. The spectrum of lung disease due to chronic occult aspiration. Ann Am Thorac Soc 2014;11(6):865–73.
29. Dal Negro RW, Turco P, Micheletto C, et al. Cost analysis of GER-induced asthma: a controlled study vs. atopic asthma of comparable severity. Respir Med 2007; 101(8):1814–20.
30. Nafe L, Grobman M, Masseau I, et al. Aspiration-related respiratory disorders in dogs. J Am Vet Med Assoc 2018;253(3):293–300.
31. Hawkins EC, Basseches J, Berry CR, et al. Demographic, clinical, and radiographic features of bronchiectasis in dogs: 316 cases (1988-2000). J Am Vet Med Assoc 2003;223(11):1628–35.
32. Johnson LR. Laryngeal structure and function in dogs with cough. J Am Vet Med Assoc 2016;249(2):195–201.

33. Stanley BJ, Hauptman JG, Fritz MC, et al. Esophageal dysfunction in dogs with idiopathic laryngeal paralysis: a controlled cohort study. Vet Surg 2010;39(2): 139–49.
34. Adhami T, Goldblum JR, Richter JE, et al. The role of gastric and duodenal agents in laryngeal injury: an experimental canine model. Am J Gastroenterol 2004; 99(11):2098–106.
35. Nafe LA, Grobman ME, Masseau I, et al. Aspiration-related respiratory disorders in dogs. J Am Vet Med Assoc 2018;253(3):292–300.
36. Hu X, Yi ES, Ryu JH. Diffuse aspiration bronchiolitis: analysis of 20 consecutive patients. J Bras Pneumol 2015;41:161–6.
37. Lee AS, Ryu JH. Aspiration pneumonia and related syndromes. Mayo Clin Proc 2018;93(6):752–62.
38. Marik PE. Pulmonary aspiration syndromes. Curr Opin Pulm Med 2011;17(3): 148–54.
39. Hunt EB, Sullivan A, Galvin J, et al. Gastric aspiration and Its role in airway inflammation. Open Respir Med J 2018;12:1–10.
40. Gleeson K, Eggli DF, Maxwell SL. Quantitative aspiration during sleep in normal subjects. Chest 1997;111(5):1266–72.
41. Troche MS, Brandimore AE, Godoy J, et al. A framework for understanding shared substrates of airway protection. J Appl Oral Sci 2014;22(4):251–60.
42. Kennedy TP, Johnson KJ, Kunkel RG, et al. Acute acid aspiration lung injury in the rat: biphasic pathogenesis. Anesth Analg 1989;69(1):87–92.
43. Määttä OM, Laurila HP, Holopainen S, et al. Reflux aspiration in lungs of dogs with respiratory disease and in healthy West Highland White Terriers. J Vet Intern Med 2018;32(6):2074–81.
44. Pauwels A, Decraene A, Blondeau K, et al. Bile acids in sputum and increased airway inflammation in patients with cystic fibrosis. Chest 2012;141(6):1568–74.
45. Grabowski M, Kasran A, Seys S, et al. Pepsin and bile acids in induced sputum of chronic cough patients. Respir Med 2011;105(8):1257–61.
46. Tobey NA, Hosseini SS, Caymaz-Bor C, et al. The role of pepsin in acid injury to esophageal epithelium. Am J Gastroenterol 2001;96(11):3062–70.
47. Kahrilas PJ, Kia L. Pepsin: a silent biomarker for reflux aspiration or an active player in extra-esophageal mucosal injury? Chest 2015;148(2):300–1.
48. Raghavendran K, Nemzek J, Napolitano LM, et al. Aspiration-Induced lung injury. Crit Care Med 2011;39(4):818–26.
49. Prather AD, Smith TR, Poletto DM, et al. Aspiration-related lung diseases. J Thorac Imaging 2014;29(5):304–9.
50. Dent J, El-Serag H, Wallander MA, et al. Epidemiology of gastro-oesophageal reflux disease: a systematic review. Gut 2005;54(5):710–7.
51. DiBardino DM, Wunderink RG. Aspiration pneumonia: a review of modern trends. J Crit Care 2015;30(1):40–8.
52. Ovbey DH, Wilson DV, Bednarski RM, et al. Prevalence and risk factors for canine post-anesthetic aspiration pneumonia (1999–2009): a multicenter study. Vet Anaesth Analg 2014;41(2):127–36.
53. Kogan DA, Johnson LR, Sturges BK, et al. Etiology and clinical outcome in dogs with aspiration pneumonia: 88 cases (2004–2006). J Am Vet Med Assoc 2008; 233(11):1748–55.
54. Krebs IA, Lindsley S, Shaver S, et al. Short- and long-term outcome of dogs following surgical correction of a persistent right aortic arch. J Am Anim Hosp Assoc 2014;50(3):181–6.

55. Ryckman LR, Krahwinkel DJ, Sims MH, et al. Dysphagia as the primary clinical abnormality in two dogs with inflammatory myopathy. J Am Vet Med Assoc 2005;226(9):1519–1523, 1501.
56. Elliott RC. An anatomical and clinical review of cricopharyngeal achalasia in the dog. J S Afr Vet Assoc 2010;81(2):75–9.
57. Reeve E, Sutton D, Friend E, et al. Documenting the prevalence of hiatal hernia and oesophageal abnormalities in brachycephalic dogs using fluoroscopy. J Small Anim Pract 2017;58(12):703–8.
58. Gasiorowska A, Fass R. The proton pump inhibitor (PPI) test in GERD: does it still have a role? J Clin Gastroenterol 2008;42(8):867–74.
59. Paul-Dauphin A, Guillemin F, Virion J-M, et al. Bias and precision in visual analogue scales: a randomized controlled trial. Am J Epidemiol 1999;150(10):1117–27.
60. Marks SL, Kook PH, Papich MG, et al. ACVIM consensus statement: support for rational administration of gastrointestinal protectants to dogs and cats. J Vet Intern Med 2018;32(6):1823–40.
61. MacPhail CM. Laryngeal disease in dogs and cats: an update. Vet Clin North Am Small Anim Pract 2020;50(2):295–310.
62. Bonadio C, Pollard RE, Dayton P, et al. Effects of body positioning on swallowing and esophageal transit in healthy dogs. J Vet Intern Med 2009;23(4):801–5.
63. Grobman ME, Schachtel J, Gyawali CP, et al. Videofluoroscopic swallow study features of lower esophageal sphincter achalasia-like syndrome in dogs. J Vet Intern Med 2019;33(5):1954–63.
64. Grobman M, Hutcheson K, Lever T, et al. Mechanical dilation, botulinum toxin A injection, and surgical myotomy with fundoplication for treatment of lower esophageal sphincter achalasia-like syndrome in dogs. J Vet Intern Med 2019;33(3):1423–33.
65. Johnson LR, Johnson EG, Vernau W, et al. Bronchoscopy, imaging, and concurrent diseases in dogs with bronchiectasis: (2003-2014). J Vet Intern Med 2016;30(1):247–54.
66. Munster M, Horauf A, Lubke-Becker A, et al. Idiopathic esophagopathies resembling gastroesophageal reflux disease in dogs. Tierarztl Prax Ausg K Kleintiere Heimtiere 2013;41(3):173–9.
67. Vaezi MF. Diagnosing gastroesophageal reflux disease with endoscopic-guided mucosal impedance. Gastroenterol Hepatol 2016;12(4):266.
68. Tolbert K, Bissett S, King A, et al. Efficacy of oral famotidine and 2 omeprazole formulations for the control of intragastric pH in dogs. J Vet Intern Med 2011;25(1):47–54.
69. Bardhan KD, Strugala V, Dettmar PW. Reflux revisited: advancing the role of pepsin. Int J Otolaryngol 2012;2012:646901.
70. Johnston N, Dettmar PW, Bishwokarma B, et al. Activity/stability of human pepsin: implications for reflux attributed laryngeal disease. Laryngoscope 2007;117(6):1036–9.
71. Sifrim D, Holloway R, Silny J, et al. Acid, nonacid, and gas reflux in patients with gastroesophageal reflux disease during ambulatory 24-hour pH-impedance recordings. Gastroenterology 2001;120(7):1588–98.
72. Kook P, Kempf J, Ruetten M, et al. Wireless ambulatory esophageal pH monitoring in dogs with clinical signs interpreted as gastroesophageal reflux. J Vet Intern Med 2014;28(6):1716–23.
73. Kempf J, Heinrich H, Reusch CE, et al. Evaluation of esophageal high-resolution manometry in awake and sedated dogs. Am J Vet Res 2013;74(6):895–900.

74. Gaynor EB. Gastroesophageal reflux as an etiologic factor in laryngeal complications of intubation. Laryngoscope 1988;98(9):972–9.
75. Carminato A, Vascellari M, Zotti A, et al. Imaging of exogenous lipoid pneumonia simulating lung malignancy in a dog. Can Vet J 2011;52(3):310–2.
76. Stadler K, Hartman S, Matheson J, et al. Computed tomographic imaging of dogs with primary laryngeal or tracheal airway obstruction. Vet Radiol Ultrasound 2011; 52(4):377–84.
77. Strøm P, Marks SL, Rivera J, et al. Dysphagia secondary to focal inflammatory myopathy and consequent dorsiflexion of the tongue in a dog. J Small Anim Pract 2018;59(11):714–8.
78. Smith MM. Surgery for cervical, sublingual, and pharyngeal mucocele. J Vet Dent 2010;27(4):268–73.
79. Pollard RE, Marks SL, Cheney DM, et al. Diagnostic outcome of contrast videofluoroscopic swallowing studies in 216 dysphagic dogs. Vet Radiol Ultrasound 2017;58(4):373–80.
80. Niimi A, Matsumoto H, Ueda T, et al. Impaired cough reflex in patients with recurrent pneumonia. Thorax 2003;58(2):152–3.

Gastroprotective Therapy

M. Katherine Tolbert, DVM, PhD, DACVIM

KEYWORDS

- Gastric ulcer • Acid suppressant • Proton pump inhibitor
- Histamine-2 receptor antagonist

KEY POINTS

- A range of gastroprotective drugs are available for the treatment of upper gastrointestinal injury, including acid suppressants, coating agents, prostaglandin analogs, and antacids.
- The choice of gastroprotective drug is guided by the cause and location of gastrointestinal injury and the potential for adverse effects.
- Proton pump inhibitors are the most effective drugs for the medical treatment of upper gastrointestinal injury.
- However, proton pump inhibitors are not effective for all causes of upper gastrointestinal injury and bleeding.

Gastric acid secretion is triggered by hormonal and neural stimulation of parietal cells, the acid-producing cells of the stomach. The predominant stimulators of acid secretion are gastrin (released from gastric G cells), acetylcholine (released from vagal inputs), and histamine (released from enterochromaffin-like cells in the gastric fundus), whereas the major inhibitors are somatostatin (released from gastric D cells) and prostaglandins. Gastric acid secretion can be characterized by the phase of acid secretion and depends on the timing of the meal. Gastric acid secretion is divided into 3 phases: (1) cephalic, in which the sight and smell of food triggers a small amount of gastric acid secretion; (2) gastric, in which gastric distension and digested food, particularly proteins, are responsible for the largest amount of gastric acid secretion; and (3) intestinal, in which gastric acid secretion is inhibited after gastric emptying and a decrease in duodenal pH. Basal acid secretion occurs during fasting periods, whereas the highest gastric acid secretion occurs after ingestion of a meal and the subsequent gastric distension. In dogs and cats, unlike studies in humans, food seems to be a strong stimulus of acid secretion and no buffering effect of food can be detected on gastric pH (**Fig. 1**).

Gastroprotectants are widely used by veterinarians for the treatment of esophagitis and gastroduodenal mucosal injury or ulceration in dogs and cats. Despite their widespread use, there are only a handful of studies investigating the use of these drugs in

Gastrointestinal Laboratory, Department of Small Animal Clinical Sciences, Texas A&M College of Veterinary, 4474 TAMU | College Station, TX 77843-4474, USA
E-mail address: ktolbert@cvm.tamu.edu

Vet Clin Small Anim 51 (2021) 33–41
https://doi.org/10.1016/j.cvsm.2020.09.001

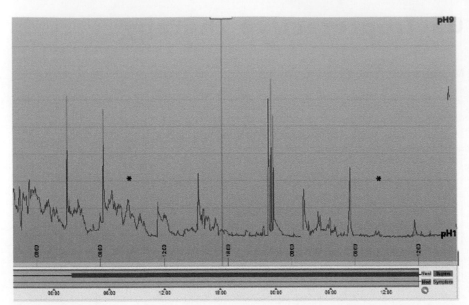

Fig. 1. Gastric pH over time in a healthy dog. Time in hours is on the x-axis and pH is on the y-axis. The asterisks (*) denote feeding times. Gastric pH is not significantly buffered by meals.

healthy cats and dogs and even fewer in those with naturally occurring disease. Most of the guidelines for therapy are derived from those established for humans, but there can be no certainty that these guidelines are appropriate for small animals. Many of the drugs are available over the counter and clients are often not provided instructions for discontinuation, which can result in months to years of inappropriate therapy. Moreover, this class of drugs is often used for dogs and cats with vomiting, presumed gastritis, or as preventative therapy for a wide range of diseases with little evidence for a benefit. Before prescribing gastroprotectants, it is important for the clinician to ask the following questions: (1) Is there an appropriate indication for the use of the drug? (2) What objective measures will be used to determine if a beneficial effect is achieved? (3) Have I provided adequate instructions for use and discontinuation of the drug? The reader is referred to the American College of Veterinary Internal Medicine consensus statement for more details on the indication and rationale for the use of gastroprotective therapy in dogs and cats.[1] A brief summary of the mechanisms for and causes of gastroduodenal ulceration as well as a review of drugs used for the treatment of gastroduodenal ulceration are provided in this article, and the recommended drug dosages are listed in **Box 1**.

GASTRODUODENAL ULCERATION IN DOGS AND CATS

Gastroduodenal ulceration results from a breakdown in the mucosal barrier either from physical disruption of the barrier, altered mucosal blood flow, or utilization of or decreased local mucus and bicarbonate secretion. Common causes of ulceration in the dog include nonsteroidal anti-inflammatory drug toxicity and gastroduodenal or pancreatic neoplasia. Although nonsteroidal anti-inflammatory drug-induced ulceration can occur in the cat, cats seem to be less susceptible than dogs. Gastroduodenal or pancreatic neoplasia is the most common cause of ulceration in the cat. Other

> **Box 1**
> **Gastroprotective drugs**
>
> H2 receptor antagonists
> - Famotidine: 1 mg/kg q 12 h PO, SC, IV (cat, dog); 8 mg/kg/d IV CRI (dog)
> - Ranitidine: 2.0 to 3.5 mg/kg PO*, SC, IV q 12 h
>
> Proton pump inhibitors
> - Omeprazole, pantoprazole: 1 mg/kg q 12 h PO, IV, SC
> - Esomeprazole: 1 mg/kg q 12 h IV, 1 mg/kg q12 to 24 h PO, SC (dog); 1 mg/kg q12 h IV, PO (cat)
>
> Coating agents
> - Sucralfate slurry (tablet crushed and dissolved in water): 0.5 to 1.0 g q 6 to 8 h PO (dog); 0.25 g q 6 to 8 h PO (cat)
> - Barium: 1 to 2 mL/kg q 8 to 12 h PO, per rectum (colorectal bleeding)
>
> Prostaglandin analogs
> - Misoprostol: 3 μg/kg q 8 to 12 PO (dog)
>
> *Abbreviations:* CRI, constant rate infusion; IV, intravenously; PO, by mouth; q, every; SC, subcutaneously.
>
> *See text regarding concerns for oral administration.

causes of ulceration in the cat or dog include advanced liver disease (ie, portal hypertension, intrahepatic portal vein shunting), high-dose corticosteroids, foreign bodies, trichobezoars inflammatory bowel disease, and severe stress (eg, critical illness, high-intensity exercise). It is important to note that gastroprotective therapy may not be effective depending on the underlying cause of ulceration (eg, portal hypertension).

ANTACIDS

Medical treatment of upper gastrointestinal (GI) ulceration can be directed toward neutralizing gastric acid, promoting prostaglandin production or action, coating and protecting denuded epithelium, and promoting clot formation and stabilization. Antacids (eg, calcium carbonate, aluminum hydroxide, and magnesium hydroxide) neutralize local gastric acid, but do not effectively inhibit gastric acid secretion and are therefore less effective than acid suppressants in treating gastric ulceration. Moreover, they need to be administered frequently to maintain their effect on gastric acid neutralization, which can be problematic in vomiting dogs and cats. Therefore, antacids are not recommended as a sole therapy for the treatment of gastric ulceration. Antacids might have a beneficial effect in dogs and cats with painful erosive or ulcerative lesions such as oral mucositis or erosive esophagitis. They can also promote local prostaglandin production. The side effects of antacid administration include constipation (aluminum preparations), diarrhea (magnesium preparations), and electrolyte derangements.

COATING AGENTS
Sucralfate

Sucralfate is composed of a polyaluminum sucrose sulfate that is divided into sucrose sulfate and aluminum salts in the presence of gastric acid. The negatively charged sulfate groups protect the ulcerated tissue from additional injury by binding electrostatically to positively charged proteins exposed in ulcerated areas. Sucralfate's affinity for abnormal, injured tissue is 5 times greater than for normal mucosa. Sucralfate also decreases pepsin activity and stimulates the release of protective prostaglandins, which in turn increases mucosal blood flow and increases mucus production and viscosity.[2] Sucralfate is particularly beneficial where pain is an anticipated sequela, such as with reflux esophagitis. In a canine ex vivo model of acid-induced injury, sucralfate was effective at restoring gastric barrier defects.[3] Based on comparative studies in humans, sucralfate might be more effective in the adjunctive treatment of duodenal ulcers compared with gastric ulcers. Importantly, it should be given as a commercially available suspension (eg, sucralfate [Carafate] suspension) or slurry rather than crushed or given as a whole tablet. A slurry may be prepared just before administration by dissolving a 1 g tablet in approximately 10 mL of water and allowing the mixture to stand for 15 to 20 minutes. The slurry should be shaken well before administration. Flavorings can be added, if needed, to improve palatability. Sucralfate is associated with very few adverse effects aside from constipation and drug interactions. However, its use, especially at high doses, is discouraged in cats with chronic kidney disease.[4] Sucralfate does change the pH of the stomach and therefore can interfere with the metabolism of drugs that are dependent on an acidic gastric pH (eg, proton pump inhibitors [PPIs]). It also interferes with drugs affected by the aluminum component of sucralfate (eg, tetracyclines, ciprofloxacin).[5,6] Therefore, these drugs (eg, acid suppressants, antibiotics) should be administered at least 2 hours before or after sucralfate administration.

Barium

Barium, like sucralfate, is proposed to have mucosal protecting effects and hemostatic properties. However, to the authors' knowledge, there are no published studies evaluating the efficacy of barium for gastric injury or bleeding. Barium enemas are effective for treatment of lower GI bleeding in people but there are no studies evaluating barium enemas in dogs or cats. The dose recommended for mucosal hemostasis (1–2 mL/kg) can be occasionally challenging to administer orally especially in a patient with a history of dysrexia or vomiting. Although barium is inert, aspiration of barium with gastric fluid contents can be fatal. Discontinue barium for at least 24 hours before GI endoscopy and do not use in animals where GI perforation is suspected.

ACID-SUPPRESSING DRUGS
Histamine Type 2 Receptor Antagonists

Gastric acid secretion is triggered by hormonal and neural stimulation of parietal cells, the acid producing cells of the stomach. Acid-suppressing drugs, which take aim at these physiologic targets on the parietal cell surface, have largely supplanted antacids (acid-neutralizing drugs) as the drugs of choice for acid-related diseases. Histamine type-2 receptor antagonists (H2RAs) were developed in the 1970s after the identification of histamine type-2 receptors and proton pumps on parietal cells.[7] Gastrin, acetylcholine, and histamine were identified as the major secretagogues of gastric acid secretion with histamine recognized as the most potent secretagogue. Healing of acid-related disorders was determined to be partially dependent on gastric acid suppression. Thus, H2RAs became the standard of care for the treatment of gastric ulcers and erosive esophagitis in humans and animals until the development of PPIs in the 1980s.

The H2RAs (eg, famotidine, ranitidine, cimetidine hydrochloride) are competitive inhibitors of the interaction of histamine with the histamine type-2 receptor on the parietal cell. They have a good safety profile and can be administered with a full meal. Cimetidine was the first H2RA to be used clinically in dogs and cats. When administered orally 3 times daily, its effect on reducing aspirin-induced gastritis is comparable to once-daily orally administered omeprazole.[8] However, its potency is diminished compared with famotidine and ranitidine. Unlike the other H2RAs, cimetidine inhibits cytochrome P450, which can result in drug interactions with other drugs influenced by the cytochrome P450 system.[9,10] Cimetidine may also decrease hepatic blood flow.[11] For these reasons, the use of cimetidine for the treatment of erosive and ulcerative diseases in dogs and cats is not recommended. Ranitidine has poor acid suppressant activity as determined by studies in both healthy cats and dogs in which it was no better than placebo in increasing the gastric pH when administered orally or intravenously, respectively, at approximately 2 mg/kg every 12 hours.[12,13] Ranitidine is more commonly used to promote GI motility, although in the majority of studies in healthy dogs the effects of ranitidine on the prevention of gastroesophageal reflux[14] and promotion of gastric emptying[15] were largely absent. More studies are needed to determine if ranitidine has a prokinetic effect in dogs with GI motility disorders. The presence of the probable human carcinogen, N-nitrosodimethylamine, in several generic and brand-name ranitidine products may limit the availability of ranitidine for veterinary practitioners.

Famotidine has good (cats) to excellent (dogs) acid suppressing activity during the first few days of intravenous or oral administration and has a good safety profile.[12,16,17] Intravenously administered famotidine was anecdotally reported to cause hemolysis in cats; however, this effect has not been documented when the drug is intravenously administered as a slow bolus over 5 minutes.[18] Repeated daily oral administration of famotidine, and likely the other H2RAs, results in a diminished effect in healthy dogs and cats,[16,17,19,20] which might occur within 2 to 3 days of therapy. In humans, a diminished effect or tachyphylaxis to the drug occurs regardless of the type of H2RA used, or dosage or frequency administered, as long as the drug is given daily. Intravenous administration of famotidine also results in tolerance in humans, but this effect has not been demonstrated in dogs and cats.

Because of their relatively weak acid-suppressing activity after several days of use, H2RAs should not supplant PPIs for the treatment of moderate to severe gastroduodenal erosion or ulceration especially those which require prolonged treatment such as ulceration secondary to gastric tumors. Moreover, H2RAs should not be combined with PPIs for the treatment of ulcerative disease as there is no benefit to this practice in raising gastric pH.[21] H2RAs are a good choice when only weak acid suppressant activity is needed, for immediate relief of symptoms when taken on an as needed basis (eg, bilious vomiting), or short-term such as in preventative therapy for esophageal reflux under anesthesia. The H2RAs are also effective against basal acid secretion and therefore have efficacy against nocturnal gastric acidity. Therefore, there might be some benefit in the combination of a PPI with nighttime famotidine for the treatment of gastroesophageal reflux. When pantoprazole shortages dictate the need for H2RA use in dogs with ulcerative disease or when more aggressive acid suppression is needed, a continuous rate infusion of famotidine at 8 mg/kg/d has been demonstrated to provide excellent acid suppression.[22] Intravenously administered esomeprazole can also be considered for these patients.[23] Famotidine is renally excreted and should be dose reduced in dogs and cats with acute kidney injury or chronic kidney disease.

Proton Pump Inhibitors

The PPIs (eg, omeprazole, esomeprazole, pantoprazole) target the final common pathway of acid production and inhibit gastric secretion regardless of the stimulus. The PPIs are lipophilic, weakly basic drugs that permeate the parietal cell membrane and become trapped in its acidic environment. Once trapped, the drug forms disulfide bonds with the active proton-pumping H^+-K-ATPase enzymes. The PPIs are more effective than H_2RAs in healing upper GI erosion and ulceration.[24] Indeed, a variety of omeprazole formulations (whole and divided enteric-coated tablet, capsule, reformulated paste, suspension) have been evaluated and demonstrated to be superior in raising the gastric pH in healthy dogs and cats compared with H_2RAs.[12,13,19,20] Although peak concentrations of H2RAs occur within hours of oral administration and the PPIs can take up to 4 days to reach peak effect, PPIs are likely as effective as H_2RAs on day 1 of administration. Orally administered PPIs should be given on an empty stomach immediately before offering a full meal. A small treat can be given with the drug if necessary to aid in oral administration.[13]

Although keeping the enteric-coated tablet intact is desired when possible, the tablet can be divided to optimize dosing for cats and small dogs. The degree of acid suppression is likely not as good on day 1 compared with an intact tablet, but provides good acid suppression over time as any drug that escapes premature gastric degradation begins to provide its own "enteric coating" by raising the gastric pH.[19] For most causes of upper GI ulceration or bleeding, dogs and cats should be treated twice daily with a PPI.[12,13,20] However, once-daily treatment may be effective for certain causes of gastric injury such as with exercise-induced gastritis.[24] Once-daily omeprazole administration is also effective for reduction of aspirin-induced gastritis, but was no better than placebo for the treatment of mechanically induced ulceration, which raises concern for once-daily administration of omeprazole for the treatment of common causes of ulceration, including gastric tumors and nonsteroidal anti-inflammatory drugs.[8] If once-daily administration of a PPI is necessary or compliance is a concern, orally administered esomeprazole seems to be an effective option even when dosed once daily.[25]

Esomeprazole might also be the preferred treatment for erosive esophagitis based on studies in people and may provide superior gastric acid suppression when intravenously administered as compared with pantoprazole.[23] Esomeprazole, in combination with cisapride, dosed 12 to 18 hours and 1.0 to 1.5 hours before induction is an effective treatment for prevention of anesthetic-induced reflux in dogs.[26] Acid suppressants should be discontinued after anesthetic recovery. Adverse effects of PPI administration in dogs and cats can include diarrhea (dogs),[12,20] induction of intestinal dysbiosis,[27,28] and hypergastrinemia and drug withdrawal-induced rebound gastric acid hypersecretion.[29] The PPIs are the medical treatment of choice for dogs and cats with documented nonsteroidal anti-inflammatory drug-induced upper GI bleeding or injury. However, omeprazole administration might induce intestinal injury when co-administered with the nonsteroidal anti-inflammatory drug, carprofen, in healthy dogs.[30] Thus, prophylactic omeprazole administration to healthy dogs receiving nonsteroidal anti-inflammatory drugs is not recommended unless other risk factors for gastric bleeding are present. Serum gastrin concentrations should normalize within 7 days after PPI or H2RA cessation.[31]

The PPIs are inhibitors of the hepatic cytochrome P450 system. Thus, drug interactions with concurrent PPI administration are possible with drugs that are affected by increased gastric pH or cytochrome P450 inhibition. Omeprazole does not diminish the antiplatelet effects of clopidogrel in healthy dogs. Over-the-counter omeprazole suspensions can contain xylitol and should not be used in dogs. Chronic use of PPIs and H2RAs or prophylactic administration for diseases in which a benefit has not been demonstrated is discouraged owing to reports of an association with a wide variety of adverse effects in people following long-term PPI use including chronic kidney disease, osteoporosis and pathologic fractures, community-acquired pneumonia, *Clostridium difficile*-associated diarrhea, and spontaneous bacterial peritonitis. However, the quality of evidence for a cause-and-effect relationship between PPIs and these adverse effects is low.

Prostaglandin Analogs

Prostaglandins play a critical role in the integrity of the GI mucosal barrier including by stimulating the secretion of bicarbonate-rich mucus, enhancing mucosal blood flow, and promoting epithelial restitution. The most commonly used prostaglandin agonist in veterinary medicine is misoprostol, a prostaglandin E_1 analog. By simulating endogenous eicosanoids, misoprostol may offer many of the protective benefits of prostaglandins. However, despite its mechanism of action, misoprostol is predominantly effective for nonsteroidal anti-inflammatory drug-induced injury[32] and has no effect with steroid-associated ulceration.[33] Misoprostol may increase GI and urogenital smooth muscle contractions leading to side effects of cramping, diarrhea, and abortions.

SUMMARY

Gastroprotectants are widely used by veterinarians for the treatment of esophagitis and gastroduodenal mucosal injury in dogs and cats. A range of gastroprotective drugs are available including acid suppressants (ie, histamine-2 receptor antagonists, PPIs), coating agents, prostaglandin analogs, and antacids. Of these, the PPIs are the most effective drugs for the medical treatment of upper GI injury. However, PPIs are not effective for all causes of upper GI injury and bleeding. The choice of gastroprotective drug should be guided by the cause and location of GI injury and the potential for adverse effects. Detailed instructions for proper use of the medication including when to discontinue the drug should be provided in all cases.

CLINICS CARE POINTS

Before prescribing gastroprotectants, it is important for the clinician to ask the following questions in order to avoid adverse effects and to ensure rationale use of drug:

- Is there an appropriate indication for the use of the drug?
- What objective measures will be used to determine if a beneficial effect is achieved?
- Have I provided adequate instructions for use and discontinuation of the drug?
- Is there a possibility of drug interactions or adverse effects for which to warn the client?

DISCLOSURE

The author is a consultant for TriviumVet, Inc. Studies performed by the author in the text above were supported by the Comparative Gastroenterology Society, American Veterinary Medical Foundation, Winn Feline Foundation (W17-017), Miller Trust (MT18-004), UTK Companion Animal Fund, and the ACVIM Foundation.

REFERENCES

1. Marks SL, Kook PH, Papich MG, et al. ACVIM consensus statement: support for rational administration of gastrointestinal protectants to dogs and cats. J Vet Intern Med 2018;32:1823–40.

2. Shorrock CJ, Rees WD. Effect of sucralfate on human gastric bicarbonate secretion and local prostaglandin E2 metabolism. Am J Med 1989;86:2–4.
3. Hill TL, Lascelles BDX, Blikslager AT. Effect of sucralfate on gastric permeability in an ex vivo model of stress-related mucosal disease in dogs. J Vet Intern Med 2018;32:670–8.
4. Quimby J, Lappin M. Evaluating sucralfate as a phosphate binder in normal cats and cats with chronic kidney disease. J Am Anim Hosp Assoc 2016;52:8–12.
5. KuKanich K, KuKanich B. The effect of sucralfate tablets vs. suspension on oral doxycycline absorption in dogs. J Vet Pharmacol Ther 2015;38:169–73.
6. KuKanich K, KuKanich B, Guess S, et al. Effect of sucralfate on the relative bioavailability of enrofloxacin and ciprofloxacin in healthy fed dogs. J Vet Intern Med 2016;30:108–15.
7. Huang JQ, Hunt RH. Pharmacological and pharmacodynamic essentials of H(2)-receptor antagonists and proton pump inhibitors for the practising physician. Best Pract Res Clin Gastroenterol 2001;15:355–70.
8. Jenkins CC, DeNovo RC, Patton CS, et al. Comparison of effects of cimetidine and omeprazole on mechanically created gastric ulceration and on aspirin-induced gastritis in dogs. Am J Vet Res 1991;52:658–61.
9. Johnson LM, Lankford SM, Bai SA. The influence of cimetidine on the pharmacokinetics of the enantiomers of verapamil in the dog during multiple oral dosing. J Vet Pharmacol Ther 1995;18:117–23.
10. Maskasame C, Lankford S, Bai SA. The effects of chronic oral diltiazem and cimetidine dosing on the pharmacokinetics and negative dromotropic action of intravenous and oral diltiazem in the dog. Biopharm Drug Dispos 1992;13: 521–37.
11. Sako J, Yasuda Y. The effect of intravenous cimetidine and histamine on splanchnic circulation in the dogs. Nihon Shokakibyo Gakkai Zasshi 1993;90: 1405–15.
12. Bersenas AM, Mathews KA, Allen DG, et al. Effects of ranitidine, famotidine, pantoprazole, and omeprazole on intragastric pH in dogs. Am J Vet Res 2005;66: 425–31.
13. Sutalo S, Ruetten M, Hartnack S, et al. The effect of orally administered ranitidine and once-daily or twice-daily orally administered omeprazole on intragastric pH in cats. J Vet Intern Med 2015;29:840–6.
14. Favarato ES, Souza MV, Costa PR, et al. Evaluation of metoclopramide and ranitidine on the prevention of gastroesophageal reflux episodes in anesthetized dogs. Res Vet Sci 2012;93:466–7.
15. Lidbury JA, Suchodolski JS, Ivanek R, et al. Assessment of the variation associated with repeated measurement of gastrointestinal transit times and assessment of the effect of oral ranitidine on gastrointestinal transit times using a wireless motility capsule system in dogs. Vet Med Int 2012;2012:938417.
16. Tolbert MK, Graham A, Odunayo A, et al. Repeated famotidine administration results in a diminished effect on intragastric pH in dogs. J Vet Intern Med 2017;31: 117–23.
17. Golly E, Odunayo A, Daves M, et al. The frequency of oral famotidine administration influences its effect on gastric pH in cats over time. J Vet Intern Med 2019;33: 544–50.
18. de Brito Galvao JF, Trepanier LA. Risk of hemolytic anemia with intravenous administration of famotidine to hospitalized cats. J Vet Intern Med 2008;22:325–9.

19. Parkinson S, Tolbert K, Messenger K, et al. Evaluation of the effect of orally administered acid suppressants on intragastric pH in cats. J Vet Intern Med 2014;29(1):104–12.
20. Tolbert K, Bissett S, King A, et al. Efficacy of oral famotidine and 2 omeprazole formulations for the control of intragastric pH in dogs. J Vet Intern Med 2011; 25:47–54.
21. Tolbert K, Odunayo A, Howell R, et al. Efficacy of intravenous administration of combined acid suppressants in healthy dogs. J Vet Intern Med 2015;29(2): 556–60.
22. Hedges K, Odunayo A, Price JM, et al. Evaluation of the effect of a famotidine continuous rate infusion on intragastric pH in healthy dogs. J Vet Intern Med 2019;33:1988–94.
23. Kuhl A, Odunayo A, Price J, et al. Comparative analysis of the effect of IV administered acid suppressants on gastric pH in dogs. J Vet Intern Med 2020;34(2): 678–83.
24. Williamson KK, Willard MD, Payton ME, et al. Efficacy of omeprazole versus high-dose famotidine for prevention of exercise-induced gastritis in racing Alaskan sled dogs. J Vet Intern Med 2010;24:285–8.
25. Hwang JH, Jeong JW, Song GH, et al. Pharmacokinetics and acid suppressant efficacy of esomeprazole after intravenous, oral, and subcutaneous administration to healthy beagle dogs. J Vet Intern Med 2017;31:743–50.
26. Zacuto AC, Marks SL, Osborn J, et al. The influence of esomeprazole and cisapride on gastroesophageal reflux during anesthesia in dogs. J Vet Intern Med 2012; 26:518–25.
27. Schmid SM, Suchodolski JS, Price JM, et al. Omeprazole minimally alters the fecal microbial community in six cats: a pilot study. Front Vet Sci 2018;5:79.
28. Garcia-Mazcorro JF, Suchodolski JS, Jones KR, et al. Effect of the proton pump inhibitor omeprazole on the gastrointestinal bacterial microbiota of healthy dogs. FEMS Microbiol Ecol 2012;80:624–36.
29. Gould E, Clements C, Reed A, et al. A prospective, placebo-controlled pilot evaluation of the effect of omeprazole on serum calcium, magnesium, cobalamin, gastrin concentrations, and bone in cats. J Vet Intern Med 2016;30:779–86.
30. Jones SM, Gaier A, Enomoto H, et al. The effect of combined carprofen and omeprazole administration on gastrointestinal permeability and inflammation in dogs. J Vet Intern Med 2020;34(5):1886–93.
31. Parente NL, Bari Olivier N, Refsal KR, et al. Serum concentrations of gastrin after famotidine and omeprazole administration to dogs. J Vet Intern Med 2014;28: 1465–70.
32. Ward DM, Leib MS, Johnston SA, et al. The effect of dosing interval on the efficacy of misoprostol in the prevention of aspirin-induced gastric injury. J Vet Intern Med 2003;17:282–90.
33. Rohrer CR, Hill RC, Fischer A, et al. Efficacy of misoprostol in prevention of gastric hemorrhage in dogs treated with high doses of methylprednisolone sodium succinate. Am J Vet Res 1999;60:982–5.

Gastric Motility Disorders in Dogs and Cats

Roman Husnik, MVDr, PhD[a],*, Frédéric Gaschen, Dr med vet, Dr habil[b]

KEYWORDS

- Gastrointestinal • Gastric emptying • Critical illness-related motility disorder
- Postoperative ileus • Ultrasound • Prokinetic

KEY POINTS

- Delayed gastric emptying (GE) usually occurs secondary to disorders affecting the gastrointestinal tract or other organs. It is the most commonly recognized manifestation of gastric motility disorders in small animals. Functional disorders are diagnosed after mechanical obstruction has been ruled out.
- Postoperative ileus is a common complication of abdominal surgery, and critical illness–related motility disorders are a prevalent concern in intensive care unit patients.
- The various methods available to investigate GE include scintigraphy, ultrasonography, radiographic contrast studies, wireless motility and endoscopy capsules, GE breath test, and measurement of gastric residual volumes.
- Therapy for nonobstructive gastric dysmotility is aimed at correcting any existing primary disorder and making judicious use of dietary modifications and prokinetic drugs.

INTRODUCTION

Canine and feline gastrointestinal (GI) motility disorders present both diagnostic and therapeutic challenges and likely are under-recognized in small animal practice. Gastric emptying (GE) is a complex process, which is controlled and affected by many physiologic, dietary, pharmacologic, and pathologic factors.[1,2] Abnormal GE is associated with clinical signs, such as vomiting, anorexia, nausea, abdominal discomfort, and abdominal distension, which are known to have a negative impact on quality of life. In people, disorders of GI motility are common reasons for patients to visit their physician.

Conflict of Interest Declaration: Authors declare no conflict of interest.
 a Department of Veterinary Clinical Sciences, College of Veterinary Medicine, Purdue University, 625 Harrison Street, West Lafayette, IN 47907, USA; b Department of Veterinary Clinical Sciences, Louisiana State University School of Veterinary Medicine, Skip Bertman Drive, Baton Rouge, LA 70803, USA
* Corresponding author.
E-mail address: husnikr@gmail.com

Vet Clin Small Anim 51 (2021) 43–59
https://doi.org/10.1016/j.cvsm.2020.09.002
0195-5616/21/© 2020 Elsevier Inc. All rights reserved.

GASTRIC EMPTYING OF SOLIDS—PHYSIOLOGY

Functionally, the stomach can be divided into the gastric reservoir and gastric pump.[3,4] The gastric reservoir consists of fundus and body. The gastric pump includes the distal part of the body and the pyloric antrum.

The main function of the gastric reservoir is to store ingesta and progressively release them into the gastric pump. With increasing volume of the stomach after meal ingestion, the internal gastric pressure increases only slightly due to gastric wall relaxation. Emptying of the reservoir includes 2 mechanisms: tonic contractions and peristaltic waves. The pyloric antrum acts as a pump from which peristaltic waves originate. Contractions occur only when excitatory neurotransmitters, such as acetylcholine, are released in response to stimulation of mechanoreceptors and chemoreceptors. The mechanical action of the antral pump is divided into 3 phases: (1) propulsion, (2) mixing and emptying of fine particles, and (3) retropulsion of particles greater than 2 mm and further grinding.

Motility of the duodenum is coordinated with gastric motility. The stomach is electrically isolated from duodenum by the pylorus; thus, the gastric electric and peristaltic waves end at the pylorus. Duodenal pacemaker potentials are more frequent than their gastric counterparts. During the emptying phase of the stomach, duodenal contractions are inhibited, and the proximal duodenum relaxes, which is described as antroduodenal coordination.

In carnivores, the daily energy requirement can be digested and absorbed within approximately 12 hours. The stomach and small intestine are empty during the remaining time. The GI tract does not remain in a state of motor quiescence between meals, however: recurring cycles of activity are the basis of the interdigestive motility, which consists of 3 phases—I (motor quiescence), II (irregular contractions), and III (migrating motor complex [MMC] in the dog or giant contractions in the cat). Motilin plasma levels increase cyclically every 90 minutes to 120 minutes during the interdigestive fasting period and are synchronous with phase III activity. This cyclical release of motilin stops after ingestion of a meal.

GI motility is coordinated so that the main priority is the protection of the duodenum: excessive distension of the stomach leads to constriction of the pylorus, which prevents large volumes of solid ingesta from being rapidly emptied into the duodenum.

After ingestion of a solid meal, gastric motility and emptying are modulated by various control mechanisms. They include gastrogastric reflexes, such as stimulation of antral contractions after filling and distention of the gastric reservoir. In addition, the activity of the pyloric sphincter is modulated by reflexes originating in the antrum and duodenum and involves the release of nitric oxide and vasoactive intestinal peptide. GE is inhibited by nutrients entering the small intestine (feedback control) through enterogastric reflexes and release of cholecystokinin from the intestinal epithelium resulting in relaxation of the gastric reservoir. Other hormones, such as glucagon-like peptide 1 and peptide YY, produced in the distal small intestine, also exert a negative feedback on GE. Additionally, the rate of GE after a solid meal is modulated by the composition of the diet and other factors, such as stress and body size.[1,2]

DISORDERS OF GASTRIC MOTILITY
Delayed Gastric Emptying

Once mechanical obstruction has been ruled out, delayed GE is the most commonly recognized manifestation of gastric motility disorders in small animals. The most common causes of nonobstructive delayed GE in dogs and cats are listed in **Box 1**.

Box 1
Causes of nonobstructive delayed gastric emptying in dogs and cats

Primary functional disorders
  GDV
  Dysautonomia
  Pyloric stenosis in young Siamese cats

Secondary functional abnormalities of GE
  Neurogenic inhibition (trauma, stress, spinal and abdominal surgery, peritonitis, and
  pancreatitis)
  Postoperative ileus (POI)
  Critical illness–related motility disorders (CIRMDs)
  Inflammatory, infiltrative, and ulcerative gastric or intestinal lesions (GI infections, parasites,
  gastric ulcers, adverse food reactions, IBD, dysbiosis, and GI neoplasia)
  Metabolic (hypokalemia, hypocalcemia, renal disease, acidosis, diabetes mellitus,
  hypoadrenocorticism, liver disease, hypothyroidism, and hypergastrinemia)
  Systemic disorders (immune-mediated diseases, abdominal inflammation, and neoplasia)
  Medications (opioid analgesics, anticholinergics, and vincristine)

Primary functional disorders appear to be rare in small animals and usually are attributed to myenteric plexus or autonomic nervous system dysfunction. So far, only a few disorders have been described that can be included into this category, such as pyloric stenosis, in young Siamese cats and diseases affecting the autonomous nervous system, such as dysautonomia.[5] The role of gastric dysmotility in the etiology of canine gastric dilatation-volvulus (GDV) has not been elucidated to date. It is unclear if the abnormal motility is at the origin of GDV or merely a complication of the disease and its surgical treatment.[6]

Secondary functional abnormalities of GE are thought to occur commonly and may be caused by many diseases. Neuromuscular gastric function may be affected by neurogenic inhibition; inflammatory, infiltrative, and ulcerative gastric or intestinal lesions; and systemic and metabolic disorders. Abnormal small intestinal and colonic motility have been documented in dogs after ablation of 66% of renal mass and associated chronic kidney disease, whereas GE seemed normal. It is possible, however, that a larger reduction of functional renal mass (>75%) as is observed in clinical chronic kidney disease cases may have negative impact on gastric motility.[7]

Delayed GE may be induced by various medications; opioid analgesics and anticholinergics may interfere with GI neurotransmitters and cause impaired smooth muscle function.[8,9] Vincristine, a frequently used chemotherapy agent, has been shown to transiently decrease gastric antral motility in dogs.[10]

Postoperative Ileus and Critical Illness–Related Gastrointestinal Motility Disorders

Postoperative ileus (POI) is a common complication of abdominal surgery in people, which may prolong the length of hospital stay and increase morbidity in affected patients.[8,11] The origin of POI in human patients is multifactorial and manipulation of the intestines, administration of opioids, and postoperative stress all contribute to the problem.[8,11] It arises from mechanisms triggered by the autonomic nervous system and hormonal responses. The pathogenesis involves 2 phases: the neurologic phase results from activation of the sympathetic nervous system after anesthesia and surgical incision. This is followed by an inflammatory phase associated with intestinal manipulation, which ultimately triggers an inflammatory cascade both in manipulated and nonmanipulated areas. In addition, permeability of the intestinal barrier is increased during this phase, which could lead to translocation of intestinal microbiota.

Hormonal responses are characterized by release of corticotropin-releasing factor and additional stimulation of proinflammatory cytokines in the bowel.[11] Finally, motility returns during and after the vagally mediated resolution phase.[8]

Even though dogs have been used as a model for POI in people for decades, clinical parameters associated with canine POI have not been well defined. Although return of appetite after abdominal surgery is rapid in most dogs, postoperative GI motility was decreased in dogs when measured with wireless motility capsules (WMCs),[12] breath test[6] or pressure transducers. Clinical signs include prolonged anorexia, nausea, vomiting and/or regurgitation, cranial abdominal discomfort, abdominal distension, and bloated abdomen. In experimental studies, epidural injection of morphine[13] and laparoscopic surgery (vs laparotomy) were shown to shorten the duration of POI in dogs.[14] Moreover, enteral supplementation of glutamine[15] and administration of GI prokinetics (metoclopramide[16] and motilin analogues[17]) were helpful in the treatment of POI.

Critical illness–related motility disorders (CIRMDs) are a common concern in human intensive care unit (ICU) patients.[18] Clinical signs include vomiting, abdominal distention, complaints of discomfort, and high gastric residual volumes (GRVs) (>500 mL total or >6.2 mL/kg). Abnormal GE compromises the effectiveness of enteral nutrition, an essential component of treatment.[18] Critical patients with CIRMD have increased GRV, which may predispose them to macroaspiration or microaspiration with resulting airway disease.[18,19] Approach of CIRMD includes use of the GI prokinetics metoclopramide and erythromycin, which have been shown to decrease feeding intolerance when used alone or in combination.[20]

There are no published data documenting the existence of CIRMD in canine and feline ICU patients. Internists and criticalists commonly manage paralytic ileus and delayed GE in critically ill dogs and cats with diseases, including severe acute pancreatitis, gastroenteritis, and peritonitis. Clinical signs are similar to those observed in POI, in addition to signs caused by the primary underlying disease. Typically, abdominal radiographs show moderately distended bowels loops filled with gas and liquid content, and abdominal ultrasound reveals distended and hypomotile stomach and intestine. As is the case in people, presence of POI or CIRMD in dogs and cats may increase morbidity and mortality and prolong the duration of hospitalization.

Retrograde Transit

Gastroesophageal reflux (GER) is a well-documented cause of morbidity and potential mortality in people, dogs, and cats.[21,22] Abnormalities in liquid or solid food emptying and in antral contractility have been observed in people with GER.[22] Delayed GE was associated with an increased rate of daily and postprandial liquid/mixed reflux events in human patients.[23] In addition, acceleration of GE with prucalopride decreased esophageal acid exposure.[24] GER may cause, trigger or exacerbate respiratory comorbidities.[19,25] Aspiration-related respiratory disorders are discussed in another article in this issue.

Diagnosis of duodenogastric reflux in dogs has been the subject of controversy because it may occur under normal circumstances. Canine bilious vomiting syndrome is a poorly defined suspected motility disorder associated with duodenogastric reflux.[26] The vomiting is thought to be a result of mucosal irritation caused by a reflux of alkaline duodenal fluid into the gastric lumen. In people, conditions with a similar pathophysiology are referred to as alkaline reflux gastritis and are thought to result from some abnormalities in the motor function of the stomach and changes in the speed of GE.[27] Dogs with a tentative diagnosis of bilious vomiting syndrome may respond to being fed a late night meal or to gastric acid reduction, antiemetic medication, and/or prokinetics.[26]

Rapid Gastric Emptying

The category of rapid GE includes dumping syndrome, mostly iatrogenic, as a result of vagotomy, pyloroplasty, partial gastrectomy, and gastroenterostomy.[28] It also may occur in feline hyperthyroidism, duodenitis, and exocrine pancreatic insufficiency and was described in a case of myenteric ganglionitis in a dog.

DIAGNOSTIC APPROACH

Signalment, history, and physical examination can be useful in prioritizing differential diagnoses and detecting underlying disorders. The most common clinical signs associated with gastric motility disorders in dogs and cats are listed in **Box 2**. Physical examination may be normal or may reveal findings associated with the underlying disease and the systemic effects of vomiting. In cases of POI or CIRMD, intestinal sounds usually are absent on abdominal auscultation. High GRV may predispose patients to macroaspiration or microaspiration with resulting airway disease.[18,19] GI dysmotility can lead to intolerance to enteral feeding, increased mucosal permeability for endoluminal mediators and bacteria, and the development of systemic inflammatory response syndrome and sepsis.[29] Radiographs are used to rule out the possibility of a GI obstruction and to evaluate if extragastric disorders are present. Abdominal ultrasound may show morphologic gastric wall abnormalities, radiolucent foreign objects, or detect nongastric causes of delayed GE. Presence of food in the stomach on radiographs or ultrasound after prolonged fasting (more than 8–12 hours) suggests delayed GE. Contrast radiography can be used to confirm suspicion of gastric obstruction when plain radiographs are inconclusive.

After mechanical obstruction has been ruled out, delayed GE can be attributed to defective propulsion. In such cases, a minimal database consisting of complete blood cell count, serum chemistry, and urinalysis is recommended to screen for underlying

---

Box 2
Clinical signs associated with delayed gastric emptying in dogs and cats

Vomiting
  The most common clinical sign, especially when it occurs long after food intake (8 hours and often 10–16 hours after a meal), when the stomach should be empty.
  Sometimes projectile vomiting may occur in the absence of a prodromal phase (nausea or salivation).
  The character of the vomitus depends on time interval since the last meal, amount of gastric secretions, degree of gastric trituration, and extent of hydrolytic digestion.

Regurgitation

Signs of nausea

Hyporexia/anorexia

Increased belching

Abdominal discomfort, cranial abdominal pain, colic

Abdominal distension, bloated abdomen

Weight loss

Melena

Hematemesis

Polydipsia

Pica

diseases and monitor for metabolic consequences of vomiting. Additional, more targeted tests can be performed based on the list of differential diagnoses applying to each particular patient (see **Box 1**). Upper GI endoscopy with collection of mucosal biopsies may be useful in identifying structural lesions associated with gastric outflow obstruction and gastric/duodenal causes of decreased propulsion. Finally, exploratory surgery may be indicated when full-thickness GI biopsies are required or when lesions of other abdominal organs are suspected.

CLINICAL EVALUATION OF GASTRIC EMPTYING

With the exception of survey and contrast radiographs and abdominal ultrasound, GE rarely is evaluated in dogs and cats. This likely is due to the lack of easily applicable methods: detailed evaluation of GE usually requires special equipment or skills that can be found only in few referral centers. Additionally, some techniques that can be performed only with manual or chemical restraint may deliver inaccurate results because stress and sedatives may interfere with gastric motility.[1,2]

Radionuclide scintigraphy (**Fig. 1**) is considered the gold standard technique in dogs and cats. Its clinical utility is limited, however, by the need for specialized equipment and radiation licensing. Consequently, availability is limited to academic institutions and a small number of specialty centers, where the method is used primarily for research rather than for clinical purposes.

Barium contrast radiography is easily available in clinical practice. Liquid barium is widely used; however, it is a poor indicator of gastric motility, and its use is limited to confirming the presence of gastric outflow obstructions that are not easily visible on survey radiographs. Barium-impregnated polyethylene spheres (BIPS) (Medical ID Systems, Grand Rapids, Michigan) have been used for evaluation of GI transit times in dogs and cats. Correlation between GE of BIPS and radionuclide scintigraphy, however, is disappointing in dogs and cats.[30,31] This probably reflects the facts that BIPS greater than 2 mm are emptied only after all solid food has left the stomach.

Qualitative transabdominal ultrasound examination of the GI tract now is a routine part of the investigation of patients with GI clinical signs. In addition to radiographs, ultrasound can be useful for evaluation of gastric filling state (**Fig. 2**), detection of morphologic gastric wall abnormalities, and measuring gastric contractile activity. A

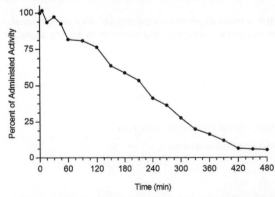

Fig. 1. Evaluation of GE by radionuclide scintigraphy in a healthy cat. Time curve of GE is shown. The Y axis represents the percentage of administered activity, and the X axis represents time. $GET_{50\%}$ is 217 minutes. $GET_{50\%}$, time when 50% of meal has left the stomach. (*Courtesy of* R. Husnik, MVDr, PhD, Guelph, Canada.)

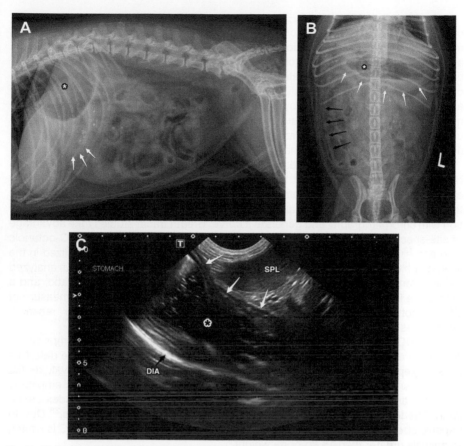

Fig. 2. Right lateral (*A*) and ventrodorsal (*B*) abdominal radiographs from a 4-year-old MC Boston terrier with acute pancreatitis. The stomach was moderately dilated with a mixed fluid and gas opacity. There was a small amount of mineral opaque content located in the antrum and proximal duodenum. The duodenum showed a rigid course to the caudal flexure. The dog responded well to a metoclopramide CRI (2 mg/kg/d). (*Asterisk*) gastric body; (*white arrows*) ventral part of the gastric antrum (lateral view), and greater curvature of the stomach (VD view); (*black arrows*) duodenum. Abdominal ultrasound (*C*): markedly fluid-distended stomach lacking peristalsis in the absence of gastric outflow obstruction. The entire pancreas was hypoechoic, mildly enlarged, irregular in shape, and surrounded by hyperechoic mesentery (not shown). (*Asterisk*) gastric lumen; (*white arrows*) greater curvature of the stomach. DIA, diaphragm; SPL, spleen. (*Courtesy of* L. Gaschen, DVM, Dr.med.-vet., Dr.habil., PhD, DECVD, Baton Rouge, LA.)

normal stomach containing some food should contract 4 times to 5 times per minute. This depends, however, on the degree of filling and time since the last meal; an empty stomach can be in a resting state and have fewer and weaker contractions.[32]

A conventional small intestinal examination can detect presence or absence of peristalsis. Contractility of the small intestine can be assessed by imaging of a region of intestine over a short period of time. Normal rates of peristalsis are 4 to 5 contractions/min for proximal duodenum and 1 to 3 contractions/min for the rest of the small intestine.

Quantitative assessment of GE and gastric motility consists of sequential evaluation of antral size after a meal. Ultrasonographic evaluation of GE relies on the postprandial measurement of the cross-sectional area or estimated volume of the relaxed pyloric antrum over time. As the stomach empties, the size of the antrum decreases and ultimately returns to the fasted state. GE times can be derived from a time plot of antral cross-sectional area (**Fig. 3**). A close correlation between the rate of both liquid-phase and solid-phase GE measured by ultrasonography and scintigraphy has been documented in people.[33] The technique allows determination of GE times as well as evaluation of motility parameters, such as frequency and amplitude of antral contractions (**Fig. 4**) and motility index, and has been validated in both dogs and cats.[34,35]

Several kinds of tracer studies, including plasma and breath tracers, have been developed for the assessment of GE and/or intestinal transit. Acetaminophen is absorbed rapidly in the duodenum as chyme exits the stomach, and its rate of absorption reflects GE. Blood samples are collected to determine acetaminophen concentration with chromatography and generate a curve. Breath tracer studies take advantage of site-specific absorption of orally administered compounds after GE. ^{13}C-octanoic acid and ^{13}C-sodium acetate are absorbed in the duodenum and metabolized in the liver, and $^{13}CO_2$ ultimately is released from the lungs.[35–37] The exhaled air is analyzed by spectrometry or spectroscopy to measure the $^{12}CO_2/^{13}CO_2$ isotope ratio, and a time curve is generated. The ^{13}C breath tests have been validated as a measure of GE in both dogs and cats and their use currently is limited to research laboratories.[35–37]

The WMC (SmartPill, Medtronic, Minneapolis, Minnesota) can record temperature, pH, and pressure during its journey through the GI tract and transmits the data to a receiver kept in a vest worn by the dog. The WMC makes it possible to evaluate GE as well as small intestinal and colonic transit times (**Fig. 5**).[38] Frequency and amplitude of gastric and intestinal contractions can be determined and a motility index calculated. The technique has been validated for measurement of GE in dogs.[38] Due to capsule size, there is a risk of gastric retention in small dogs and the WMC is limited to animals greater than 15 kg body weight.

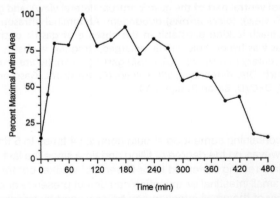

Fig. 3. Evaluation of GE by ultrasonography in a healthy cat. Time curve of GE is shown. The Y axis represents the percentage of maximal antral area, and the X axis represents time. GET$_{50\%}$ is 222 minutes. GET$_{50\%}$, time when 50% of meal has left the stomach, respectively. (*Courtesy of* R. Husnik, MVDr, PhD, Guelph, Canada.)

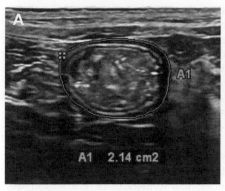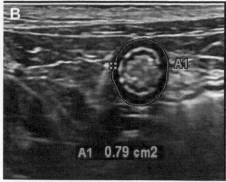

Fig. 4. Evaluation of GE by ultrasonography in a healthy cat. Ultrasound images of the transverse section of the gastric antrum in the cat taken 150 minutes after ingestion of a meal. The test meal provided approximately 20% of the estimated daily energy requirement of the cat. (*A*) Maximal gastric antrum relaxation. (*B*) Maximal gastric antrum contraction. The yellow line in the images follows the serosal side of the antrum, and is used to compute the cross-sectional antral area. A1 represents the cross-sectional area of the gastric antrum. (*Courtesy of* R. Husnik, MVDr, PhD, Guelph, Canada.)

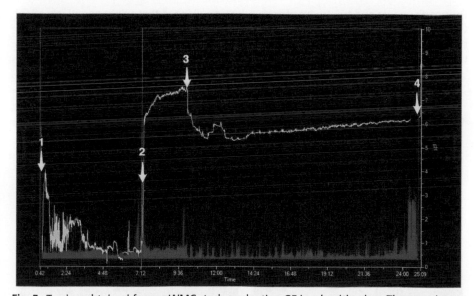

Fig. 5. Tracing obtained from a WMC study evaluating GE in a healthy dog. The capsule was administered with a test meal, which provided approximately 30% of the daily estimated energy requirement. The dark blue line shows temperature (°C), the green line shows pH, and the red line shows intraluminal pressure. The X axis represents time (hours: minutes). 1, Capsule enters the stomach (low pH); 2. capsule exits the stomach (rise in pH by >3 units); 3, capsule enters large bowel (drop in pH by approximately 1 unit); and 4, capsule exits the rectum (drop in the temperature curve). The gastric emptying time (GET) (time 2 minus time 1) is 6 hours and 28 minutes. Small bowel transit time (time 3 minus time 2) is approximately 2 hours and 30 minutes. Large bowel transit time (time 4 minus time 3) is approximately 15 hours and 15 minutes. Total transit time (time 4 minus time 1) is a little longer than 24 hours. (*Courtesy of* F. Gaschen, Dr. med. vet., Dr. habil., Baton Rouge, LA.)

Video capsule endoscopy (Alicam, Infiniti Medical, Redwood City, California; Pillcam SB3, Medtronic) is an easy-to-use, novel GI imaging technique performed by oral administration of a fully automated capsule-sized camera device that is propelled by natural peristalsis. The time required for passage of the capsule through the stomach and small intestine can be determined based on correlation of images with an internal clock (**Fig. 6**).[39] A limitation of video capsules is that they are administered to fasted dogs, and it is not sure how fasted GE is correlated to postprandial GE of solids. Video capsule endoscopy was used to assess gastric and small intestinal transit times in healthy dogs[39] but the method has not been validated for measurement of GE.

GRVs measured intermittently are common practice for evaluation of gastric motility and feeding tolerance in human ICU patients. The utility and the significance of GRV, however, remain controversial because substantial evidence for correlation with gastric motility is lacking. Moreover, measurement of GRV is not standardized and results can be affected by patient positioning, technique, tube location and diameter, use of prokinetic drugs, and composition of the liquid diet.[18] In a veterinary study, no direct association between GRV, the occurrence of vomiting or regurgitation, or incidences of aspiration could be found.[40] Therefore, the use of GRV to guide treatment strategies should be approached with caution.

MANAGEMENT OF GASTROINTESTINAL MOTILITY DISORDERS

Proper diagnosis and treatment of any underlying disease that might negatively affect GI motility are an essential premise. Therapy for functional nonobstructive gastric motility disorders is based on 2 main interventions: dietary modifications and judicious use of prokinetic drugs.

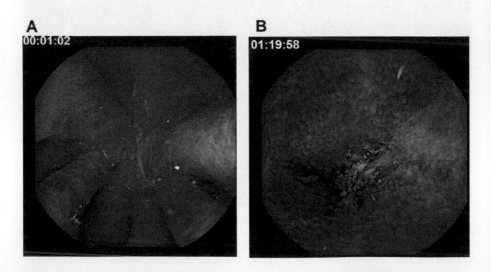

Fig. 6. Evaluation of GE by video capsule endoscopy in a 4-year-old Boston terrier presented for mast cell tumor and intermittent upper GI signs. Capsule was administered after 12-hour fast for GI cleanse. First gastric (A) and first duodenal images (B) are shown. The time required for passage of the capsule through the stomach can be determined based on correlation of images with an internal clock of the capsule. The gastric transit time is 1 hour, 18 minutes, and 56 seconds. (*Courtesy of* R. Husnik, MVDr, PhD, Guelph, Canada.)

Dietary Modifications

Dietary modifications are an essential part of the management of GI motility disorders and are based on physiologic principles. First, GE of liquid food is faster than that of solid foods. Also, diets with high caloric density tend to remain longer in the stomach. In addition, GE of fat is slower than that of proteins, which is slower than that of carbohydrates. Consequently, feeding liquid or semiliquid diet of low caloric density and low in fat and protein should maximize GE. In addition, increasing meal frequency and decreasing meal size also are beneficial.

Prokinetic Drugs

They should be administered only after a GI obstruction has been definitely ruled out. Clinicians need to remember that the available evidence on the effects of prokinetic drugs in healthy dogs and cats is tenuous, whereas it is almost nonexistent for dogs and cats with GI dysmotility. Therefore, collective clinical experience plays an important role in most recommendations for drug usage and dosage (**Table 1**). It is the authors' conviction that timely recognition and appropriate management of GI hypomotility are essential for successful treatment of diseases, such as acute pancreatitis, peritonitis, and severe gastroenteritis or enterocolitis. In dogs and cats receiving opiate analgesics, strong consideration should be given in using alternate methods for analgesia without negative impact on GI motility, such as lidocaine (discussed later) and possibly ketamine constant-rate infusions (CRIs). Abrupt discontinuation of analgesia is not recommended because pain is another possible cause of GI hypomotility.

Table 1
Mode, site of action, and dosage recommendation for commonly used prokinetics in small animals

Name	Mode of Action	Site of Action	Dose (for Dogs and Cats Unless Specified)
Metoclopramide	Serotonergic (5-HT$_4$ receptors) Dopamin-antagonist (D$_2$ receptors)	Pyloric antrum Duodenum (?)	0.5 mg/kg q 8 h, PO, SC CRI: 1–2 mg/kg/24 h
Cisapride	Serotonergic (principally 5-HT$_4$ receptors)	LES Pyloric antrum Small intestine Colon	0.5 mg/kg PO, q 8–12 h
Mosapride	Serotonergic (5-HT$_4$ receptor-specific)	Pyloric antrum	0.5–2 mg/kg PO q 12–24 h (dog). Only available in Japan
Prucalopride	Serotonergic (5-HT$_4$ receptor-specific)	Pyloric antrum Small intestine (?) Colon	0.05–0.5 mg/kg PO q 12–24 h
Erythromycin	Motilin analogue	Pyloric antrum Small intestine Colon	0.5–1.0 mg/kg IV, PO q 8 h
Azithromycin	Motilin analogue	Unknown, probably similar to erythromycin	2.0 mg/kg IV q 8 h (dog) 3.5 mg/kg PO q24 h (cat)

Abbreviations: LES, lower esophageal sphincter; PO, by mouth; SC, subcutaneous.
? indicates that it is controversial if the drug works on the duodenum

Serotonergic drugs

Serotonergic drugs act on presynaptic 5-hydroxytryptamine (5-HT) receptors of different types.

Metoclopramide is an antagonist of dopamine-2 and 5-HT$_3$ receptors and an agonist of 5-HT$_4$ receptors. 5-HT$_4$ receptors are located on enteric cholinergic neurons that innervate intestinal smooth muscle. Their activation results in release of acetylcholine in the synaptic cleft and excitation of the postsynaptic cell membrane. In addition, D$_2$ receptor blockade on the same neurons is thought to counteract the inhibitory effect of dopamine on the release of acetylcholine. These effects ultimately stimulate contraction of smooth muscle cells of the stomach and proximal small intestine. Metoclopramide was shown to shorten the time to restoration of GI motility after surgery in dogs.[16] A recent study in healthy cats showed that metoclopramide shortens GE time and increases the motility index of antral contractions.[41] In the authors' clinical experience, intravenous (IV) administration using a CRI of 1 mg/kg/d to 2 mg/kg/d is the most efficient option in dogs and cats with paralytic ileus. In people, the treatment can become less effective over days to weeks, due to tachyphylaxis.[42,43]

Cisapride is another serotonergic drug that was withdrawn from the pharmaceutical market due to its cross-reactivity with serotonergic receptors on the myocardium and associated risk of lethal re-entry cardiac arrhythmias in people. Cisapride, however, does not cause prolongation of the QT interval and polymorphic ventricular arrhythmia in cats unless administered at doses 20-times higher than currently recommended.[44] In North America, it currently is available from compounding pharmacies. The principal mode of action of cisapride is its ability to bind to 5-HT$_4$ receptors and to stimulate smooth muscle contractions.

Prucalopride (Motegrity, Takeda Pharmaceuticals, Lexington, Massachusetts) is a novel, highly selective 5-HT$_4$ agonist that is approved for use in people under different brand names in many countries. In people with idiopathic gastroparesis, prucalopride significantly improved symptoms and quality of life and enhanced GE compared with placebo.[45] It has prokinetic properties on the canine pyloric antrum, small intestine, and canine and feline colon.[46] Prucalopride has been used anecdotally with some success in dogs with GI hypomotility.

Mosapride is a selective 5HT$_4$ agonist that is approved for use in dogs in Japan and other Asian countries. It has been reported to be helpful in constipated cats and showed a prokinetic effect in the stomach of healthy dogs.[10]

Motilin agonists

Erythromycin is a macrolide antibiotic. At reduced doses, it exerts gastrokinetic effects similar to those of motilin, the hormone that triggers the onset of MMC type III, the motility pattern responsible for cleaning the canine stomach and small intestine during the interdigestive phase. The administration of erythromycin to dogs stimulates GE without any attention to particle size. Cats do not display well-organized interdigestive motility patterns; however, motilin receptors are present in their GI tract. Erythromycin recently was shown to shorten GE times and increase the motility index of antral contractions in healthy cats.[41] Erythromycin is an inhibitor of the cytochrome p450 enzyme CYP3A, and it increases the risk of cardiac arrhythmias in people. Tachyphylaxis due to down-regulation of motilin receptors has been reported after approximately 1 week of treatment in people treated with motilin agonists.[42,43]

Azithromycin, another macrolide antibiotic, shares the motilin agonist properties of erythromycin. It has been recommended as a good GI prokinetic in people, although large-scale studies on its effects still are missing.[47] Following recent price increases in erythromycin, azithromycin has been used anecdotally with good success in small animals with GI hypomotility by both authors. Additionally, it was recently shown to be as effective as erythromycin in accelerating GE in healthy cats (Rutherford S. et al., personal communication).

Acetylcholinesterase inhibitors
Ranitidine and nizatidine, in addition to their H_2-receptor blocking properties, also have an acetylcholinesterase inhibitor effect, which results in increased acetylcholine concentration in the synaptic cleft between postganglionic myenteric neurons and GI smooth muscle cells. A WMC study done in healthy dogs, however, could not detect any significant effect of ranitidine on GI motility parameters.[48]

Acotiamide is a novel selective acetylcholinesterase inhibitor approved for use as a GI prokinetic in people in Japan. It enhanced postprandial gastroduodenal and colonic motor activity in healthy dogs after IV and oral administration.[49]

Drugs with potential gastrointestinal prokinetic effect in dogs and cats
Ghrelin-agonists: ghrelin is a GI hormone with multiple effects. It is thought to influence GI motility through stimulation of central nervous system receptors and activation of efferent vagal pathways. In phase II studies, the ghrelin agonist relamorelin has shown value in the treatment of diabetic gastroparesis in people.[50] Capromorelin is a ghrelin agonist approved for treatment of anorexia in dogs. Its prokinetic properties, however, have not been investigated to date, and it cannot be recommended for treatment of GI hypomotility at this time.

L-arginine and L-glutamate administered as a mixture orally (L-arginine, L-glutamate pharmaceutical amino acid salt [20 mM; 1:1]; 30 mg/kg) before a meal to healthy dogs reversed clonidine-induced gastroparesis as successfully as cisapride. The effect of the oral arginine/glutamate mixture is thought to be vagally mediated.[51]

Drugs with questionable or no gastrointesintal prokinetic effect in dogs and cats
Lidocaine: a CRI of lidocaine during any surgical intervention is thought to decrease the severity of POI through the drug's antinociceptive, antihyperalgesic, and anti-inflammatory properties. Lidocaine CRI, however, does not appear to have any direct effect on GI motility in dogs.[52]

Mirtazapine is an inhibitor of central presynaptic α_2-adrenergic receptors (resulting in increased central release of noradrenaline) and a potent inhibitor of 5-HT_2 and 5-HT_3 receptors. The drug often is used as an appetite stimulant and antinausea drug. Mirtazapine at a very high dose of 45 mg/dog, administered orally 1.5 hours before a meal, accelerated GE and colonic transit in healthy beagles.[53] A recent study evaluating low doses, medium doses, and high doses of mirtazapine in healthy dogs using the ^{13}C-sodium acetate breath test, could not duplicate these results.[54] Therefore, the drug cannot be recommended for use as a GI prokinetic at this time.

Maropitant, the NK1-receptor antagonist antiemetic drug commonly used in dogs and cats, did not show any prokinetic effect in healthy dogs using 2 different methods.[55]

Bethanechol directly stimulates cholinergic receptors. At therapeutic doses, its effects usually are limited to muscarinic receptors; however, nicotinic stimulation may occur with higher doses. Bethanechol has significant stimulating effects on the GI and urinary tracts. It has been recommended for treatment of feline dysautonomia. In people, however, bethanechol evokes fundoantral contractions but does not induce propulsive contractions or accelerate GE.[56]

Combination Prokinetic Therapy

Combination prokinetic therapy with 2 different agents may be useful to accelerate GE and reduce symptoms in some refractory gastroparetic patients. Prokinetic agents that enhance GE through different mechanisms may work synergistically when combined. Recent studies in critically ill people support the efficacy of a combination of different prokinetics as first-line therapy for feeding intolerance.[18] In human ICU patients, the combination of erythromycin and metoclopramide has been shown to achieve the highest efficacy in the treatment of feeding intolerance, best facilitates GE in critically ill, and is associated with a lesser degree of drug tachyphylaxis.[57]

SUMMARY

The most commonly recognized manifestation of gastric dysmotility in small animals is delayed GE secondary to disorders originating in the GI tract or other organs. POI and CIRMDs occur commonly and must be recognized in a timely manner. Routine abdominal imaging allows ruling out a GI obstruction, to qualitatively assess GI motility and to evaluate if other abdominal disorders are present. Quantitative evaluation of GE is not easily available for clinical canine and feline cases. Therapy for functional disorders is based on treatment of any underlying disorder, dietary modifications, and use of prokinetics.

REFERENCES

1. Warrit K, Boscan P, Ferguson LE, et al. Effect of hospitalization on gastrointestinal motility and pH in dogs. J Am Vet Med Assoc 2017;251(1):65–70.
2. Mistiaen W, Blockx P, Van Hee R, et al. The effect of stress on gastric emptying rate measured with a radionuclide tracer. Hepatogastroenterology 2002;49(47): 1457–60.
3. Camilleri M. Gastric motility and gastric emptying. In: Podolsky DK, Camilleri M, Fitz JG, et al, editors. Yamada's textbook of gastroenterology. 6th edition. Chichester (UK): Wiley-Blackwell; 2016. p. 348–66.
4. Ehrlein H, Schemann M. Gastrointestinal motility, Technical University Munich. 2007. Available at: https://www.humanbiology.wzw.tum.de.
5. Clarke KE, Sorrell S, Breheny C, et al. Dysautonomia in 53 cats and dogs: retrospective review of clinical data and outcome. Vet Rec 2020.
6. Schmitz S, Jansen N, Failing K, et al. 13C-sodium acetate breath test for evaluation of gastric emptying times in dogs with gastric dilatation-volvulus. Tierarztl Prax Ausg K Kleintiere Heimtiere 2013;41(2):87–92.
7. Lefebvre HP, Ferre JP, Watson AD, et al. Small bowel motility and colonic transit are altered in dogs with moderate renal failure. Am J Physiol Regul Integr Comp Physiol 2001;281(1):R230–8.
8. Venara A, Neunlist M, Slim K, et al. Postoperative ileus: pathophysiology, incidence, and prevention. J Visc Surg 2016;153(6):439–46.
9. Ketwaroo GA, Cheng V, Lembo A. Opioid-induced bowel dysfunction. Curr Gastroenterol Rep 2013;15(9):344.
10. Tsukamoto A, Ohno K, Tsukagoshi T, et al. Ultrasonographic evaluation of vincristine-induced gastric hypomotility and the prokinetic effect of mosapride in dogs. J Vet Intern Med 2011;25(6):1461–4.
11. Augestad KM, Delaney CP. Postoperative ileus: impact of pharmacological treatment, laparoscopic surgery and enhanced recovery pathways. World J Gastroenterol 2010;16(17):2067–74.

12. Boscan P, Cochran S, Monnet E, et al. Effect of prolonged general anesthesia with sevoflurane and laparoscopic surgery on gastric and small bowel propulsive motility and pH in dogs. Vet Anaesth Analg 2014;41(1):73–81.

13. Nakayoshi T, Kawasaki N, Suzuki Y, et al. Epidural administration of morphine facilitates time of appearance of first gastric interdigestive migrating complex in dogs with paralytic ileus after open abdominal surgery. J Gastrointest Surg 2007;11(5):648–54.

14. Tittel A, Schippers E, Anurov M, et al. Shorter postoperative atony after laparoscopic-assisted colonic resection? An animal study. Surg Endosc 2001; 15(5):508–12.

15. Ohno T, Mochiki E, Ando H, et al. Glutamine decreases the duration of postoperative ileus after abdominal surgery: an experimental study of conscious dogs. Dig Dis Sci 2009;54(6):1208–13.

16. Graves GM, Becht JL, Rawlings CA. Metoclopramide reversal of decreased gastrointestinal myoelectric and contractile activity in a model of canine postoperative ileus. Vet Surg 1989;18(1):27–33.

17. Furuta Y, Takeda M, Nakayama Y, et al. Effects of SK-896, a new human motilin analogue ([Leu13]motilin-Hse), on postoperative ileus in dogs after laparotomy. Biol Pharm Bull 2002;25(8):1063–71.

18. Ladopoulos T, Giannaki M, Alexopoulou C, et al. Gastrointestinal dysmotility in critically ill patients. Ann Gastroenterol 2018;31(3):273–81.

19. Nafe LA, Grobman ME, Masseau I, et al. Aspiration-related respiratory disorders in dogs. J Am Vet Med Assoc 2018;253(3):292–300.

20. Lewis K, Alqahtani Z, McIntyre L, et al. The efficacy and safety of prokinetic agents in critically ill patients receiving enteral nutrition: a systematic review and meta-analysis of randomized trials. Crit Care 2016;20(1):259.

21. Garcia RS, Belafsky PC, Della Maggiore A, et al. Prevalence of gastroesophageal reflux in cats during anesthesia and effect of omeprazole on gastric pH. J Vet Intern Med 2017;31(3):734–42.

22. Mikami DJ, Murayama KM. Physiology and pathogenesis of gastroesophageal reflux disease. Surg Clin North Am 2015;95(3):515–25.

23. Gourcerol G, Benanni Y, Boueyre E, et al. Influence of gastric emptying on gastroesophageal reflux: a combined pH-impedance study. Neurogastroenterol Motil 2013;25(10):800-e634.

24. Kessing BF, Smout AJ, Bennink RJ, et al. Prucalopride decreases esophageal acid exposure and accelerates gastric emptying in healthy subjects. Neurogastroenterol Motil 2014;26(8):1079–86.

25. Kogan DA, Johnson LR, Jandrey KE, et al. Clinical, clinicopathologic, and radiographic findings in dogs with aspiration pneumonia: 88 cases (2004-2006). J Am Vet Med Assoc 2008;233(11):1742–7.

26. Ferguson L, Wennogle SA, Webb CB. Bilious vomiting syndrome in dogs: retrospective study of 20 cases (2002-2012). J Am Anim Hosp Assoc 2016;52(3): 157–61.

27. McCabe MEt, Dilly CK. New causes for the old problem of bile reflux gastritis. Clin Gastroenterol Hepatol 2018;16(9):1389–92.

28. Vavricka SR, Greuter T. Gastroparesis and dumping syndrome: current concepts and management. J Clin Med 2019;8(8).

29. Ukleja A. Altered GI motility in critically III patients: current understanding of pathophysiology, clinical impact, and diagnostic approach. Nutr Clin Pract 2010; 25(1):16–25.

30. Goggin JM, Hoskinson JJ, Kirk CA, et al. Comparison of gastric emptying times in healthy cats simultaneously evaluated with radiopaque markers and nuclear scintigraphy. Vet Radiol Ultrasound 1999;40(1):89–95.

31. Lester NV, Roberts GD, Newell SM, et al. Assessment of barium impregnated polyethylene spheres (BIPS) as a measure of solid-phase gastric emptying in normal dogs–comparison to scintigraphy. Vet Radiol Ultrasound 1999;40(5): 465–71.

32. Sanderson JJ, Boysen SR, McMurray JM, et al. The effect of fasting on gastrointestinal motility in healthy dogs as assessed by sonography. J Vet Emerg Crit Care (San Antonio) 2017;27(6):645–50.

33. Szarka LA, Camilleri M. Gastric emptying. Clin Gastroenterol Hepatol 2009;7(8): 823–7.

34. Husnik R, Fletcher JM, Gaschen L, et al. Validation of ultrasonography for assessment of gastric emptying time in healthy cats by radionuclide scintigraphy. J Vet Intern Med 2017;31(2):394–401.

35. McLellan J, Wyse CA, Dickie A, et al. Comparison of the carbon 13-labeled octanoic acid breath test and ultrasonography for assessment of gastric emptying of a semisolid meal in dogs. Am J Vet Res 2004;65(11):1557–62.

36. Schmitz S, Failing K, Neiger R. Solid phase gastric emptying times in the dog measured by 13C-sodium-acetate breath test and 99mTechnetium radioscintigraphy. Tierarztl Prax Ausg K Kleintiere Heimtiere 2010;38(4):211–6.

37. Schmitz S, Gotte B, Borsch C, et al. Direct comparison of solid-phase gastric emptying times assessed by means of a carbon isotope-labeled sodium acetate breath test and technetium Tc 99m albumin colloid radioscintigraphy in healthy cats. Am J Vet Res 2014;75(7):648–52.

38. Boillat CS, Gaschen FP, Gaschen L, et al. Variability associated with repeated measurements of gastrointestinal tract motility in dogs obtained by use of a wireless motility capsule system and scintigraphy. Am J Vet Res 2010;71(8):903–8.

39. Pomrantz J, Lidbury J, Hardy B, et al. Feasibility of measuring gastrointestinal transit time in healthy dogs using ALICAM. J Vet Intern Med 2016;30:1461.

40. Holahan M, Abood S, Hauptman J, et al. Intermittent and continuous enteral nutrition in critically ill dogs: a prospective randomized trial. J Vet Intern Med 2010; 24(3):520–6.

41. Husnik R, Gaschen FP, Fletcher JM, et al. Ultrasonographic assessment of the effect of metoclopramide, erythromycin and exenatide on solid phase gastric emptying in healthy cats. J Vet Intern Med 2020;34(4):1440–6.

42. Nguyen NQ, Chapman MJ, Fraser RJ, et al. Erythromycin is more effective than metoclopramide in the treatment of feed intolerance in critical illness. Crit Care Med 2007;35(2):483–9.

43. Nguyen NQ, Chapman M, Fraser RJ, et al. Prokinetic therapy for feed intolerance in critical illness: one drug or two? Crit Care Med 2007;35(11):2561–7.

44. Kii Y, Nakatsuji K, Nose I, et al. Effects of 5-HT(4) receptor agonists, cisapride and mosapride citrate on electrocardiogram in anaesthetized rats and guinea-pigs and conscious cats. Pharmacol Toxicol 2001;89(2):96–103.

45. Carbone F, Van den Houte K, Clevers E, et al. Prucalopride in gastroparesis: a randomized placebo-controlled crossover study. Am J Gastroenterol 2019; 114(8):1265–74.

46. Wong BS, Manabe N, Camilleri M. Role of prucalopride, a serotonin (5-HT(4)) receptor agonist, for the treatment of chronic constipation. Clin Exp Gastroenterol 2010;3:49–56.

47. Larson JM, Tavakkoli A, Drane WE, et al. Advantages of azithromycin over erythromycin in improving the gastric emptying half-time in adult patients with gastroparesis. J Neurogastroenterol Motil 2010;16(4):407–13.
48. Lidbury JA, Suchodolski JS, Ivanek R, et al. Assessment of the variation associated with repeated measurement of gastrointestinal transit times and assessment of the effect of oral ranitidine on gastrointestinal transit times using a wireless motility capsule system in dogs. Vet Med Int 2012;2012:938417.
49. Nagahama K, Matsunaga Y, Kawachi M, et al. Acotiamide, a new orally active acetylcholinesterase inhibitor, stimulates gastrointestinal motor activity in conscious dogs. Neurogastroenterol Motil 2012;24(6):566–574, e256.
50. Chedid V, Camilleri M. Relamorelin for the treatment of gastrointestinal motility disorders. Expert Opin Investig Drugs 2017;26(10):1189–97.
51. Ishibashi-Shiraishi I, Shiraishi S, Fujita S, et al. L-arginine L-glutamate enhances gastric motor function in rats and dogs and improves delayed gastric emptying in dogs. J Pharmacol Exp Ther 2016;359(2):238–46.
52. Johnson RA, Kierski KR, Jones BG. Evaluation of gastric emptying time, gastrointestinal transit time, sedation score, and nausea score associated with intravenous constant rate infusion of lidocaine hydrochloride in clinically normal dogs. Am J Vet Res 2017;78(5):550–7.
53. Yin J, Song J, Lei Y, et al. Prokinetic effects of mirtazapine on gastrointestinal transit. Am J Physiol Gastrointest Liver Physiol 2014;306(9):G796–801.
54. Schleifenbaum N, Salavatl S, Neiger R. Effect of mirtazapine on canine emptying assessed by 13c-sodium acetate breath test (13c-sabt). J Vet Intern Med 2018; 32:535–6.
55. Schmitz S, Fink T, Failing K, et al. Effects of the neurokinin-1 antagonist maropitant on canine gastric emptying assessed by radioscintigraphy and breath test. Tierarztl Prax Ausg K Kleintiere Heimtiere 2016;44(3):163–9.
56. McCallum RW, Fink SM, Lerner E, et al. Effects of metoclopramide and bethanechol on delayed gastric emptying present in gastroesophageal reflux patients. Gastroenterology 1983;84(6):1573–7.
57. Hersch M, Krasilnikov V, Helviz Y, et al. Prokinetic drugs for gastric emptying in critically ill ventilated patients: Analysis through breath testing. J Crit Care 2015;30(3):655.e7-13.

Digestive Diseases in Brachycephalic Dogs

Valérie Freiche, DVM, PhD[a],*, Alexander J. German, BVSc, PhD, CertSAM, SFHEA, FRCVS[b]

KEYWORDS

- Brachycephalic airway obstructive syndrome • Endoscopy • Vomiting • Stomach
- Duodenum • Esophagus • Lymphofollicular gastritis • Hiatal hernia

KEY POINTS

- Primary conformation anomalies in brachycephalic dogs have arisen as a result of inbreeding, resulting in a high prevalence of chronic respiratory and digestive clinical signs.
- As a result, many dogs that present for evaluation of brachycephalic airway obstruction syndrome also have concomitant gastrointestinal signs.
- Digestive diseases should be carefully characterized in brachycephalic dogs because several abnormalities may coexist.
- Many diagnostic procedures are required for a full assessment of the extent of the syndrome, including clinicopathologic analyses, thoracic radiography, fluoroscopy, abdominal ultrasound imaging, and endoscopy.
- Most brachycephalic dogs with digestive diseases are managed medically, although surgery may be necessary if hiatal hernia or pyloric stenosis are confirmed. Upper airway surgery can often significantly improve digestive clinical signs in brachycephalic dogs.

 Video content accompanies this article at http://www.vetsmall.theclinics.com.

INTRODUCTION

The number of dogs affected by brachycephalic airway obstructive syndrome (BAOS) has increased dramatically over the 2 past decades, likely as a result of the increasing popularity of brachycephalic breeds including bulldogs and pugs.[1] Over the years, these dogs have been bred to accentuate features desirable to the owner (eg, brachycephalic features), but this has likely had a detrimental repercussion on their health. Most previous publications describe the respiratory consequences of BAOS, but many of the dogs also present with alimentary tract signs including ptyalism,

[a] Ecole Nationale Vétérinaire d'Alfort, CHUVA, 7 Avenue du Général de Gaulle, Maisons Alfort Cedex 94074, France; [b] Institute of Life Course and Medical Sciences, University of Liverpool, Leahurst Campus, Chester High Road, Neston, Merseyside CH64 7TE, UK
* Corresponding author.
E-mail address: valerie.freiche@vet-alfort.fr

Vet Clin Small Anim 51 (2021) 61–78
https://doi.org/10.1016/j.cvsm.2020.09.006
0195-5616/21/© 2020 Elsevier Inc. All rights reserved.
vetsmall.theclinics.com

excessive swallowing attempts, regurgitation, eructation, vomiting, and changes in appetite. A systematic approach is needed to characterize the nature of the problem and determine the most appropriate treatment and follow-up.

BACKGROUND: BRACHYCEPHALIC DOGS: ANATOMIC AND PATHOPHYSIOLOGIC CHARACTERISTICS

There are many brachycephalic dog breeds, all of which display particular anatomic and pathophysiologic changes owing to their wide and short skull (**Box 1**). However, problems are most commonly reported in French bulldogs, English bulldogs, and pugs.[2–4] In addition to alterations in the shape of their skull, these dogs have abnormalities in soft tissue structures, including an elongated soft palate, macroglossia, stenotic nares, undersized nasal chambers, malformed and aberrantly growing nasal conchae, tracheal hypoplasia, and acquired laryngeal complications.[5,6] The most common clinical manifestations relate to the respiratory tract, with signs including exercise and heat intolerance, frequent sleep disruption, and syncope, which can sometimes be life threatening (**Fig. 1**). However, digestive signs are also commonly reported,[7] and their severity correlates strongly with that of the respiratory signs.[8] In 1 study, alimentary tract signs occurred more frequently in French bulldogs compared with pugs and English bulldogs,[5] although this finding was not confirmed in another study.[3] The association between digestive and respiratory signs in brachycephalic dogs is further supported by clinical improvement and decrease in postsurgical complications when digestive signs are treated, even in dogs initially presenting with respiratory tract signs.[8] Lesions of the upper digestive tract are often detected (eg, using endoscopy), even in dogs without any alimentary tract signs. It has been suggested that increased negative pressure within the upper airways in brachycephalic dogs might promote secondary respiratory abnormalities (eg, everted tonsils, laryngeal and tracheal collapse, and everted laryngeal saccules) and digestive tract lesions, such as hiatal hernia (HH) or gastroesophageal reflux.[9] More recently, studies have examined swallowing, sliding HH and postoperative regurgitation in brachycephalic dogs, emphasizing the fact that gastroesophageal junction abnormalities and HH

Box 1
Most commonly encountered brachycephalic dog breeds

- English bulldog
- French bulldog
- Pug
- Boston terrier
- Mixed breeds
- Shih tzu
- Cavalier King Charles
- Pekingese
- Boxer
- Dogue de Bordeaux
- Bullmastiff
- Chinese Shar Pei

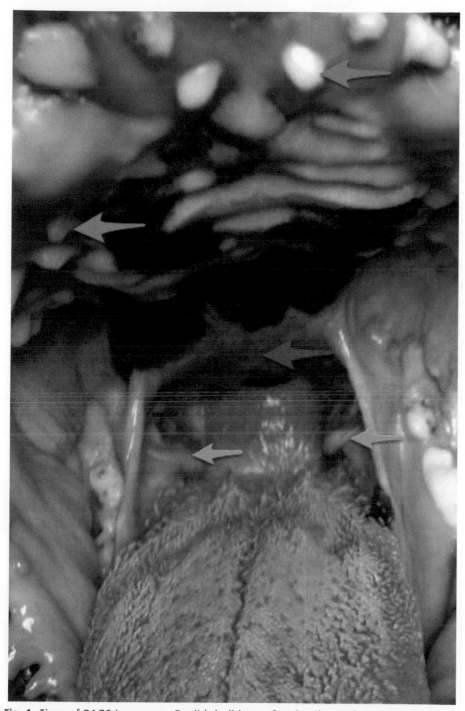

Fig. 1. Signs of BAOS in a young English bulldog; soft palate hyperplasia (*red arrow*) and everted tonsils are present (*green arrows*). Note also hyperplasia of the mucosal folds and aberrant tooth implantation (*orange arrows*). The dog also had macroglossia and everted laryngeal saccules, but these entities are not clearly evident in the photograph.

have been underestimated in brachycephalic dogs.[10–13] Videofluoroscopic swallowing studies have documented the presence of esophageal dysmotility with prolonged esophageal transit time and gastroesophageal reflux in brachycephalic dogs.[13]

DIGESTIVE SIGNS IN BRACHYCEPHALIC DOGS

Alimentary tract signs reported in brachycephalic dogs are listed in **Box 2**, the most common of which are regurgitation and vomiting. Different grading schemes have been published for assessing the dogs before and after surgery, including both respiratory (snoring, inspiratory efforts, exercise intolerance, syncope) and digestive signs (ptyalism, regurgitations, vomiting), with frequency and scaling from 1 (mild) to 3 (marked).[7] Brachycephalic dogs can also suffer from chronic enteropathy, and pugs are affected by a particularly severe form of protein-losing enteropathy.[14] French bulldogs and English bulldogs might also be predisposed to food responsive diarrhea and chronic flatulence (V. Freiche, unpublished observations, 2013-2020). However, none of these conditions seem to be related to BAOS.

DIAGNOSIS OF DIGESTIVE DISEASES IN BRACHYCEPHALIC DOGS

BAOS is known to be a progressive disease.[6] Age at presentation ranges from a few months to a few years, although BAOS is unlikely to develop for the first time in dogs older than 5 years of age.[9] A definitive diagnosis requires a systematic approach, including history, physical examination, detailed clinicopathologic investigations, diagnostic imaging, and finally endoscopy to examine both the upper airways and the digestive tract. The main diseases affecting the digestive system in brachycephalic dogs are listed in **Box 3**.

History and Physical Examination

Brachycephalic dogs can present with different combinations of clinical signs and, as a result, a detailed history is essential to accurately characterize the problem. Note that owner perception of the clinical signs in brachycephalic dogs is often unreliable,[2,15] not least because owners often consider stertor, loud breathing, and regurgitation to be normal for their dog. Clinical signs can be predominantly respiratory or consist of a mix of respiratory and digestive signs. Respiratory signs include

---

Box 2
Digestive signs observed in brachycephalic dogs

- Ptyalism
- Regurgitation[a]
- Retching
- Vomiting
- Dysphagia
- Aerophagia
- Gastroesophageal reflux
- Pica
- Pain-relieving positioning (including "prayer" posture)

[a] May be exacerbated by exercise.

Box 3
Main alimentary tract diseases affecting brachycephalic dogs

- Redundant esophagus (deviation)
- Esophagitis
- Gastroesophageal reflux
- Sliding HH (type 1)
- Delayed gastric emptying
- Gastritis (potentially lymphofollicular)
- Pyloric mucosal folds hypertrophy
- Pyloric stenosis
- Duodenitis

---

dyspnea, stertor, stridor, increased respiratory effort, exercise intolerance, heat or stress intolerance, and even cyanosis and collapse.[2,4,7,9] Digestive signs are listed in **Box 2**. Acute vomiting and regurgitation episodes can occasionally be suggestive of pseudo-obstruction, where the clinical picture suggests mechanical obstruction of the digestive tract, but there is no demonstrable evidence of any such obstruction in the intestine.

It is important to specifically question owners about the presence of digestive signs, even if they do not volunteer this information, because these signs are usually present in most of the cases.[5,7,9,10]

The physical examination should include an initial observation to determine the dog's phenotype (eg, examining the overall morphology of the dog, including skull dimensions and nares, such as the degree of stenosis), to evaluate of the respiratory cycle (especially the inspiratory effort), and to listen for spontaneous respiratory noises. Tachypnea can often be noted at this stage.[9] Next, the head and neck should be examined carefully. Given the particular anatomic conformation of brachycephalic dogs, it can be difficult to examine their oral cavity because they often struggle to breathe with their mouth wide open. Thoracic auscultation should then be performed, although this step can be challenging owing to the presence of loud referred upper respiratory tract noises. Finally, the rest of the body should be examined, although specific abnormalities are rarely identified on physical examination in brachycephalic dogs with alimentary tract disease.

Diagnostic Approach

Detailed diagnostic investigations are usually required to accurately diagnose alimentary tract disease in brachycephalic dogs. They include clinical pathology, thoracic radiographs, fluoroscopic assessment of swallowing function, and upper airway and gastrointestinal endoscopy.

Clinical Pathology

Hematologic and biochemical assessments are recommended routinely. Arterial blood analysis may be important when severe concurrent upper airway disease is present; however, in most cases partial pressure of carbon dioxide, blood pH, and bicarbonate concentration obtained by venous sample are sufficient.[9] In a recent prospective study, the systemic inflammatory response and metabolic profile were evaluated in 30 brachycephalic dogs presenting with BAOS. Digestive signs were present in many (77%) of these dogs; however, although there were variable alterations both in their inflammatory and metabolic profiles (eg, C-reactive protein, beta lipoproteins, chylomicrons, fructosamine, and cholesterol), these alterations were not associated with either clinical signs or the anatomic abnormalities present.[7] In conclusion, no specific laboratory changes could be identified in brachycephalic dogs with digestive disease.

Diagnostic Imaging

Radiographs

Thoracic radiographs are indicated to assess for possible lower airway changes that, in brachycephalic dogs, can include hypoplastic trachea and also pulmonary lesions (eg, noncardiogenic pulmonary edema and concurrent aspiration pneumonia). Alimentary tract abnormalities such as esophageal deviation or dilation and HH can also be identified. A contrast study may be useful although fluoroscopy is far more valuable than standard radiography, not least if esophageal dilation is subtle or when sliding HH is suspected (**Fig. 2**).[10] Finally, although unrelated to respiratory or alimentary tract signs, vertebral malformations are also commonly observed.

Fluoroscopy

Video fluoroscopic swallow studies are the gold standard test to investigate esophageal motility disorders, and HH (Video 1).[10,11,13,16,17] In one study, esophageal dysmotility was found to be more common in young brachycephalic dogs when compared with nonbrachycephalic dogs.[13] The most common abnormalities identified by video fluoroscopic swallow studies include prolonged esophageal transit time, morphologic esophageal variations, decreased propagation of secondary peristaltic waves, gastroesophageal reflux, and HH.[13] Another study found that esophageal abnormalities and HH were more common in French bulldogs than in brachycephalic dogs of other breeds.[10]

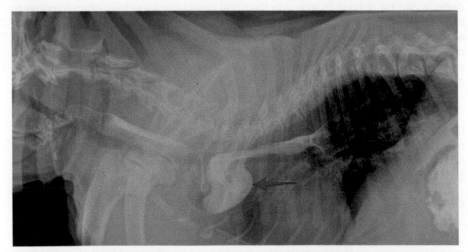

Fig. 2. Severe redundant esophagus in an English Bulldog (*red arrow*). Despite the tortuous nature of the esophagus in the cranial mediastinum, no persistent right aortic arch was detected in this dog. (*Courtesy of* J. Hernandez is DVM, PhD, Nantes, France.)

Abdominal ultrasound examination

Abdominal ultrasound examination is usually recommended in brachycephalic dogs to assess gastric wall characteristics, particularly mucosal folds and the pyloric muscular layer (**Fig. 3**), whereas gastric motility can be assessed at the same time. Delayed vomiting of food might suggest gastric retention and/or pyloric stenosis (**Fig. 4**). Gastric stasis was present in 32% of the cases in a prospective study recruiting 73 brachycephalic dogs with upper respiratory syndrome.[7]

Endoscopy

Endoscopy of both the upper respiratory and digestive tracts is required to obtain a complete overview of abnormalities and to help guide management. As discussed elsewhere in this article, concurrent digestive abnormalities can be found, even in dogs that do not present with any alimentary tract signs.[7,9] Delayed gastric emptying is often present even in the absence of pyloric stenosis.[7] As a result, it is advisable to withhold food for at least 14 hours before esophagogastroduodenoscopy. For the procedure, it is important to place the dog in left lateral recumbency because this positioning will aid in the intubation of the antrum and pylorus. Endoscopic examination enables direct examination of the digestive mucosa and collection of standardized gastric and duodenal biopsy samples. At least 6 biopsies per site are needed for histopathologic analysis. Esophageal biopsies are usually not feasible in dogs with a normal or only mildly abnormal mucosa. It is advisable to formally record any findings and use of the World Small Animal Veterinary Association endoscopic scoring system is recommended.[18] **Table 1** summarizes the alimentary tract endoscopic findings in brachycephalic dogs.

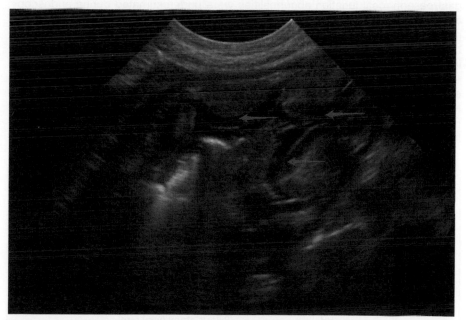

Fig. 3. Abdominal ultrasound imaging in a 3-year-old spayed female Boston Terrier presented with chronic vomiting. The gastric wall is thickened and mucosal folds (*red arrows*) are prominent. (*Courtesy* ENVA Diagnostic Imaging Department, Maisons Alfort Cedex. France.)

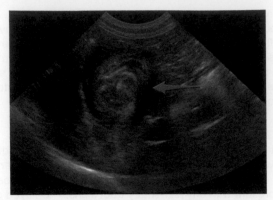

Fig. 4. Ultrasound appearance of the pylorus (*red arrow*) in a young brachycephalic dog that presented with chronic vomiting containing partially digested food. Pyloric stenosis was confirmed at exploratory celiotomy.

Esophageal lesions Esophageal inflammatory lesions are most frequently localized and display a "star pattern" as illustrated in **Fig. 5**. They reflect both chronic gastro-esophageal reflux and atony of the lower esophageal sphincter (Video 2). Esophageal luminal contents are often present, including food, gastric juice and saliva (Video 3). Esophageal redundancy is quite common in brachycephalic dogs and, in some cases, deviation is so pronounced that existence of a persistent fourth aortic arch may be suspected.

In a recent pilot study of 20 BAOS dogs, the presence of both sliding HH and gastroesophageal junction abnormalities were underestimated during endoscopy, although performing manipulations to increase the transdiaphragmatic pressure gradient (eg, manual pressure on the cranial abdomen, moving into the Trendelenburg position [30° angle], or temporary complete endotracheal tube obstruction) during endoscopy improved the chances of identifying them.[10,11] Of the manipulations evaluated, temporary complete endotracheal tube obstruction was the most likely to enable identification of gastroesophageal junction abnormalities including sliding HH. Although no complications were identified in the study, some anesthetists have been concerned about the safety of such a manipulation (A.J. German, unpublished observations).

Table 1			
Endoscopic lesions identified in brachycephalic dogs			
	Esophagus	**Stomach**	**Duodenum**
Inflammatory lesions	Esophagitis (mainly distal)	Nonspecific gastritis(localized or diffuse) Lymphofollicular gastritis	Nonspecific duodenitis
Anatomic or functional disorder	Redundant esophagus Gastroesophageal reflux (frequent) HH	Cardiac atony (rare) Delayed gastric emptying Pyloric mucosal hyperplasia Pyloric stenosis Pyloric atony (very rare)	None

Adapted from Poncet, CM, Dupre GP, FreicheVG, et al. Prevalence of gastrointestinal tract lesions in 73 brachycephalic dogs with upper respiratory syndrome. J Small Anim Pract. 2005; 46(6);273–279; with permission.

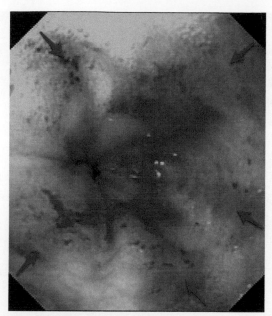

Fig. 5. Upper digestive endoscopy in an English bulldog dog with chronic vomiting and regurgitation. There is evidence of a "star pattern" in the distal esophagus, where stripes of hyperemia can be seen radiating outward from the lower esophageal sphincter (*blue arrows*).

Gastric lesions Diffuse, nonspecific inflammatory lesions are often reported. Various degrees of discoloration, erythema, or edema of the gastric mucosa can be observed. In a recent study, a strong positive association was established between inspiratory dyspnea and chronic gastritis with lymphofollicular hyperplasia in dogs.[19] Lymphofollicular hyperplasia was also recently reported in another study.[7] Characteristic gastric lesions are illustrated in **Figs. 6** and **7**. It is also common to identify differences in pyloric conformation in brachycephalic dogs, compared with other breeds, most notably prominent mucosal folds surrounding the pyloric canal, even without any confirmed pyloric stenosis (**Fig. 8**). This finding is reported to occur in brachycephalic dogs presented with frequent vomiting of food, retarded growth, and chronic gastric dilation.[20] In such cases, retrograde peristaltic waves can be identified during the endoscopic procedure (Video 4).

Duodenal lesions Although duodenal lesions can be observed, the duodenal mucosa is usually unremarkable in brachycephalic dogs (**Fig. 9**). In the authors' experience, a "rice grain" appearance to the mucosa attributed to dilated lacteals is often seen, even though the dogs do not show any clinical sign of protein-losing enteropathy, such as diarrhea or hypoalbuminemia. The significance of this finding is unclear.

TREATMENT OF DIGESTIVE DISEASES IN BRACHYCEPHALIC DOGS

The management of brachycephalic dogs with digestive signs typically involves medical management (including dietary modifications and pharmaceutical agents) and surgical management in cases of HH that remains unresponsive to medical management.

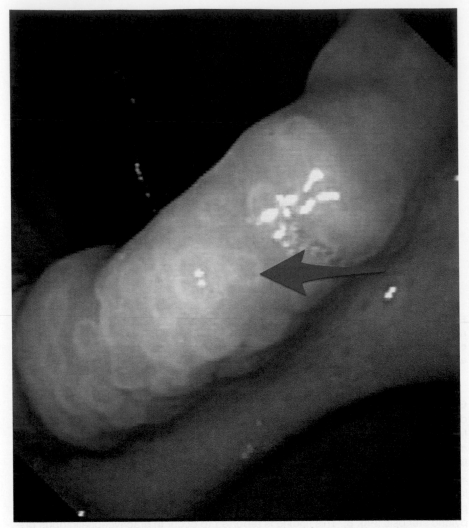

Fig. 6. Gastroscopy image from a French bulldog presented for BAOS upper airway surgery. Although no alimentary tract signs were reported, severe edema is evident in the mucosa of the lesser curvature (*red arrow*).

Medical Treatment

Dietary modifications that can be helpful include altering the type of food (eg, wet food rather than dry food; feeding food with less fiber and fat), its consistency (eg, adding water), and meal pattern (eg, feeding the daily requirement over a number of small meals). These adjustments are designed to promote passage of food through the digestive tract, thereby decreasing the tendency for regurgitation, vomiting, or gastro-esophageal reflux.

The drugs most often used in brachycephalic dogs with alimentary tract disease include antiemetics, acid-blocking drugs, mucosal "protectants" and prokinetic agents. Because robust clinical trials on the efficacy of these drugs have not yet been performed, therapies are usually a matter of personal preference of the attending

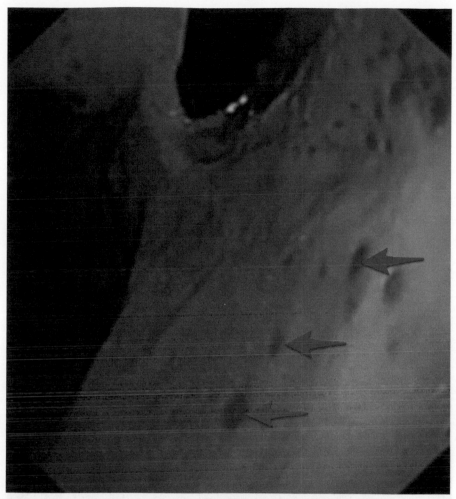

Fig. 7. Gastroscopy performed in a 3-year-old male French bulldog. Multiple small gray-to-red punctiform areas are present (*red arrows*) scattered over the gastric mucosal surface. This pattern is consistent with lymphofollicular hyperplasia.

clinician. Where there is evidence of esophagitis (eg, secondary to gastroesophageal reflux or HH), acid-blocking drugs and mucosal protectants (eg, sucralfate) are indicated. The authors favor proton pump inhibitors (eg, omeprazole at 1 mg/kg every 12 hours by mouth) over H_2 antagonists for gastric acid suppression. Occasionally, ranitidine is recommended based on its putative gastric prokinetic activity on account of the fact that they inhibit acetylcholinesterase activity.[21] However, it is unlikely to have any effect in the esophagus given the predominance of skeletal muscle in this site.[22] Antiemetics, usually either maropitant or metoclopramide, can be used in dogs with confirmed vomiting. The use of metoclopramide is controversial given the reported effects on lower esophageal sphincter tone,[23] although this effect has not been confirmed in other work.[24] It is unclear as to whether such effects will be of benefit or detrimental. **Table 2** summarizes the options available to medically manage digestive diseases in brachycephalic dogs.

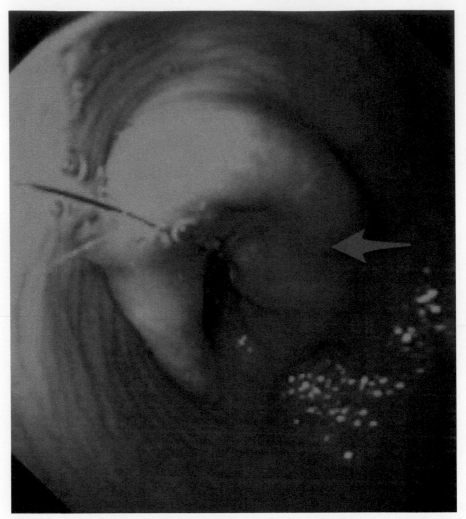

Fig. 8. Typical endoscopic appearance of the pylorus in brachycephalic dogs. The pylorus is protuberant and thickened (*red arrow*), but no stenosis is evident. Despite this, it can often be difficult to pass an endoscope through to the duodenum.

Whatever treatments are selected, care should be taken with owners administering pills orally, because many brachycephalic dogs do not like having their mouth opened. Forcible drug administration might also cause nausea, salivation, or vomiting. A further problem with administering medications orally is that transit might be impaired in the presence of esophageal dysmotility and HH, so that orally administered drugs might be retained within the esophagus for prolonged periods.

Surgical Treatment

Surgical treatment of digestive diseases is rarely needed. As mentioned elsewhere in this article, BAOS corrective surgery is followed by improvement of digestive clinical signs in many cases.[3,8,9,15] The 2 main indications for surgery include pyloric stenosis and permanent HH. In the first case, clinical signs include gastric dilation or distention

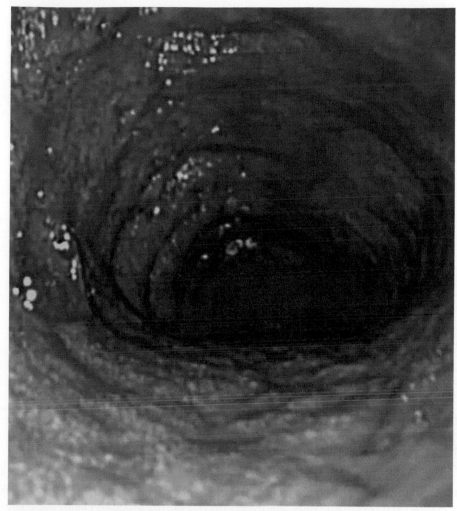

Fig. 9. Duodenoscopy in a brachycephalic dog with BAOS and presented for investigation of the alimentary tract. There is marked thickening and granularity of the gastric mucosa.

and frequent vomiting of food long after a meal that do not respond to medical treatment.

Hiatal hernia
As mentioned elsewhere in this article, HH can be an acquired condition owing to BAOS. The main clinical signs include chronic vomiting, regurgitation, weakness, odynophagia, and other complications, such as aspiration pneumonia.

Pyloric stenosis surgical treatment
Pyloric stenosis in brachycephalic dogs results from a benign outlet gastric obstruction. As illustrated elsewhere in this article, brachycephalic dogs generally show a typical pylorus, surrounded with hyperplastic mucosal folds. During an endoscopic procedure, passing through the pylorus is often challenging in these breeds, even in

Table 2
Medical treatments usually recommended for digestive diseases in brachycephalic dogs

Molecule	Pharmacologic Class	Dosage	Potential Side Effects
Metoclopramide	Dopamine (D2) receptor antagonist Antiemetic	0.25–0.50 mg/kg PO q8h	Extrapyramidal neurologic signs (rare)
Maropitant citrate	NK-1 receptor antagonist Antiemetic	2 mg/kg PO q24h 1 mg/kg SC, IV q24h	Transient pain at injection site
Aluminum hydroxide Sodium alginate Sucralfate	Mucosal protectants	0.5–1.0 mL/kg PO q8h 1 mL/kg PO q8h	Constipation Ptyalism
Cimetidine[a] Ranitidine Famotidine	H2 antagonists	5 mg/kg q8h PO 2 mg/kg PO q8–12h 0.5–1.0 mg/kg PO q12–24h	Drug interactions[b]
Omeprazole Pantoprazole Esomeprazole	Proton pump inhibitors	0.5-1.5 mg/kg	Intestinal dysbiosis

Abbreviations: IV, intravenous; PO, by mouth; SC, subcutaneous; TID, 3 times per day.
 [a] Although cimetidine is not commonly used in most countries, it is licensed for use in dogs in Europe. As such, veterinarians in the UK are obliged to use it as a first-line agent according to the prescribing cascade for veterinary medicines.
 [b] H2 antagonists can decrease hepatic microsomal enzyme systems to varying degrees and, theoretically at least might decrease hepatic metabolism of drugs including: benzodiazepines, barbiturates, propranolol, calcium channel blockers, metronidazole, phenytoin, theophylline, and warfarin. However, the clinical significance of this effect has not been established.

the absence of stenosis. In a small percentage of cases, clinical signs and ultrasound imaging confirm the stenosis. Different surgical procedures are performed, depending on the severity of the disease but all the procedure focused on removing outflow obstruction, normalizing gastric outflow, and decreasing gastric emptying time.[13,25]

Corrective surgical techniques include Y-U pyloroplasty and modified Finney Jabouley pyloroplasty.[16] Y-U pyloroplasty is generally indicated in cases of mucosal or combined mucosal and muscular hypertrophy (**Fig. 10**). Modified Finney Jabouley pyloroplasty can be performed after exclusion of pyloric neoplastic lesions.[25] It provides a direct communication between the antrum and the duodenum (antroduodenostomy without pylorectomy) and is indicated in case of severe thickening and inflammation of the pylorus (Video 5).

Hiatal hernia surgical treatment
Several surgical techniques are described for HHs surgical treatment. The most commonly used technique in combination or alone are left-sided gastropexy, esophagopexy, and phrenoplasty (diaphragmatic hiatal reduction).[25] Postoperative medical therapy include proton pump inhibitors, sucralfate, and maropitant or metoclopramide to prevent vomiting and/or nausea (see **Table 2**). In a prospective study, some dogs still displayed digestive clinical signs postoperatively.[16]

FOLLOW-UP AND PROGNOSIS

The prognosis of brachycephalic dogs with alimentary tract disease is difficult to determine precisely owing to the variability in their presentation and the concurrent

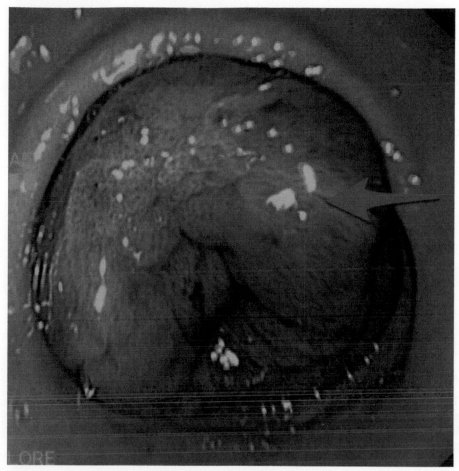

Fig. 10. Pyloric stenosis in a 2-year-old female French bulldog that was vomiting on a daily basis. During the endoscopic procedure, the pylorus seemed hyperplastic and abnormal (*red arrow*) and neoplasia was excluded on the basis of histopathologic examination.

respiratory pathology.[2,3,12,15] All features of each individual case should be considered. The overall prognosis depends on both the severity and the extent of all identified lesions. The digestive signs of dogs with BAOS usually respond well to medical treatment. Further, studies have reported improvement of respiratory and digestive signs following airway corrective surgery in about 90% of dogs.[2,3,8] However, transient postoperative vomiting, dyspnea, and regurgitation have also been reported after BAOS-corrective surgery[3,7,12,19]; therefore, the owners need to be advised of the possible complications before providing their consent.

SUMMARY

Brachycephalic dogs are predisposed not only to upper respiratory tract disease, but also to diseases affecting the alimentary tract. Association of respiratory and digestive signs is owing to breed-related anatomic characteristics (eg, esophageal redundancy) and to increased negative intrathoracic pressure that occurs during the breathing cycle. It is important for the veterinarian to perform a detailed diagnostic investigation in brachycephalic dogs presenting with either respiratory signs, digestive signs or both, to design a plan to optimally manage each individual patient. Although medical management to treat esophagitis is often the mainstay for digestive signs, a surgical approach may be required for treatment of HH in dogs that do not respond well to medical therapy. In addition, BAOS corrective surgery often has beneficial effects on digestive signs as well in brachycephalic dogs.

CLINICS CARE POINTS

- Lesions of the upper digestive tract need to be investigated in brachycephalic dogs, even if digestive clinical signs are not outlined by the owners, as respiratory and digestive lesion frequently coexist in these dogs.
- As BAOS is unlikely to develop for the first time in dogs older than 5 years of age, recent respiratory and/or digestive clinical signs require extensive investigations to rule out other diseases.
- Video fluoroscopic swallow studies are far more valuable than X-rays. They may be mandatory to investigate precisely esophageal motility disorders in brachycephalic dogs.
- A delayed gastric emptying identified during endoscopy does not necessary mean that a pyloric stenosis is present in a brachycephalic dog.
- Owners need to be advised about administrating pills orally in brachycephalic dogs as these dogs often struggle to breathe with their mouth open and are prone to regurgitations and impaired swallowing.

ACKNOWLEDGMENTS

The authors thank Dr Mathieu Manassero, DVM, PhD, ECVS Dipl. Ecole Nationale Vétérinaire d'Alfort Surgery Department for his kind contribution to the digestive surgery treatment part of the article and Alfort Vet School diagnostic imaging Department for providing illustrations.

DISCLOSURE

V. Freiche: None. A.J. German: Prof. German is an employee of the University of Liverpool, but his position is financially supported by Royal Canin, which is owned by Mars Petcare. Prof. German has also received financial remuneration from Mars Petcare for providing educational material, speaking at conferences, and consulting. None of this remuneration was for projects related to this article.

SUPPLEMENTARY DATA

Supplementary data related to this article can be found online at https://doi.org/10.1016/j.cvsm.2020.09.006.

REFERENCES

1. Packer RM, Tivers MS. Strategies for the management and prevention of conformation-related respiratory disorders in brachycephalic dogs. Vet Med (Auckl) 2015;6:219–32.
2. Dupré G, Heidenreich D. Brachycephalic Syndrome. Vet Clin North Am Small Anim Pract 2016;46:691–707.

3. Haimel G, Dupré G. Brachycephalic airway syndrome: a comparative study between pugs and French bulldogs. J Small Anim Pract 2015;56:714–9.

4. Fasanella FJ, Shivley JM, Wardlaw JL, et al. Brachycephalic airway obstructive syndrome in dogs: 90 cases (1991-2008). J Am Vet Med Assoc 2010;237: 1048–51.

5. Kaye BM, Rutherford L, Perridge DJ, et al. Relationship between brachycephalic airway syndrome and gastrointestinal signs in three breeds of dog. J Small Anim Pract 2018;59:670–3.

6. Roedler FS, Pohl S, Oechtering GU. How does severe brachycephaly affect dog's lives? Results of a structured preoperative owner questionnaire. Vet J 2013;198: 606–10.

7. Poncet CM, Dupre GP, Freiche VG, et al. Prevalence of gastrointestinal tract lesions in 73 brachycephalic dogs with upper respiratory syndrome. J Small Anim Pract 2005;46:273–9.

8. Poncet CM, Dupre GP, Freiche VG, et al. Long-term results of upper respiratory syndrome surgery and gastrointestinal tract medical treatment in 51 brachycephalic dogs. J Small Anim Pract 2006;47:137–42.

9. Lodato DL, Hedlund CS. Brachycephalic airway syndrome: pathophysiology and diagnosis. Compend Contin Educ Vet 2012;34:E3.

10. Reeve EJ, Sutton D, Friend EJ, et al. Documenting the prevalence of hiatal hernia and oesophageal abnormalities in brachycephalic dogs using fluoroscopy. J Small Anim Pract 2017;58:703–8.

11. Broux O, Clercx C, Etienne AL, et al. Effects of manipulations to detect sliding hiatal hernia in dogs with brachycephalic airway obstructive syndrome. Vet Surg 2017;47:243–51.

12. Fenner JVH, Quinn RJ, Demetriou JL. Postoperative regurgitation in dogs after upper airway surgery to treat brachycephalic obstructive airway syndrome: 258 cases (2013-2017). Vet Surg 2019;49:53–60.

13. Eivers C, Rueda RC, Liuti T, et al. Retrospective analysis of esophageal imaging features in brachycephalic versus non-brachycephalic dogs based on videofluoroscopic swallowing studies. J Vet Intern Med 2019;33:1740–6.

14. SS, DJB, SC, et al. The pug breed demonstrates a worse response to treatment of protein-losing enteropathy than other breeds of dog. JVIM 2020.

15. Poncet C, Freiche V. Brachycephalic Airway Obstruction Syndrome. In: Bonagura JD, Twedt DC, editors. Kirk's Current Veterinary Therapy XV (2014). Section VII, Respiratory Diseases; 649-652. Elsevier Saunders, St Louis, Missouri.

16. Mayhew PD, Marks SL, Pollard R, et al. Prospective evaluation of surgical management of sliding hiatal hernia and gastroesophageal reflux in dogs. Vet Surg 2017;46:1098–109.

17. Pollard RE, Johnson LR, Marks SL. The prevalence of dynamic pharyngeal collapse is high in brachycephalic dogs undergoing videofluoroscopy. Vet Radiol Ultrasound 2018;59:529–34.

18. Washabau RJ, Day MJ, Willard MD, et al. Endoscopic, Biopsy, and Histopathologic Guidelines for the Evaluation of Gastrointestinal Inflammation in Companion Animals. J Vet Intern Med 2010;24(1):10–26.

19. Faucher MR, Biourge V, German AJ, et al. Comparison of clinical, endoscopic, and histologic features between dogs with chronic gastritis with and without lymphofollicular hyperplasia. J Am Vet Med Assoc 2020;256:906–13.

20. Aslanian ME, Sharp CR, Garneau MS. Gastric dilatation and volvulus in a brachycephalic dog with hiatal hernia. J Small Anim Pract 2014;55:535–7.

21. Washabau RJ. Gastrointestinal motility disorders and gastrointestinal prokinetic therapy. Vet Clin Small Anim 2003;33:1007–28.
22. Mann CV, Shorter RG. Structure of the canine esophagus and its sphincters. J Surg Res 1964;4:160–3.
23. Dowling PM. Prokinetic drugs: metoclopramide and cisapride. Can Vet J 1995; 36:115–6.
24. Kempf J, Lewis F, Reusch CE, et al. High-resolution manometric evaluation of the effects of cisapride and metoclopramide hydrochloride administered orally on lower esophageal sphincter pressure in awake dogs. Am J Vet Res 2014;75: 361–6.
25. Cornell K. Stomach. In: Tobias KM, Johnston SA, editors. Veterinary Surgery Small Animals. Volume 2 (2012), Soft Tissue Surgery, Section VII, Digestive System; 1484-1512. Elsevier Saunders, St Louis, Missouri.

Acute Hemorrhagic Diarrhea Syndrome in Dogs

Stefan Unterer, DVM, Dr med vet, Dr habil*, Kathrin Busch, DVM, Dr med vet

KEYWORDS

- Hemorrhagic gastroenteritis • Gastrointestinal bleeding • *Clostridium perfringens*
- Pore-forming toxin • NetF • Dog

KEY POINTS

- Canine acute hemorrhagic diarrhea syndrome (AHDS) is characterized by a sudden onset of severe bloody diarrhea frequently associated with vomiting as first clinical sign.
- Clinical and laboratory findings reflect hypovolemia due to a dramatic loss of fluid into the intestinal lumen.
- Because mucosal lesions are restricted to the small and large intestine, the previously used term "hemorrhagic gastroenteritis" implying the presence of gastric inflammation is inaccurate.
- Diagnosis is based on the typical clinical course and ruling out other known causes of acute hemorrhagic diarrhea. In addition, a positive polymerase chain reaction for *Clostridium perfringens* encoding for the pore-forming toxin NetF supports the diagnosis of AHDS.
- Rapid volume replacement and symptomatic treatment usually results in a short course of the disease lasting from 24 to 72 hours. Only dogs with signs of systemic inflammation should be treated with antibiotics.

INTRODUCTION

Acute hemorrhagic diarrhea syndrome (AHDS) is defined as sudden onset of severe bloody diarrhea with significant loss of fluid into the intestinal lumen and frequently associated with vomiting as first clinical sign observed by the owner. There is strong evidence that clostridial overgrowth and toxin release may be responsible for the intestinal epithelial necrosis.[1] Fecal culture for *Clostridium* spp. or other potential enteric pathogens is not diagnostic, because many of these bacteria can be found in feces of healthy dogs.[2] A positive fecal polymerase chain reaction (PCR) for *Clostridium perfringens* type A strains, which are encoding for the pore-forming toxin NetF,[3] suggests AHDS, but diagnosis is still mainly based on observing the unique clinical features and

Clinic of Small Animal Medicine, Centre for Clinical Veterinary Medicine, Ludwig-Maximilians-University, Veterinärstr. 13, München 80539, Germany
* Corresponding author.
E-mail address: s.unterer@medizinische-kleintierklinik.de

Vet Clin Small Anim 51 (2021) 79–92
https://doi.org/10.1016/j.cvsm.2020.09.007

excluding other known causes of acute hemorrhagic diarrhea. The spectrum of clinical severity ranges from trivial signs of acute gastroenteritis with mild dehydration to life threatening conditions due to hypovolemic shock, sepsis from translocated intestinal bacteria, and significant hypoproteinemia. In most cases, however, clinical recovery with fluid and symptomatic therapy occurs within 24 to 72 hours. Mortality rate can be high if left untreated but is less than 10% in hospitalized dogs. Repeated occurrences of episodes with acute hemorrhagic diarrhea is observed only in few dogs, but about 30% of dogs develop chronic diarrhea later in life.[4]

CLINICAL AND CLINICOPATHOLOGIC ABNORMALITIES

Dogs of any age and breed can be affected, but the incidence of AHDS is greater in middle aged (median 5.0 years, range 0.3–16) and small breed (median 9.8 kg, range 1.5–55.2) dogs. The disease is characteristically acute to peracute, with vomiting as first clinical sign in about 50% of cases followed by watery hemorrhagic diarrhea. A diet change or dietary indiscretion is not associated with the onset of the disease, but one study showed that AHDS was significantly more likely to occur during winter than during other seasons. Thus, cold environment or ingestion of snow might be predisposing factors. Some dogs have a history of chronic intestinal signs, which might also represent a predisposing factor of AHDS (Kauf Maww E, unpublished data, 2019).

Physical examination findings usually reflect hypovolemia (eg, lethargy, weakness, tachycardia, prolonged capillary refill time, and weak pulse pressure). Because of the peracute onset and the lag time in compartmental fluid shifts, skin turgor may seem normal in some cases. Severe abdominal pain is uncommon, and affected dogs are usually normo- or hypothermic.

Historically, a packed cell volume (PCV) greater than 60% was used to define AHDS; however, a study including 108 dogs with AHDS showed that the median PCV at presentation is 57% with a range of 33% to 76%.[5] That means dogs with AHDS usually have a high, normal, or mildly to moderately increased PCV, but nearly never show an initial PCV less than the reference range. Thus, the presence of anemia at presentation in a dog with bloody diarrhea always indicate true intestinal bleeding (eg, hemostatic disorders, ulceration, intestinal neoplasia). Leukogram changes reflect typical changes of a stress response (mild neutrophilia, lymphopenia, eosinopenia). Because of the extensive mucosal damage, a mild left shift can be observed in about 50% of dogs with an uncomplicated clinical course and without signs of sepsis. Consequently, neutropenia, several segmented neutrophils greater than 20,000/μL or band neutrophils greater than 2500/μL, should always prompt the clinician to look for other causes of acute hemorrhagic diarrhea or to suspect an enteropathogenic bacterial infection, bacterial translocation, and sepsis. Parvovirus infection should always be considered in a neutropenic young and/or inadequately vaccinated dog. Hypoadrenocorticism should be ruled out in dogs lacking a stress leukogram and showing lymphocytosis and eosinophilia or characteristic electrolyte changes (eg, hyperkalemia, hyponatremia).

A low albumin concentration at presentation/prior rehydration can be observed in less than 10% of dogs with AHDS, which indicates a significant intestinal loss of plasma proteins. Especially in these dogs the degree of hypoalbuminemia should be reassessed after rehydration to identify the very severe cases, which require additional treatment (eg, fresh frozen plasma, albumin solutions). Despite severe dehydration, most dogs with AHDS do not experience prerenal azotemia. Therefore, in every dog with azotemia, assessment of urine-specific gravity before fluid therapy is mandatory to differentiate dehydration and renal dysfunction. Additional serum biochemistry changes are uncommon, except for mild to moderate alanine aminotransferase elevation, lower venous blood pH and bicarbonate concentration, and a significantly higher lactate concentration, which is explainable due to decreased perfusion of liver and musculature in hypovolemic states.

RECENT DISCOVERIES

In necropsy examinations, mucosal necrosis and an overgrowth of *C perfringens* was described in the intestinal tract from dogs with fatal AHDS. A prospective study confirmed these findings by analyzing endoscopically collected samples from 10 dogs with AHDS. It was shown that the principal intestinal lesions reflect an acute necrotizing and neutrophilic enterocolitis without involvement of the stomach. In all dogs with AHDS, clostridial strains could be identified on the small intestinal mucosa (**Fig. 1**), either by culture or immunohistopathology, whereas a weak growth of a clostridial strain could be detected only in 1/11 control dogs.[6] Clostridial strains isolated from the duodenum of dogs with AHDS were identified as *C perfringens* by mass spectrometry using MALDI-TOF. In 5 dogs the clostridial isolate was classified as *C perfringens* type A based on detection of the cpa gene and negative results for the other major toxins.[6] Because of the immediate vicinity of bacterial layers and epithelial lesions, the well-known prolific toxin-producing ability of *C perfringens,* as well as the fact that no other underlying cause for the necrosis of the superficial intestinal epithelium was identified in these prospectively collected cases, enterotoxemia due to *C perfringens* was suspected. It was speculated that *C perfringens* enterotoxin (CPE) was responsible, because more AHDS dogs had CPE enzyme-linked immunosorbent assay (ELISA) positive feces than healthy control dogs.[2,7] However, in a study including 54 dogs with AHDS, only 13 dogs (24%) had a CPE-positive fecal ELISA

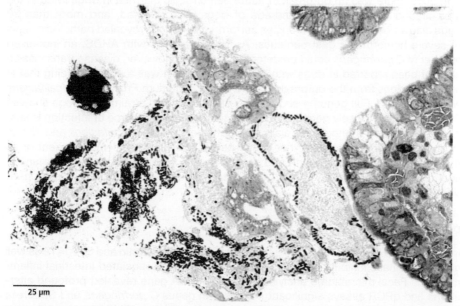

25 µm

Fig. 1. Plump, rod-shaped, gram-positive bacteria identified as *C perfringens* on the necrotic villus tip in the ileum of a dog with AHDS. (*Courtesy of* Institute of Veterinary Pathology, Ludwig-Maximilians-University, Munich, Germany.)

test result.[8] This result made it unlikely that CPE was the only toxin causing mucosal lesions and hemorrhagic diarrhea, and a search for other toxins was performed. In 2015, genome sequencing of a toxigenic type A *C perfringens* strain that was isolated from a fatal case of AHDS revealed 3 novel putative toxin genes designated as NetE (32.9 kDa), NetF (31.7 kDa), and NetG (31.7 kDa).[9] These toxins belong to the leukocidin/hemolysin superfamily and are capable to form pores in susceptible cells leading to plasma membrane destruction and eventually osmotic cell lysis. Multiple in vitro experiments were conducted and showed that the NetF toxin is highly cytotoxic in an equine ovarian cell line, and the toxic effect could be blocked by inserting a *netF* inactivation mutant. In addition, antiserum against NetF toxin neutralized the cytotoxicity of wild-type NetF-producing strains.[9]

Several studies showed a higher prevalence of *C perfringens* encoding the *netF* gene in fecal samples from dogs with AHDS compared with healthy dogs and dogs with different other intestinal diseases.[3,6,10] For years, it was speculated that overgrowth of clostridial strains might only be a secondary consequence. Therefore, it is of special interest that in a group of dogs with parvovirus infection that had intestinal lesions similar to those of dogs with AHDS, no *C perfringens* strains encoding *netF* could be detected. Thus, a generalized secondary overgrowth of these clostridial strains in dogs with acute hemorrhagic diarrhea is unlikely. Summarizing all current information, it can be assumed that NetF is likely a major virulence factor responsible for AHDS. However, *C perfringens* produces numerous extracellular enzymes and minor toxins, such as collagenase (κ-toxin), neuraminidase, caseinase (λ-toxin), deoxyribonuclease (η-toxin), hyaluronidase (μ-toxin), and urease. Individually, each of these toxins may play a minor role in the pathogenesis of *C perfringens*–associated diseases, but their cumulative effect is likely profound. Further studies are needed to define the exact role of pore forming toxins and CPE in the pathogenesis of AHDS and to discover novel toxins responsible for virulence.

In 2019, there was an outbreak of acute hemorrhagic diarrhea in dogs living in the area around Oslo, Norway. Hundreds of dogs were affected, and more than 20 dogs died across Norway. Necropsies performed in 10 dogs revealed pathologic signs of severe hemorrhagic gastroenteritis. As shown in dogs with AHDS, an increased number of *C perfringens* could be detected in the gut. However, disease transmission has not been reported in dogs with AHDS. Therefore, it was a striking finding that in many sick dogs from the outbreak in Norway the bacterium *Providencia alcalifaciens* was discovered. Full genome sequencing of this bacterial strain in 22 dogs showed that many are so closely genetically related that a common source of infection is suspected. Research is ongoing to clarify the pathogenicity of *P alcalifaciens* and its role in dogs with hemorrhagic diarrhea either as a single primary infectious agent or as trigger for clostridial overgrowth and secondary toxin release (Personal communication Dr. Ellen Skancke; https://www.vetinst.no/en/news/normalized-situation-in-dogs-in-norway, 2019).

DIAGNOSTIC STRATEGY

In dogs with AHDS, increased fecal markers such as calprotectin and S100A12 as well as α1-proteinase inhibitor reflect intestinal damage and associated intestinal inflammation.[11] Fecal microbiome analysis of the 16S rRNA gene revealed profound alterations and qPCR assays significant increases in genus *C perfringens* and *Sutterella* in dogs with AHDS when compared with healthy dogs.[12] Fecal ELISA test for detection of CPE is often positive, and on fecal cultures growth of *C perfringens* can be consistently documented.[2] However, these results can also be seen in dogs with other gastrointestinal diseases and even in healthy dogs (eg, positive fecal culture for *C perfringens*).[2] Confirming the presence of *C perfringens* encoding for NetF suggests AHDS, but a few healthy dogs can harbor these strains in their large intestine. This means, that there is currently no noninvasive test to diagnose AHDS. Therefore, diagnosis of AHDS is mainly based on the typical clinical presentation and clinical course together with exlusion of other known causes of acute intestinal signs associated with significant damage of the intestinal mucosa (**Box 1**).

As the first diagnostic test, a PCV is very helpful to differentiate between AHDS and gastrointestinal bleeding as well as to assess the severity of dehydration and must be determined in every dog with blood in its feces. A complete blood count (CBC) and serum biochemistry profile should routinely be performed to identify potential causes and complications of the disease (**Tables 1** and **2**). Rarely dogs with hypoadrenocorticism can be presented with acute hemorrhagic diarrhea without classic electrolyte changes at presentation.[13] Because these patients cannot be differentiated from dogs with AHDS based on history, CBC, and serum biochemistry profile including electrolytes, it is advisable to include a serum basal cortisol level in the routine diagnostic workup. The necessity to perform other additional tests depends on the observation of untypical clinical findings (eg, severe abdominal pain, fever) or an unexpected clinical course (eg, inadequate improvement on fluid therapy and pain management over the first 24 hours) (**Figs. 2** and **3**).

TREATMENT AND CLINICAL COURSE

The peracute loss of intestinal mucosal integrity in AHDS results in a rapid movement of fluid and electrolytes into the gut lumen, leading to significant dehydration and hypovolemic shock. Dogs suspected of having AHDS might not show obvious clinical signs of dehydration, if they are presented early in the disease course. Despite this fact they should be hospitalized and treated aggressively because clinical deterioration is often rapid and can be fatal (**Table 3**). Depending on severity of clinical signs, rapid volume replacement with balanced electrolyte solutions are given as shock bolus as fast as 30 mL/kg in 10 minutes repeated up to 3 times if needed or as continuous intravenous (IV) infusion with the rate of up to 40 to 60 mL/kg/h IV until the PCV is in the mid-normal range. Response to fluid therapy should be reassessed every hour with the clinical goal of a heart rate less than 120/min in small breed dogs and less than 100/min in large breed dogs, as well as a capillary refill time less than 2 seconds,

---

Box 1
Differential diagnoses for dogs with acute hemorrhagic diarrhea

- Drugs/toxins causing mucosal irritation (eg, doxycycline, NSAIDs)
- Previous event causing intestinal damage (eg, hypovolemia, blood loss, hypotension, heat stroke)
- Acute liver or kidney failure
- Acute pancreatitis
- Hypoadrenocorticism
- Intestinal foreign body, intussusception, or mesenteric volvulus
- Intestinal infection (eg, canine parvovirus, *Salmonella* spp., *Campylobacter* spp.)

Abbreviation: NSAID, nonsteroidal antiinflammatory drug.

Table 1
Further considerations and diagnostic approach in case of complications in dogs with acute hemorrhagic diarrhea syndrome

Complication	Possible Findings	Further Diagnostic Tests

Bacterial translocation/sepsis	• Fever or hypothermia
	• Hypotension
	• Neutrophils
	   >20,000 or
	   <3000 cells/µL
	• Band neutrophils
	   >2500 cells/µL
	• Hypoglycemia
	• Hyperbilirubinemia
		• Blood culture
		• Abdominal ultrasound
		• Consider culture from enlarged lymph nodes and abdominal fluids if present
		• Fecal culture

DIC	• Petechiae • Thrombocytopenia	• Coagulation profile • D-dimers
Severe intestinal protein loss	• Peripheral edema • Low-protein abdominal or pleural effusion • Albumin <2 g/dL	• Urine protein creatine ratio to rule out renal loss • Serum bile acids to rule out liver dysfunction • Protein concentration in effusion fluid if present to rule out loss over body cavities
No improvement after 24–48 h of treatment	• Vomiting • Reduced mental status • Abdominal pain	• Abdominal imaging • Serum bile acids to rule out liver dysfunction • Repeat CBC and serum biochemistry profile

Abbreviation: DIC, disseminated intravascular coagulation.

Table 2
Further considerations and diagnostic approach in case of atypical findings in dogs with acute hemorrhagic diarrhea syndrome

Atypical Findings in AHDS	Differential Diagnosis	Further Diagnostic Tests
Significant abdominal pain	• Foreign body • Intussusception • Acute pancreatitis • Mesenteric volvulus	• Abdominal ultrasound • Abdominal radiographs • Pancreatic lipase test (quantitative, if SNAP cPL is positive)
Neutropenia	• CPV infection	• Fecal PCR for CPV
Neutrophilia, left shift, fever	• Primary bacterial enteropathogen • Bacterial translocation	• Blood culture • Culture of aspirated abdominal fluid/lymph node • Fecal culture
ALT/AP enzyme activity >3 × upper reference interval	• Primary liver disease	• Serum bile acids elevated: workup liver disease • Serum bile acids normal: recheck liver enzymes after 2 wk
Azotemia + urine specific gravity <1.030	• Kidney dysfunction	• Work-up kidney disease
Positive fecal tests for protozoa and helminths	• Acute parasitic/protozoal infection/coinfection	• Recheck after anthelmintic treatment
Serum basal cortisol level <2 µg/dL	• Hypoadrenocorticism	• ACTH stimulation test

Abbreviations: ALP, alkaline phosphatase; ALT, alanine aminotransferase; CPV, canine parvovirus.

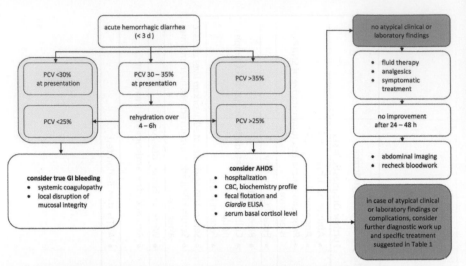

Fig. 2. Decision tree for the diagnostic approach of acute hemorrhagic diarrhea in dogs and the identification of possible complications. CBC, complete blood count; GI, gastrointestinal; PCV, packed cell volume. Reference interval for PCV: 35% to 58%.

normal pulse pressure, and mental status. After a few hours of adequate fluid therapy, dogs should be able to urinate when walked outside. Fluid therapy addressing maintenance requirements (about 50 mL/kg/24 h) and ongoing losses (up to 10 mL/kg/h in severely affected dogs) has to be continued until the dog is able to sustain a normal

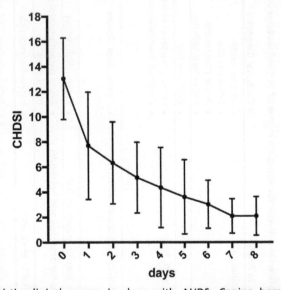

Fig. 3. Characteristic clinical course in dogs with AHDS. Canine hemorrhagic diarrhea severity index (CHDSI) was calculated as the sum of the scoring of the following parameters: attitude, appetite, vomiting, stool consistency, stool frequency, and dehydration. Each parameter was scored (0 = normal, 1 = mild, 2 = moderate, 3 = severe) in 24 dogs with AHDS on each treatment day, and the sum of scores (max. 18) yielded a total cumulative score. Clinical significance of disease: 0 to 3: clinical insignificant, 4 to 5: mild, 6 to 8: moderate, greater than 9 severe. Error bars show mean + standard deviation.

Table 3
Overview of frequently used drugs in dogs with acute hemorrhagic diarrhea syndrome

Medication	Dosage	Route	Frequency	Indication	Remarks
Isotonic crystalloid fluids (eg, lactated or acetated Ringer's solution)	40–60 mL/kg/d + losses + rehydration in hypovolemic shock: 30 mL/kg in 10 min repeated up to 3 times if needed	IV	CRI	Rehydration, fluid substitution, treatment of shock	Substitute potassium (avoid arrhythmogenic risks of rapid supplementation) and glucose as necessary
Synthetic colloids (eg, HES, succinylated gelatin)	1. Bolus: 5–15 mL/kg maybe repeated 2. Bolus followed by CRI: 1–2 mL/kg/h	IV	CRI	1. Hypovolemia <20 g/L 2. Hypoalbuminemia <15 g/L and clinical signs (edema, effusions, hypovolemia)	Consider side effects (coagulopathies, acute kidney injury) When administering synthetic colloid fluids reduce crystalloids by 40%–60%
Plasma	1. DIC: 10–20 mL/kg; 2. Hypoalbuminemia: 20–25 mL/kg to increase plasma level by 5 g/L	IV		DIC (fresh frozen), hypoalbuminemia <15 g/L and clinical signs (edema, effusions, hypovolemia)	Preferred over human albumin; in anemic patients whole blood transfusion is recommended additionally
Canine albumin (5%)	Albumin (g) = deficit^a x 0,1 x kg over 10 h	IV	CRI	Hypoalbuminemia <15 g/L and clinical signs (edema, effusions, hypovolemia)	Preferred over human albumin; transfusion reaction possible
Human albumin (25%)	Albumin (g) = deficit^a x 0,1 x kg over 10 h	IV	CRI	Hypoalbuminemia <15 g/L and clinical signs (edema, effusions, hypovolemia)	Type III hypersensitivity possible even after weeks
Amoxicillin/clavulanate	20 mg/kg (amoxicillin) + 2.5 mg/kg (clavulanate)	IV (SC, PO)	q8–12h	See **Box 2**	Broad-spectrum antibiotic
Cefotaxime	50 mg/kg	IV	q8h	See **Box 2**	Covers especially gram-negative spectrum

(continued on next page)

Table 3
(continued)

Medication	Dosage	Route	Frequency	Indication	Remarks
Maropitant	1 mg/kg	IV, SC	q24 h	Vomiting, nausea	Contraindicated in the presence of GI obstruction or some toxicoses
Metoclopramide	0.2–0.5 mg/kg 1–2 mg/kg/d (CRI)	IV, SC, PO	q8h or CRI	Vomiting	Contraindicated in the presence of GI obstruction or some toxicoses
Sucralfate	20–40 mg/kg or 0.5–1 g per dog	PO	q8–12h	Prevention or treatment of esophageal injury in case of frequent vomiting	Potentially less negative side effects compared with proton pump inhibitors, administer 2 h after meal and avoid simultaneous administration with other medication
Buprenorphine	5–20 µg/kg	IV, SC	q6–8h	Analgesia	May decrease gastrointestinal motility
Metamizole (not available in the United States)	20–50 mg/kg	IV, IM, PO	q6–8h	Analgesia	Analgesic without negative impact on mucosal perfusion
Enteral nutrition	Glutamine, low fat diet, hydrolyzed diet	PO or feeding tube	Multiple small meals per day, CRI (feeding tube)	Anorexia, hyporexia, hypoalbuminemia	Early enteral nutrition might improve intestinal barrier function Hydrolyzed diet might prevent sensitization to food antigens
Probiotics	Follow manufacturer's instructions	PO		Stabilization of the intestinal microbiome	High dose of multistrain products
Fecal microbiota transplantation (FMT)	5 g/kg recipient (diluted)	Rectal	q48 h	Stabilization of the intestinal microbiome	Follow donor screening guidelines, benefit not proven in prospective studies

Abbreviations: CRI, constant rate infusion; DIC, disseminated intravascular coagulopathy; HES, hydroxyethyl starch solution; IV, intravenous; PO, per os; SC, subcutaneous; SIRS, systemic inflammatory response syndrome

[a] Albumin deficit is calculated by deducting the actual from the desired albumin concentration (eg, 20 g/L–14 g/L = 6 g/L).

fluid balance by oral intake. Dogs with an uncomplicated course of AHDS characteristically and consistently show a very rapid improvement over the first 24 to 48 hours (**Fig. 3**). A lack of clinical improvement should prompt clinicians to reevaluate the patient for other causes of hemorrhagic diarrhea (eg, acute pancreatitis) or for possible complications such as severe hypoalbuminemia, bacterial translocation/sepsis, and disseminated intravascular coagulation. Few dogs develop significant hypoalbuminemia and require synthetic colloids, plasma, or albumin solutions preferably of canine rather than human origin, if available.

The prevalence of bacteremia in dogs with AHDS is low and not different from those of healthy control dogs.[14] Two prospective studies showed that in dogs with aseptic AHDS, antibiotics do not change outcome or time to recovery.[15,16] Another study showed that there is no benefit in the addition of metronidazole to amoxicillin-clavulanic acid for treatment of severe cases of AHDS.[17] Antibiotics can disrupt the protective intestinal microbiota, potentially stimulate toxin production and release, and lead to the development of resistant bacteria and long-term dysbiosis. Therefore, their use should be restricted to situations outlined in **Box 2**. However, the decision to administer antibiotics should not be based on a positive fecal PCR for toxin-encoding bacterial strains (eg, CPE A gene) and potential enteropathogenic bacteria. Fecal cultures, ideally in combination with blood cultures and cultures from aspirated material from enlarged abdominal lymph nodes, are only indicated in dogs with signs of systemic illness/inflammation in order to identify a causative enteropathogen (eg, *Campylobacter* spp., *Salmonella* spp.) or translocated bacteria. In these cases, the ultimate goal of these additional tests is to select an appropriate antibiotic based on sensitivity testing.

About 50% of dogs show vomiting as first clinical signs, and most dogs do not start to eat until day 3 or 4. Therefore, an antiemetic such as maropitant (1 mg/kg q24 h IV) should be administered to control nausea. Although obvious signs of abdominal pain are not always detected on physical examination, analgesics not affecting intestinal

---

Box 2
Criteria justifying administration of antibiotics in dogs with acute hemorrhagic diarrhea syndrome

- Systemic signs of illness that persist after rehydration, pain management, and symptomatic treatment, for example,
  - Depressed mental status
  - Tachycardia: HR >120/min small breed dogs; >100/min large breed dogs
  - Tachypnea: RR >30/min
  - Hypotension: BP MAP <80 mm Hg

- Signs of systemic inflammation at presentation, for example,
  - Rectal temperature greater than 39.5°C or 103.1°F
  - WBC less than 4000 or greater than 25,000/μL
  - Band neutrophils greater than 2500/μL

- Presence of an immunocompromising underlying disease, for example,
  - Immunosuppressive treatment
  - Neutropenia

- High probability of ineffective clearance of bacteria by the liver, for example,
  - Portosystemic shunt flow
  - Liver dysfunction

Abbreviations: BP, blood pressure; HR, heart rate; MAP, mean arterial pressure; RR, respiratory rate.

integrity and minimally suppressing intestinal motility (eg, buprenorphine, 5-20 μg/kg, IV q6–8h; metamizole, 20-50 mg/kg q8h., Caution: nonsteroidal antiiflammatory drugs [NSAIDs] and pure μ receptor agonists should be avoided) should routinely be administered.

POTENTIAL STRATEGIES FOR PREVENTION OF LONG-TERM PROBLEMS

Acute enteritis is a well-recognized trigger of chronic diseases in humans. Similarly, 2 independent studies showed that dogs with an episode of severe acute intestinal damage are at increased risk for developing chronic gastrointestinal disorders later in life.[18] Forty-two percent of dogs that survived a canine parvovirus infection and about 30% of dogs with an episode of AHDS develop chronic diarrhea later in life, which is significantly higher compared with age and breed matched control groups (control group for canine parvovirus infection 12%, for AHDS 14%). There is evidence that in acute disease, barrier dysfunction and dysbiosis can lead to loss of oral tolerance and sensitize the immune system to food components and to the intestinal microbiota. Therefore, new treatment strategies with the aim to rapidly restore intestinal barrier function and normobiosis might be considered. Early enteral nutrition, mucosal nutrients (eg, glutamine), and addition of dietary fiber as source of short-chain fatty acids might help to improve intestinal barrier integrity. In addition, further studies need to evaluate if restricting the diet to one protein source or feeding a hydrolyzed diet in the acute phase might help avoid sensitizing the immune system to different antigens. Drugs with the potential to affect integrity of the tight junction complex such as NSAIDs and proton pump inhibitors (PPIs)[19] and, unless specific criteria are met, antibiotics causing dysbiosis have to be avoided. Positive modulation of the intestinal microbiota might become a main focus of treatment in acute intestinal disease. Specific probiotics might strengthen tight junctions and downregulate existing pathogens or inhibit their adherence to the intestinal mucosa.[20–23] In humans, a meta-analysis determined that probiotic administration has the potential to reduce the risk of atopic sensitization.[24] Compared with dogs that were only treated symptomatically, dogs with AHDS that received a high dose of a multistrain probiotic had accelerated normalization of bacterial groups considered to have a beneficial influence (eg, *Blautia* spp., *Clostridium hiranonis*) and downregulation of toxigenic *C perfringens* strains.[25] Future studies need to determine if the administration of probiotics or fecal transplantation as an additional microbiome-modulating strategy might help to rapidly improve gut homeostasis and thus have a positive long-term impact on host health.

SUMMARY

Although most dogs with AHDS have an uncomplicated course of the disease and recover very rapidly, complications can develop in a nonnegligible number of dogs. Currently, the main challenge for clinicians is to make a definitive diagnosis of AHDS after exclusion of other known causes of acute hemorrhagic diarrhea and to identify patients requiring antibiotic treatment. Based on systemic inflammatory response-syndrome criteria defined by de Laforcade and colleagues[26] (2003) and Hauptman and others (1997),[27] dogs with AHDS and signs of hypovolemic shock cannot be differentiated from dogs with sepsis at presentation. Therefore, clinical reassessment after fluid therapy is an essential step to correctly categorize patients as septic versus nonseptic. Future research should aim to discover parameters that can help to identify patients with sepsis or high risk to become septic already at presentation or at an early stage of the disease and to establish clear criteria for antibiotic use.

There is preliminary evidence that after an episode with AHDS, dogs have an increased risk to develop chronic diarrhea later in life. Thus, the focus of simply managing problems during the acute phase of the disease should be adjusted to include treatment strategies preventing progression to chronicity. Therefore, the hypothesis that sensitization to food antigens and to intestinal microbiota may take place during the phase of barrier dysfunction has to be confirmed. In addition, factors increasing the risk for development of long-term complications have to be identified.

DISCLOSURE

The authors have nothing to disclose.

REFERENCES

1. Unterer S, Busch K, Leipig M, et al. Endoscopically visualized lesions, histologic findings, and bacterial invasion in the gastrointestinal mucosa of dogs with acute hemorrhagic diarrhea syndrome. J Vet Intern Med 2014;28(1):52–8.
2. Marks SL, Rankin SC, Byrne BA, et al. Enteropathogenic bacteria in dogs and cats: diagnosis, epidemiology, treatment, and control. J Vet Intern Med 2011; 25(6):1195–208.
3. Sindern N, Suchodolski JS, Leutenegger CM, et al. Prevalence of Clostridium perfringens netE and netF toxin genes in the feces of dogs with acute hemorrhagic diarrhea syndrome. J Vet Intern Med 2019;33(1):100–5.
4. Kaufmann EB, Busch K, Suchodolski JS, et al. Long-term consequences of acute hem- orrhagic diarrhea syndrome in dogs (Abstract DVG). Tierarztl Prax Ausg K Klein- tiere Heimtiere 2020;48(01):67.
5. Mortier F, Strohmeyer K, Hartmann K, et al. Acute haemorrhagic diarrhoea syndrome in dogs: 108 cases. Vet Rec 2015;176(24):627.
6. Leipig-Rudolph M, Busch K, Prescott JF, et al. Intestinal lesions in dogs with acute hemorrhagic diarrhea syndrome associated with netF-positive Clostridium perfringens type A. J Vet Diagn Invest 2018;30(4):495–503.
7. Weese JS, Staempfli HR, Prescott JF, et al. The roles of Clostridium difficile and enterotoxigenic Clostridium perfringens in diarrhea in dogs. J Vet Intern Med 2001;15(4):374–8.
8. Busch K, Suchodolski JS, Kuhner KA, et al. Clostridium perfringens enterotoxin and Clostridium difficile toxin A/B do not play a role in acute haemorrhagic diarrhoea syndrome in dogs. Vet Rec 2015;176(10):253.
9. Mehdizadeh Gohari I, Parreira VR, Nowell VJ, et al. A novel pore-forming toxin in type A Clostridium perfringens is associated with both fatal canine hemorrhagic gastroenteritis and fatal foal necrotizing enterocolitis. PLoS One 2015;10(4): e0122684.
10. Mehdizadeh Gohari I, Unterer S, Whitehead AE, et al. NetF-producing Clostridium perfringens and its associated diseases in dogs and foals. J Vet Diagn Invest 2020;32(2):230–8.
11. Heilmann RM, Guard MM, Steiner JM, et al. Fecal markers of inflammation, protein loss, and microbial changes in dogs with the acute hemorrhagic diarrhea syndrome (AHDS). J Vet Emerg Crit Care (San Antonio) 2017;27(5):586–9.
12. Suchodolski JS, Markel ME, Garcia-Mazcorro JF, et al. The fecal microbiome in dogs with acute diarrhea and idiopathic inflammatory bowel disease. PLoS One 2012;7(12):e51907.

13. Busch K, Wehner A, Dorsch R, et al. [Acute haemorrhagic diarrhoea as a presenting sign in a dog with primary hypoadrenocorticism]. Tierarztl Prax Ausg K Kleintiere Heimtiere 2014;42(5):326–30.
14. Unterer S, Lechner E, Mueller RS, et al. Prospective study of bacteraemia in acute haemorrhagic diarrhoea syndrome in dogs. Vet Rec 2015;176(12):309.
15. Israiloff J. Comparison of different treatment options in dogs with idiopathic hemorrhagic gastroenteritis [scientific monograph]. Vienna (Austria): Veterinary Medicine University of Vienna; 2009.
16. Unterer S, Strohmeyer K, Kruse BD, et al. Treatment of aseptic dogs with hemorrhagic gastroenteritis with amoxicillin/clavulanic acid: a prospective blinded study. J Vet Intern Med 2011;25(5):973–9.
17. Ortiz V, Klein L, Channell S, et al. Evaluating the effect of metronidazole plus amoxicillin-clavulanate versus amoxicillin-clavulanate alone in canine haemorrhagic diarrhoea: a randomised controlled trial in primary care practice. J Small Anim Pract 2018;59(7):398–403.
18. Kilian E, Suchodolski JS, Hartmann K, et al. Long-term effects of canine parvovirus infection in dogs. PLoS One 2018;13(3):e0192198.
19. Gabello M, Valenzano MC, Zurbach EP, et al. Omeprazole induces gastric transmucosal permeability to the peptide bradykinin. World J Gastroenterol 2010;16(9):1097–103.
20. Rossi G, Pengo G, Caldin M, et al. Comparison of microbiological, histological, and immunomodulatory parameters in response to treatment with either combination therapy with prednisone and metronidazole or probiotic VSL#3 strains in dogs with idiopathic inflammatory bowel disease. PLoS One 2014;9(4):e94699.
21. De Keersmaecker SC, Verhoeven TL, Desair J, et al. Strong antimicrobial activity of Lactobacillus rhamnosus GG against Salmonella typhimurium is due to accumulation of lactic acid. FEMS Microbiol Lett 2006;259(1):89–96.
22. Neeser JR, Granato D, Rouvet M, et al. Lactobacillus johnsonii La1 shares carbohydrate-binding specificities with several enteropathogenic bacteria. Glycobiology 2000;10(11):1193–9.
23. Fujiwara S, Hashiba H, Hirota T, et al. Inhibition of the binding of enterotoxigenic Escherichia coli Pb176 to human intestinal epithelial cell line HCT-8 by an extracellular protein fraction containing BIF of Bifidobacterium longum SBT2928: suggestive evidence of blocking of the binding receptor gangliotetraosylceramide on the cell surface. Int J Food Microbiol 2001;67(1–2):97–106.
24. Plunkett CH, Nagler CR. The Influence of the Microbiome on Allergic Sensitization to Food. J Immunol 2017;198(2):581–9.
25. Ziese AL, Suchodolski JS, Hartmann K, et al. Effect of probiotic treatment on the clinical course, intestinal microbiome, and toxigenic Clostridium perfringens in dogs with acute hemorrhagic diarrhea. PLoS One 2018;13(9):e0204691.
26. de Laforcade AM, Freeman LM, Shaw SP, et al. Hemostatic changes in dogs with naturally occurring sepsis. J Vet Intern Med 2003;17(5):674–9.
27. Hauptman JG, Walshaw R, Olivier NB. Evaluation of the sensitivity and specificity of diagnostic criteria for sepsis in dogs. Vet Surg 1997;26(5):393–7.

Differentiating Inflammatory Bowel Disease from Alimentary Lymphoma in Cats: Does It Matter?

Sina Marsilio, Dr med vet, PhD

KEYWORDS

- Feline chronic enteropathy • Inflammatory bowel disease • Small cell lymphoma

KEY POINTS

- Differentiation of feline inflammatory bowel disease (IBD) from small cell lymphoma (SCL) can be challenging and often requires ancillary testing, such as immunohistochemistry and clonality testing.
- It is still unclear whether IBD and SCL represent 2 distinct disease processes or whether they are part of a disease spectrum.
- Further research on these diseases is required to improve understanding of etiopathogenesis, progression, alternative treatment modalities, and prognosis.

INTRODUCTION

Feline chronic enteropathy (FCE) is among the most common disorders in the elderly cat population, with rising incidence over the past decades.[1,2] The disorder is defined as the presence of clinical signs of gastrointestinal disease for more than 3 weeks, while extragastrointestinal diseases as well as infectious intestinal diseases have been excluded. Although there is no uniform classification scheme for chronic enteropathies, most investigators subclassify cases based on the response to treatment into food-responsive enteropathy, inflammatory bowel disease (IBD) (often used interchangeably with steroid-responsive enteropathy), and small cell lymphoma (SCL). The most common underlying diseases for FCE, especially in elderly cats, are IBD and alimentary SCL.

Although the etiopathogenesis is unknown, IBD is thought to occur as a result of perturbations in the cross-talk between the environment, the immune system, and the microbiome in a genetically susceptible host. Histopathologically, small mature lymphocytes and plasma cells dominate the inflammatory infiltrate.

Department of Veterinary Medicine and Epidemiology, UC Davis School of Veterinary Medicine, Tupper Hall, 1275 Med Science Drive, Davis, CA 95616, USA
E-mail address: SMarsilio@UCDavis.edu

Vet Clin Small Anim 51 (2021) 93–109
https://doi.org/10.1016/j.cvsm.2020.09.009
0195-5616/21/© 2020 Elsevier Inc. All rights reserved.

The term, *lymphoma*, refers to the clonal expansion of 1 (or sometimes a few) lymphocytic clones. Even in the post–feline leukemia virus era, lymphomas remain the most common feline neoplasms,[2–7] with the alimentary tract affected in 42% to 52% of cases.[3–5,8–10]

Gastrointestinal lymphomas can be classified by their morphology (small cell vs large cell), distribution within the mucosa (eg, epitheliotropism), immunophenotype (B cell, T cell, and natural killer [NK] cell), anatomic location, histopathologic appearance, and biological behavior (low grade vs high grade). Three main types of feline gastrointestinal lymphoma can be differentiated that vary in appearance, treatment, and prognosis: low-grade SCL; intermediate to large cell lymphoma (LCL); and large granular lymphocyte (LGL) lymphomas.

SCLs are the most common form of gastrointestinal lymphoma in cats, accounting for up to 75% of all gastrointestinal lymphomas in feline patients. They consist of small lymphocytes that represent a mature, well-differentiated population of cells with low mitotic rates. Clinical progression is usually slow, with clinical signs often present over weeks to month. Thus, these lymphomas are classified as low-grade SCLs. More than 90% of SCLs are of T-cell origin and usually they arise in the jejunum, duodenum, and ileum in descending order of occurrence.[11]

intermediate to large cell lymphoma (LCL) represent a progressively more immature and less differentiated cell population. Mitotic rates are higher and they are more aggressive tumors, following a more acute and rapid clinical course. LGL lymphoma is a separate form of gastrointestinal lymphoma in cats, which may show variable cell size but generally is considered a high-grade, aggressive neoplasm. From a clinical perspective, these differentiations are important because signalment, clinical findings, biologic behavior, therapy, and, most importantly, prognosis differ significantly between the different forms of gastrointestinal lymphoma. Although LCLs and LGL lymphomas have a guarded to poor prognosis, the prognosis for SCL is good to excellent.

Some clinicians argue that the differentiation of IBD and SCL is unnecessary because treatment often is the same for refractory IBD and SCL. Although this might be true for many individual patients, the author disagrees with this dismissive approach to the medical profession and to science in general. It was not until the late 1990s that feline intestinal lymphoma was even recognized as a distinct disease process.[8,12,13] Most publications did not differentiate, however, between SCL and LCL or between intestinal and extraintestinal lymphoma, and feline leukemia virus–associated lymphomas dominated the study populations. Since then, more than 50 studies were published on FCE and lymphoma. In 2005, Louwerens and colleagues[2] published a large retrospective case series of 477 cats with retroviral-negative lymphoma and showed a marked increase in the incidence of feline lymphomas between 1984 and 2003. In the same year, Moore and colleagues[14] characterized the feline T-cell receptor and laid the fundament for clonality testing. Finally, between 2005 and 2009, the first studies were published that actively differentiated between SCL and LCL.[6,7,15,16] This shows that without scientific curiosity and research advancing the field, the profession will be lost and unfit for future challenges. As part of the medical profession, I believe it is a privilege and obligation to contribute to the body of medical knowledge. Although first-class medicine may not be able to be applied to every patient, at the very least doing so should be striven for.

SIGNALMENT

Both signalment and clinical signs are not suitable differentiators between feline IBD and SCL. Although cats with IBD tend to be younger, with a median reported age of approximately 8 years,[17–20] compared with cats with SCL, with an approximate median age of 12.5 years,[15,21,22] the age ranges overlap significantly (IBD range, 1.3–16 years, vs SCL range, 4–20 years). Domestic shorthair cats are affected most commonly in both groups and, although Siamese cats have been found to be overrepresented in cats with FCE in some studies, this again is true for SCL and IBD alike.

CLINICAL SIGNS AND PHYSICAL EXAMINATION

Similarly, clinical signs are indistinguishable between feline IBD and SCL. Weight loss is the most common clinical sign in cats with FCE (80%–90%), followed by vomiting (70%–80%), anorexia (60%–70%), and diarrhea (50%–65%).[7,23,24] This is in contrast to dogs, where diarrhea is by far the most common presenting complaint. In the author's and others' experience,[25] weight loss often is overlooked due to its very gradual progression over weeks to months. Cats often lose muscle tissue first and may develop significant sarcopenia, particularly appreciable along the spine, before adipose tissue is lost. Abdominal fat pads often are preserved even in otherwise cachectic cats. Beside sarcopenia and a generally low body condition score, physical examination may reveal segmental or diffusely thickened intestinal loops (ropy loops) and abdominal discomfort/pain often located in the cranial abdomen, possibly related to concurrent pancreatitis and/or cholangiohepatitis.

In contrast to IBD and SCL, cats with intermediate to large cell lymphoma usually show more acute onset and rapidly progressive clinical signs. Abdominal masses, intussusception, obstruction, or even perforation mostly are associated with this more aggressive form of alimentary lymphoma.

MINIMALLY INVASIVE DIAGNOSTIC TESTS

Several studies have investigated the use of minimally invasive diagnostic tests as means to diagnose FCE and differentiate IBD from SCL. Today, however, there is no single biomarker that reliably distinguishes IBD from SCL. Nevertheless, laboratory tests and imaging studies still are extremely helpful tools to localize and characterize lesions and decide further diagnostic steps.

Laboratory Tests

Although significant protein loss and the development of protein-losing enteropathy are rare in cats, hypoalbuminemia is a common finding in both disease entities, with up to 100% of cats with severe IBD or SCL affected.[18,23] In contrast, total protein often is normal or increased due to concurrent hyperglobulinemia and an increased total protein concentration is part of the Feline Chronic Enteropathy Activity Index.[20] Hypoglobulinemia and panhypoproteinemia, however, are not uncommon findings either and are described in both IBD (39%) and SCL (55%).[23] Other laboratory tests with potential diagnostic as well as therapeutic and prognostic value are serum folate, cobalamin, and inorganic phosphorus concentrations, and deficiencies previously have been associated with disease severity in cats with chronic enteropathy.[26] Cobalamin is a water-soluble vitamin present in dietary proteins. In the small intestinal tract, it is bound to intrinsic factor, which, in cats, stems exclusively from pancreatic secretion. Cobalamin is absorbed in the distal small intestinal tract, especially the ileum, through binding of intrinsic factor to its respective receptors. Similarly, folate is a water-soluble vitamin present in a wide variety of food sources and also can be produced by certain bacteria. Folate is absorbed mainly in the proximal small intestinal tract. Serum folate concentrations can be increased in FCE as a result of dysbiosis or decreased due to mucosal infiltration and subsequent malabsorption. Both folate and cobalamin are essential for DNA synthesis. Besides the bone marrow, enterocytes are among the most rapidly dividing cells in the body, with a high level of DNA turnover. Therefore, hypocobalaminemia and hypofolatemia can affect gastrointestinal integrity, and supplementation has been shown to be beneficial in cats[27] and in people.[28] Studies in cats with gastrointestinal signs have shown rising serum concentrations of methylmalonic acid, with cobalamin concentrations less than 400 ng/L, indicating cellular cobalamin deficiencies (Steiner, personal communication). Therefore, the author recommends cobalamin supplementation in cats with signs of chronic enteropathy with serum cobalamin concentrations of less than or equal to 400 ng/L.

Other micronutrients found to be decreased in cats with chronic enteropathy are inorganic phosphorus[26] and vitamin D.[29] Even though supplementation of deficient micronutrients might be beneficial, the author views these deficiencies primarily as surrogate markers of malabsorption due to a primary underlying pathology (**Table 1**). Hence, treating the underlying disease is key to regaining control of metabolic perturbations. Besides information on malabsorption, cobalamin and folate also can provide some clues on the disease location. In the presence of hypocobalaminemia, ileal biopsies are essential to maximize the likelihood of collecting samples that are representative of the disease process. In addition to serum cobalamin and folate, the measurements of feline pancreatic lipase immunoreactivity (fPLI) and feline trysin-like immunoreactivity (fTLI) have value in cats with chronic enteropathy. Concurrent chronic pancreatitis often is observed in cats with CE. Thus, FCE should be considered a differential concurrent diagnosis in cats with increased fPLI. Addressing the underlying enteropathy often improves chronic pancreatitis but the same is not necessarily true vice versa. Exocrine pancreatic insufficiency (EPI) increasingly is recognized in cats.[30] Although canine EPI commonly is caused by pancreatic acinar atrophy in young dogs, cats with EPI often are older and sometimes have a history of pancreatitis. It has been hypothesized that EPI in cats may be a consequence of chronic pancreatitis causing fibrosis and severe loss of functional tissue. Therefore, measurements of fPLI and fTLI in cats with signs of chronic gastrointestinal disease are necessary to identify of concurrent pancreatic disorders.

Abdominal Ultrasound

The normal intestinal wall consists of 4 main layers: the mucosa (with the epithelium and lamina propria), the submucosa, the lamina muscularis (ie, muscularis propria), and the serosa. The mucosa, submucosa, and muscularis can be visualized using a high-frequency transducer. Common ultrasonographic abnormalities in IBD and SCL are thickened muscularis propria, loss of wall layering, and lymphadenopathy. A muscularis-to-submucosa ratio of greater than 1 is suggestive of an abnormal bowel segment (**Fig. 1**).[15,31] Several studies have attempted to differentiate IBD from SCL using ultrasonography.[31,32] Although older cats with thickening of the muscularis mucosa and cats with abdominal lymphadenopathy were more likely to have a diagnosis of lymphoma, there was substantial overlap between SCL and IBD or even with findings in healthy cats.[31,32] One of these studies found that none of the cats showed that infiltrates in the muscularis layer and thickening of the muscularis layer were not common histopathologic findings in cats with IBD or SCL.[32] Another recent study in 169 cats that underwent abdominal ultrasound and full-thickness biopsies found the ability of ultrasound to predict mucosal lesions as high but low for submucosal or muscularis lesions.[33] Both studies suggest that the ultrasonographic appearance of a thickened muscularis layer may be an epiphenomenon that is not correlated with histopathologic tissue changes. Exceptions may be eosinophilic enteritis or the feline gastrointestinal eosinophilic sclerosing fibroplasia, where the

Table 1
Biochemical parameters that can serve as surrogate markers in cats with clinical signs of chronic enteropathy

Parameter	Location	Parameter Concentration Trend	Surrogate Marker for	Differential Diagnoses
Albumin	Liver (production), intestinal tract (loss)	↓	Negative acute-phase protein, intestinal loss	• Loss/malabsorption: infiltrative mucosal disease (inflammatory cells (eg, IBD), neoplastic cells (eg, lymphoma), infectious agents (eg, fungal disease) • Decreased production: hepatopathy • Illness: decreased DNA transcription, shift of amino acids toward production of positive acute phase proteins
Globulin	Liver (production), intestinal tract (loss)	↓	Intestinal loss	• Infiltrative mucosal disease • Hepatopathy
		↑	Chronic antigenic stimulation	• Infiltrative mucosal disease
Cobalamin	Distal small intestine/ileum	↓	Malabsorption	• EPI • Infiltrative mucosal disease • Receptor defect (not described in cats)
Folate	Proximal small intestine	↑ ↓	Dysbiosis Malabsorption	• Primary dysbiosis • Infiltrative mucosal disease
fPLI	Exocrine pancreas	↑	Pancreatitis	• Primary acute pancreatitis • Chronic pancreatitis • Chronic pancreatitis concurrent to CE
fTLI	Exocrine pancreas	↑	Pancreatitis	• See fPLI
		↓	EPI	• Secondary to chronic pancreatitis/CE • Pancreatic acinar atrophy (very uncommon)

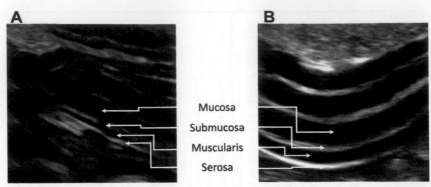

Fig. 1. Sagittal ultrasound images of a cat with normal small intestine (*left*) and a cat presented for signs of chronic enteropathy (*right*). The mucosal, submucosal, muscularis, and serosal layers are indicated with arrows in the far field. Compared with normal intestines, the muscularis propria is thickened in the cat affected with SCL. (*Courtesy of* A. LaPorte, Vacaville, CA., E. McLarty, DVM, DACVR, Davis, CA. and M. Wanamaker, DVM, DACVR, Victoria, Canada.)

muscularis layer often is found to be thickened both on ultrasound and histopathology.[34,35] Ultrasonographic findings still should be interpreted carefully, and IBD and SCL cannot be differentiated using ultrasonography.

Ultrasound, however, still plays an important role in the diagnosis of FCE as guidance on the best next diagnostic step. Cats with diffuse changes in the duodenum and proximal jejunum and/or the ileum may be good candidates for gastroduodenoscopy and ileocolonoscopy. By contrast, patients with localized and/or extramural changes, changes outside the range of the endoscope, and changes in other organs should undergo laparotomy or laparoscopy with collection of full-thickness biopsies. Patients with LCL or fungal disease often show localized mass lesions, lymphadenopathy, hepatosplenomegaly, or splenomegaly. In these cases, a diagnosis often can be made using fine-needle aspirates.[36] Fine-needle aspirates, however, are unhelpful in differentiating IBD from SCL (discussed later).

BIOPSY COLLECTION

Every biopsy collection method has advantages and disadvantages and it is important to realize those in order to best advise cat owners on this crucial diagnostic step.

The main disadvantages of endoscopic biopsies over surgical biopsies are that they are limited to the mucosa and occasionally submucosa, that they have a limited range (ie, lesions in the mid to distal jejunum or usually out of the endoscopic range), and that extramural lesions cannot be biopsied. Therefore, patients with these types of lesions should undergo laparoscopy or laparotomy and with sampling of surgical biopsies. The collection of endoscopic biopsies, however, is minimally invasive and fast, recovery time is very short, and therapy can be started immediately after the procedure without the risk of wound dehiscence. In addition, the mucosal surface can be visualized and targeted biopsies can be obtained from visually affected areas. Using appropriate endoscopic equipment, advancement of the insertion tube well into the duodenum is easily accomplished, often reaching the proximal jejunum.[37] Current guidelines recommend collecting a minimum of 6 mucosal biopsies of adequate quality from the feline duodenum and 3 to 5 from the ileum for a reliable histopathologic assessment.[38] The author, however, usually collects 10 to 15 samples per location utilizing the entire endoscopic range. Ideally, ileocolonoscopy also should be performed in all cats, particularly in those with hypocobalaminemia. Adequate endoscopic biopsies can provide a minimally invasive method to acquire substantial data representative of a large portion of the small intestinal mucosa. This is especially advantageous because mucosal areas can be affected in a patchy fashion.

In contrast, surgical biopsies, even if taken from every section of the small intestines (ie, the duodenum, jejunum, and ileum), are representative of only a single site within each section. A recent, yet unpublished, study at the Gastrointestinal Laboratory at Texas A&M University revealed that the diagnostically available mucosal surface can be reduced substantially in full-thickness compared with endoscopic biopsies due to the number of specimens available (please add something like: Study author, personal communication. If you are the author, add Marsilio and colleagues, unpublished data). An overwhelming majority of diffuse small intestinal lesions start in or involve the mucosa and thus can be detected on adequate endoscopic biopsies.[7,11,19] In the end, taking samples that are representative of the disease process is key, regardless of the technique used, and every technique is prone to failure if used incorrectly. Endoscopic biopsies can be too superficial (often containing only crushed villi), too small, or too few. Surgical biopsies are taken blindly and might not be representative of the disease. Sometimes surgical biopsies are taken as a wedge, with a large serosal area that funnels down through the muscularis into the mucosa; thus, while the biopsy appears large, the most important part of the biopsy, the mucosa, is small, damaged, or even absent. Besides technical errors made by the biopsy collector, other errors, such as over-fixation and misorientation, can decrease the diagnostic value of the sample.[39] Samples should be orientated ensuring that the slides show a transversal plane through the intestinal wall. Misorientation can lead to diagnostically suboptimal or even inadequate hematoxylin-eosin (H&E) slides, despite adequately collected samples (**Fig. 2**). Some laboratories orientate the samples before paraffinization with the help of a microscope. Not every pathology laboratory, however, performs sample orientation. A recent study compared diagnostic utility of mounting intestinal biopsies on cucumber slices or moisturized synthetic foam sponges compared with free flotation

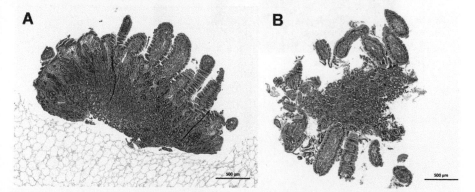

Fig. 2. Endoscopic biopsy specimens from the duodenum [Stain, H&E]. (*A*) Section from specimen submitted freely floating in formalin. Note the small size, inappropriate orientation, and crush artifacts. (*B*) Section from sample mounted on synthetic sponge. (*From* Ruiz GC, Reyes-Gomez E, Hall, EJ et al. Comparison of 3 handling techniques for endoscopically obtained gastric and duodenal biopsy specimens: a prospective study in dogs and cats. J Vet Intern Med. 2016;30(4):1014-1021; with permission.)

in formalin (see **Fig. 2**; **Fig. 3**).[39] Mounted biopsy specimens had significantly fewer artifacts and pathologists had higher confidence in their interpretation and diagnosis. If in doubt, the pathologists should be contacted and biopsy reorientation requested.

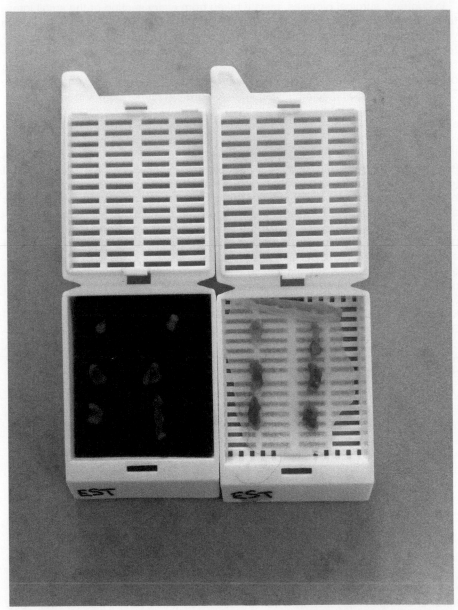

Fig. 3. Endoscopic biopsy specimens mounted and oriented on the synthetic foam sponge (*left cassette*) and on the thin cucumber slice (*right cassette*). (*From* Ruiz GC, Reyes-Gomez E, Hall, EJ et al. Comparison of 3 handling techniques for endoscopically obtained gastric and duodenal biopsy specimens: a prospective study in dogs and cats. J Vet Intern Med. 2016;30(4):1014-1021; with permission.)

HISTOPATHOLOGY

The gut-associated lymphoid tissue (GALT) is the largest immune organ in the body.[40] It consists of 2 compartments—the organized lymphoid tissue, such as lymphoid follicles, Peyer patches, and mesenteric lymph nodes; and scattered lymphocytes in the lamina propria and the epithelium.[40,41] These 2 compartments actually represent 2 opposite sides of the immune response. The organized lymphoid tissue is the induction site of an immune response. Epithelial microfold (M) cells and dendritic cells of the lamina propria collect luminal antigens and present them to naïve T cells and B cells in lymphoid follicles and Peyer patches. Activated lymphocytes migrate through draining lymph nodes and the thoracic duct into the blood stream. In a final step, these activated lymphocytes eventually become part of the effector site of the GALT, represented by scattered lamina propria and epithelial lymphocytes, through a process called homing. Circulating lymphocytes express homing factors, such as integrins, that bind to addressins expressed by the intestinal vascular endothelium. After binding, lymphocytes migrate through the vascular wall into the lamina propria and the epithelium. Hence, even though the induction and the effector site of the GALT are in close proximity, scattered lymphocytes of the lamina propria originate from the organized lymphoid compartment and have circulated in the blood stream before homing into the effector site of the lamina propria and epithelium. Faced with myriad antigens, the GALT has the herculean task of preventing disease caused by harmful pathogens while at the same time counterbalancing exaggerated inflammatory responses and ensuring mucosal tolerance to beneficial antigens, such as the healthy intestinal microbiota and proteins from nutrients. To ensure a proper immune response, the diffuse lymphoid tissues of the lamina propria contain a large number of lymphocytes, plasma cells, macrophages, dendritic cells, and stromal cells. It comes as no surprise that these cell numbers can vary; hence, a definition of normal has proved challenging. A study published in 2002 showed that histopathology has an inherently high interobserver variability.[42] The study investigated the agreement between 5 different board-certified pathologists reviewing slides from gastrointestinal specimens from dogs and cats.[42] Results showed a poor agreement between pathologists and triggered the formation of the World Small Animal Veterinary Association (WSAVA) Gastrointestinal Standardization Group.[43] The group was formed in an attempt to standardize histopathologic assessment of gastrointestinal biopsies. The WSAVA group also was first to recognize the importance of architectural changes over cellular infiltrates in the definition of gastrointestinal inflammation. The group published a standard form for pathologists that included a grading scheme for the cellular infiltrate as well as for morphologic abnormalities, such as epithelial injury, villus blunting, crypt distention, fibrosis, and lacteal dilation. Findings are graded on a scale of 0 (normal) to 3 (severe). In addition, the group published pictorial templates of normal and abnormal as a visual guide for pathologists (**Fig. 4**).[43,44]

Subsequent studies, however, have shown that interobserver variability still persists and, since then, other investigators have attempted to simplify the grading scheme.[45] Another flaw of the current WSAVA guidelines concerns the demographic characteristic of the group of cats that served as examples for the definition of the normal baseline. These samples were collected from a group of mostly young (approximately 1.5 years old), specific pathogen–free, colony cats. This group is hardly representative, however, of the group of cats that is presented for signs of chronic enteropathy in clinical practice. A recent study by the author investigated histopathologic findings in endoscopic gastric and duodenal biopsies of 20 healthy, client-owned cats with demographic characteristics similar to those of cats presented for chronic enteropathy

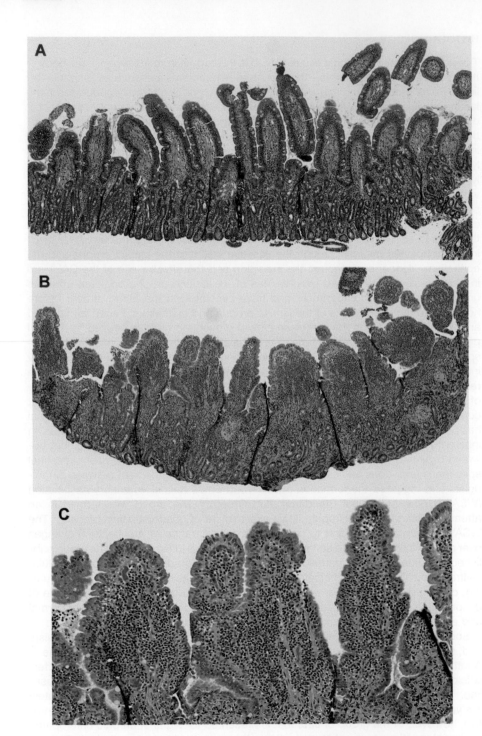

(median age 9.5 years, range 3–18 years).[46] All cats showed histopathologic findings considered to be abnormal based on the current WSAVA criteria. Only 3 cats, however, went on to develop gastrointestinal disease. The remaining 17 cats were clinically unchanged after a median follow-up time of 709 days.

Despite all flaws, histopathology still is the most reliable diagnostic test for a diagnosis chronic enteropathy currently available.

Histopathologically, the most common form of feline IBD is lymphoplasmacytic enteritis (LPE). Inflammation is found in the mucosa and sometimes extends to the epithelium and is characterized by increased numbers of well-differentiated lymphocytes and plasma cells accompanied by destruction of the normal architecture. SCL is characterized by epithelial/mucosal ± transmural infiltration with well-differentiated lymphocytes often accompanied by lymphoplasmacytic inflammation in the same and/or other parts of the intestinal tract.[11,14,25,47,48] Not surprisingly, severe cases of LPE can be difficult to distinguish from IBD, and progression of LPE into SCL has been suspected. For these reasons, the degree of architectural changes always should be assessed and viewed in combination with the cellular infiltrate. Advanced diagnostics, such as immunohistochemistry (IHC) and polymerase chain reaction (PCR)-based methods, also may be needed to identify SCL in equivocal cases.[11,49] Fine-needle aspirates lack the architectural context required for a correct diagnosis and generally are unhelpful for the differentiation of these 2 disease entities. Finally, a diagnosis of LPE is not equivalent to a diagnosis of IBD. LPE may be associated with intestinal parasites, food hypersensitivity, or even hyperthyroidism. This illustrates why other differential diagnoses need to be excluded before tissue sampling.[50]

Although architectural changes are a good indicator of the severity of intestinal disease, cellular infiltrates still are valuable because they may give clues about the underlying etiology. A prominent eosinophilic inflammatory component may be associated with parasites, food hypersensitivity, or T-cell lymphoma[51] or occur as a part of the hypereosinophilic syndrome. This systemic eosinophilic disorder is characterized by an increased production of eosinophilic precursors in the bone marrow. Patients display peripheral (mature) eosinophilia and eosinophilic infiltration in multiple tissues (eg, gastrointestinal tract, spleen, liver, lymph nodes, heart, and lungs) with subsequent organ damage.[52–54] Neutrophilic (suppurative) and/or histiocytic infiltration may suggest an infectious cause and indicates the need for additional testing, including special staining, and possibly fluorescence in situ hybridization.

ANCILLARY TESTING FOR FELINE CHRONIC ENTEROPATHY

Despite all attempts, there is no clear distinction between IBD and SCL based on histopathology alone and thus there are many ambiguous cases. Until now, IHC and clonality assays have been used to differentiate IBD from SCL. In neoplastic lesions, lymphocytes are derived from a single (or few) precursor cell(s); thus, the daughter cells show the same receptor specificity (clonal). In reactive processes, lymphocytes

Fig. 4. H&E-stained endoscopic biopsy specimens from cats with chronic enteropathy. (*A*) Mild LPE. Mild villus stunting and crypt hyperplasia. Mildly increased infiltration with lymphocytes and plasma cells. (*B*) Epitheliotropic SCL. Severe architectural changes, including villus stunting, villus fusion, and fibrosis. The lamina propria is infiltrated by a dense infiltrate of small lymphocytes. (*C*) The infiltrate is present predominantly in the lamina propria of the villi and also forms nests and plaques in the epithelium.

are derived from multiple precursor cells that differ in their antigen receptor specificity (polyclonal). By contrast, inflammatory responses comprise a mixture of T cells, B cells, and possibly other immune cells. This concept is the basis of IHC and PCR-based analysis.

Immunohistochemistry

If a sample is suspicious for SCL on H&E staining, the first step for further differentiation is IHC and specific staining, such as CD3 for T cells, and CD20, CD 79a, or PAX-5 for B cells and potentially other cells. In this step, the pathologist tries to determine whether all lymphocytes seen on regular H&E stain are of a single lineage or whether the infiltrate consists of a mixture of T cells, B cells, and plasma cells, the former supporting a diagnosis of lymphoma and the latter a diagnosis of inflammation, that is, IBD. A comprehensive study on the mucosal architecture, phenotype, and clonality of feline gastrointestinal lymphoma, published in 2012 by Moore and colleagues,[11] showed that only approximately 16% of alimentary lymphomas were of B-cell origin and of those all were considered LCL. A majority of approximately 84% of intestinal lymphomas were T-cell lymphomas and of those approximately 85% were considered SCLs. Of 11 T-cell lymphomas considered LCLs, 9 were LGL lymphomas. This form may be of cytotoxic T-cell or NK-cell origin because both cell types display intracytoplasmic eosinophilic granules. A vast majority of LGL lymphomas arise in the gastrointestinal tract, causing segmental or centrifugal thickening or multiple masses within the small intestine. The jejunum, ileum, ileocolic junction and duodenum, and large intestine are affected in descending order of frequency. Extragastrointestinal involvement is common and includes abdominal or extra-abdominal lymph nodes, liver, spleen, or kidneys. LGL lymphomas often are diagnosed readily on cytologic examination of slides acquired by fine-needle aspiration and usually do not require biopsy collection. On H&E stain, eosinophilic granules are obvious and granzyme B can be used as a special stain for final diagnosis.

SCLs often can be accompanied by inflammation; thus, a diagnosis can be difficult even with IHC. Therefore, other methods to assess the clonality of the lymphocyte receptors have been developed.[14]

Clonality Testing

The most commonly applied clonality assay is the PCR for receptor antigen rearrangement (PARR) because it can be performed on formalin-fixed, paraffin-embedded tissue samples.[14]

Virtually any substance can be the target of an immune response, and immune responses are mediated by the antigen receptor. Therefore, antigen receptors have an extremely high diversity. In fact, the diversity of B-cell immunoglobin receptors (Ig) or T-cell receptors (TCR) is estimated to be in the order of 10^{12}.

This diversity is made possible by the somatic rearrangement of germline DNA sequences inside the lymphocytes. Clonality assays permit visualization of the diversity of the antigen receptors. Presence of diverse receptors suggests the existence of inflammatory lesions (ie, polyclonal), whereas uniform receptors indicate neoplastic lesions (ie, clonal). Even though the primers used in the PARR assays are specific for T cells or B cells, the cell lineage cannot be determined by PARR. In up to 10% of cases, T cells can rearrange B-cell receptor genes and vice versa in a process of cross-lineage rearrangement.[55] Therefore, clonality assays should not be used to determine the lineage of the clone.

Clonality often implies immortality and uninhibited mitosis, as seen in cases of lymphoma. Clonality is not always equal to malignancy, however. Benign clonal expansions have been described in various diseases in humans[56,57] and dogs[58] and it is even a well-documented phenomenon in elderly otherwise healthy people.[59] Similarly, recent studies evaluating clonality assays in humans and cats found specificities as low as 54.3% in humans[60] and 33.3% in cats.[46,61] Therefore, IHC and PARR always should be interpreted together and in the context of all available data, ideally in the same laboratory.

Additional Ancillary Tests

A recent study by the author investigated the diagnostic utility of histology-guided mass spectrometry for the differentiation of lymphoplasmacytic enteritis from SCL. The study showed promising results with sensitivity of 86.7 and specificity of 91.7% for this novel diagnostic test.[61] Another study characterized the fecal microbiome of cats with IBD and SCL.[17] Although there was a serial increase or decrease of the abundance of certain members of the microbiome between healthy cats, cats with IBD, and cats with SCL, no differentiating biomarker was identified.

THERAPEUTIC MANAGEMENT AND PROGNOSIS OF INFLAMMATORY BOWEL DISEASE AND SMALL CELL LYMPHOMA

From a therapeutic standpoint, differentiation of feline IBD and SCL currently does not necessarily lead to different therapeutic plans. Common differential diagnoses for IBD and SCL, however, include intermediate to large cell lymphoma, eosinophilic syndrome, fungal disease, and other gastrointestinal neoplasia for which therapy and prognosis are vastly different. Hence, the collection of biopsies is required for the diagnosis and exclusion of other diseases. Treatment of feline IBD usually involves steroids with or without a concurrent dietary trial using a novel protein or hydrolyzed diet. Cats with IBD commonly are treated with prednisolone, at 2 mg/kg/d, which can be divided every 12 hours, depending on the tolerance of the patient. The prednisolone dose usually is tapered by 50% every 3 weeks to 4 weeks until the lowest effective dose is identified. Even though cats usually are tolerant to steroid side effects, budesonide (3 mg/m^2 every 24 hours) can be a useful alternative in patients intolerant to systemic steroids (eg, cats with diabetes mellitus). On the other hand, cats with severe malabsorption can benefit from initial treatment with subcutaneous injections of dexamethasone until the disease is better controlled. In the author's experience, many cats with SCL lymphoma initially respond to treatment with steroids as well. In cases of refractory IBD or SCL, chlorambucil can be added to the treatment regime. Chlorambucil can be administered continuously, at a dose of 2 mg per cat orally, every 48 hours to every 72 hours (usually at home), or as a pulse-dose protocol, at 20 mg/m^2 every 2 weeks (eg, for fractious cats, usually in the hospital). The median survival time of cats with SCL is reported to be between 1.5 years and 3 years.[15,21,22,62] There are only few data on the survival time of cats with IBD. In a recent study with a median follow-up time of approximately 3 years, median survival time was not reached for cats diagnosed with LPE.[63]

SUMMARY

Differentiation of feline IBD from SCL remains challenging. This is complicated further by the fact that it may be a moving target, with the possibility of IBD progressing to SCL over time. From therapeutic and prognostic points of view, differentiation currently might not alter either approach or outcome. Many questions remain unanswered, however, such as whether there are different forms of SCL (epitheliotropic vs lamina propria, mucosal vs transmural location within the small intestine, lymph node involvement, and so forth) and whether those need to be approached differently. What roles do the microbiome and metabolome play and can the microenvironment be modulated to alter the outcome? Can IBD and SCL potentially even be cured? These questions need to continue to be asked and these disorders studied in order to further expand knowledge, refine treatment modalities, and ultimately improve outcome.

DISCLOSURE

The author has no disclosures.

REFERENCES

1. Richter KP. Feline gastrointestinal lymphoma. Vet Clin North Am Small Anim Pract 2003;33:1083–98, vii.
2. Louwerens M, London CA, Pedersen NC, et al. Feline lymphoma in the post-feline leukemia virus era. J Vet Intern Med 2005;19:329–35.
3. Sato H, Fujino Y, Chino J, et al. Prognostic analyses on anatomical and morphological classification of feline lymphoma. J Vet Med Sci 2014;76:807–11.
4. Vail DM, Moore AS, Ogilvie GK, et al. Feline Lymphoma (145 Cases): Proliferation Indices, Cluster of Differentiation 3 Immunoreactivity, and Their Association with Prognosis in 90 Cats. J Vet Intern Med 1998;12:349–54.
5. Vezzali E, Parodi AL, Marcato PS, et al. Histopathologic classification of 171 cases of canine and feline non-Hodgkin lymphoma according to the WHO. Vet Comp Oncol 2010;8:38–49.
6. Pohlman LM, Higginbotham ML, Welles EG, et al. Immunophenotypic and histologic classification of 50 cases of feline gastrointestinal lymphoma. Vet Pathol 2009;46:259–68.
7. Waly NE, Gruffydd-Jones TJ, Stokes CR, et al. Immunohistochemical diagnosis of alimentary lymphomas and severe intestinal inflammation in cats. J Comp Pathol 2005;133:253–60.
8. Gabor LJ, Malik R, Canfield PJ. Clinical and anatomical features of lymphosarcoma in 118 cats. Aust Vet J 1998;76:725–32.
9. Milner RJ, Peyton J, Cooke K, et al. Response rates and survival times for cats with lymphoma treated with the University of Wisconsin-Madison chemotherapy protocol: 38 cases (1996-2003). J Am Vet Med Assoc 2005;227:1118–22.
10. Chino J, Fujino Y, Kobayashi T, et al. Cytomorphological and immunological classification of feline lymphomas: clinicopathological features of 76 cases. J Vet Med Sci 2013;75:701–7.
11. Moore PF, Rodriguez-Bertos A, Kass PH. Feline gastrointestinal lymphoma: mucosal architecture, immunophenotype, and molecular clonality. Vet Pathol 2012;49:658–68.
12. Rassnick KM, Mauldin GN, Moroff SD, et al. Prognostic Value of Argyrophilic Nucleolar Organizer Region (AgNOR) Staining in Feline Intestinal Lymphoma. J Vet Intern Med 1999;13:187.
13. Fondacaro JV, Richter KP, Carpenter JL, et al. Feline gastrointestinal lymphoma: 67 cases (1988–1996). Eur J Comp Gastroenterol 1999;4:5–11.
14. Moore PF, Woo JC, Vernau W, et al. Characterization of feline T cell receptor gamma (TCRG) variable region genes for the molecular diagnosis of feline intestinal T cell lymphoma. Vet Immunol Immunopathol 2005;106:167–78.

15. Lingard AE, Briscoe K, Beatty JA, et al. Low-grade alimentary lymphoma: clinico-pathological findings and response to treatment in 17 cases. J Feline Med Surg 2009;11:692–700.

16. Cesari A, Bettini G, Vezzali E. Feline Intestinal T-Cell Lymphoma: Assessment of Morphologic and Kinetic Features in 30 Cases. J Vet Diagn Invest 2009;21(2): 277–9.

17. Marsilio S, Pilla R, Sarawichitr B, et al. Characterization of the fecal microbiome in cats with inflammatory bowel disease or alimentary small cell lymphoma. Sci Rep 2019;9:19208.

18. Janeczko S, Atwater D, Bogel E, et al. The relationship of mucosal bacteria to duodenal histopathology, cytokine mRNA, and clinical disease activity in cats with inflammatory bowel disease. Vet Microbiol 2008;128:178–93.

19. Waly NE, Stokes CR, Gruffydd-Jones TJ, et al. Immune cell populations in the duodenal mucosa of cats with inflammatory bowel disease. J Vet Intern Med 2004;18:816–25.

20. Jergens AE, Crandell JM, Evans R, et al. A clinical index for disease activity in cats with chronic enteropathy. J Vet Intern Med 2010;24(5):1027–33.

21. Kiselow MA, Rassnick KM, McDonough SP, et al. Outcome of cats with low-grade lymphocytic lymphoma: 41 cases (1995-2005). J Am Vet Med Assoc 2008;232: 405–10.

22. Stein TJ, Pellin M, Steinberg H, et al. Treatment of feline gastrointestinal small-cell lymphoma with chlorambucil and glucocorticoids. J Am Anim Hosp Assoc 2010; 46(6):413–7.

23. Burke KF, Broussard JD, Ruaux CG, et al. Evaluation of fecal α1-proteinase inhibitor concentrations in cats with idiopathic inflammatory bowel disease and cats with gastrointestinal neoplasia. Vet J 2013;196:189–96.

24. Norsworthy GD, Estep JS, Hollinger C, et al. Prevalence and underlying causes of histologic abnormalities in cats suspected to have chronic small bowel disease: 300 cases (2008-2013). J Am Vet Med Assoc 2015;247:629–35.

25. Norsworthy GD, Scot Estep J, Kiupel M, et al. Diagnosis of chronic small bowel disease in cats: 100 cases (2008-2012). J Am Vet Med Assoc 2013;243:1455–61.

26. Reed N, Gunn-Moore D, Simpson K. Cobalamin, folate and inorganic phosphate abnormalities in ill cats. J Feline Med Surg 2007;9:278–88.

27. Ruaux CG, Steiner JM, Williams DA. Early Biochemical and Clinical Responses to Cobalamin Supplementation in Cats with Signs of Gastrointestinal Disease and Severe Hypocobalaminemia. J Vet Intern Med 2005;19:155–60.

28. Habibi F, Habibi ME, Gharavinia A, et al. Quality of life in inflammatory bowel disease patients: A cross-sectional study. J Res Med Sci 2017;22:104.

29. Lalor S, Schwartz AM, Titmarsh H, et al. Cats with Inflammatory Bowel Disease and Intestinal Small Cell Lymphoma Have Low Serum Concentrations of 25-Hydroxyvitamin D. J Vet Intern Med 2014;28(2):351–5.

30. Xenoulis PG, Zoran DL, Fosgate GT, et al. Feline Exocrine Pancreatic Insufficiency: A Retrospective Study of 150 Cases. J Vet Intern Med 2016;30:1790–7.

31. Daniaux LA, Laurenson MP, Marks SL, et al. Ultrasonographic thickening of the muscularis propria in feline small intestinal small cell T-cell lymphoma and inflammatory bowel disease. J Feline Med Surg 2014;16:89–98.

32. Zwingenberger AL, Marks SL, Baker TW, et al. Ultrasonographic evaluation of the muscularis propria in cats with diffuse small intestinal lymphoma or inflammatory bowel disease. J Vet Intern Med 2010;24:289–92.

33. Guttin T, Walsh A, Durham AC, et al. Ability of ultrasonography to predict the presence and location of histologic lesions in the small intestine of cats. J Vet Intern Med 2019;33:1278–85.
34. Tucker S, Penninck DG, Keating JH, et al. Clinicopathological and ultrasonographic features of cats with eosinophilic enteritis. J Feline Med Surg 2014;16: 950–6.
35. Linton M, Nimmo JS, Norris JM, et al. Feline gastrointestinal eosinophilic sclerosing fibroplasia: 13 cases and review of an emerging clinical entity. J Feline Med Surg 2015;17:392–404.
36. Barrs VR, Beatty JA. Feline alimentary lymphoma: 1. Classification, risk factors, clinical signs and non-invasive diagnostics. J Feline Med Surg 2012;14:182–90.
37. Jergens AE, Willard MD, Allenspach K. Maximizing the diagnostic utility of endoscopic biopsy in dogs and cats with gastrointestinal disease. Vet J 2016;214: 50–60.
38. Willard MD, Moore GE, Denton BD, et al. Effect of tissue processing on assessment of endoscopic intestinal biopsies in dogs and cats. J Vet Intern Med 2010; 24:84–9.
39. Ruiz GC, Reyes-Gomez E, Hall EJ, et al. Comparison of 3 Handling Techniques for Endoscopically Obtained Gastric and Duodenal Biopsy Specimens: A Prospective Study in Dogs and Cats. J Vet Intern Med 2016;30(4):1014–21.
40. Murphy K, Weaver C. Janeway's Immunobiology. New York: W.W. Norton & Company; 2017.
41. Fagarasan S, Honjo T. Intestinal IgA synthesis: regulation of front-line body defences. Nat Rev Immunol 2003;3(1):63–72.
42. Willard MD, Jergens AE, Duncan RB, et al. Interobserver variation among histopathologic evaluations of intestinal tissues from dogs and cats. J Am Vet Med Assoc 2002;220(8):1177–82.
43. Day MJ, Bilzer T, Mansell J, et al. Histopathological standards for the diagnosis of gastrointestinal inflammation in endoscopic biopsy samples from the dog and cat: a report from the World Small Animal Veterinary Association Gastrointestinal Standardization Group. J Comp Pathol 2008;138 Suppl 1:S1–43.
44. Washabau RJ, Day MJ, Willard MD, et al. Endoscopic, biopsy, and histopathologic guidelines for the evaluation of gastrointestinal inflammation in companion animals. J Vet Intern Med 2010;24:10–26.
45. Jergens AE, Evans RB, Ackermann M, et al. Design of a simplified histopathologic model for gastrointestinal inflammation in dogs. Vet Pathol 2014;51:946–50.
46. Marsilio S, Ackermann MR, Lidbury JA, et al. Results of histopathology, immunohistochemistry, and molecular clonality testing of small intestinal biopsy specimens from clinically healthy client-owned cats. J Vet Intern Med 2019;33:551–8.
47. Jergens AE, Moore FM, Haynes JS, et al. Idiopathic inflammatory bowel disease in dogs and cats: 84 cases (1987-1990). J Am Vet Med Assoc 1992;201:1603–8.
48. Dennis JS, Kruger JM, Mullaney TP. Lymphocytic/plasmacytic gastroenteritis in cats: 14 cases (1985-1990). J Am Vet Med Assoc 1992;200:1712–8.
49. Kiupel M, Smedley RC, Pfent C, et al. Diagnostic algorithm to differentiate lymphoma from inflammation in feline small intestinal biopsy samples. Vet Pathol 2011;48(1):212–22.
50. Jergens AE. Feline idiopathic inflammatory bowel disease: what we know and what remains to be unraveled. J Feline Med Surg 2012;14:445–58.
51. Barrs VR, Beatty JA, McCandlish IA, et al. Hypereosinophilic paraneoplastic syndrome in a cat with intestinal T cell lymphosarcoma. J Small Anim Pract 2002;43: 401–5.

52. Hendrick M. A spectrum of hypereosinophilic syndromes exemplified by six cats with eosinophilic enteritis. Vet Pathol 1981;18:188–200.
53. Takeuchi Y, Matsuura S, Fujino Y, et al. Hypereosinophilic syndrome in two cats. J Vet Med Sci 2008;70:1085–9.
54. McEwen SA, Valli VE, Hulland TJ. Hypereosinophilic syndrome in cats: a report of three cases. Can J Comp Med 1985;49:248–53.
55. Andrews C, Operacz M, Maes R, et al. Cross Lineage Rearrangement in Feline Enteropathy-Associated T-cell Lymphoma. Vet Pathol 2016;53:559–62.
56. Alaibac M, Daga A, Harms G, et al. Molecular analysis of the gamma delta T-cell receptor repertoire in normal human skin and in Oriental cutaneous leishmaniasis. Exp Dermatol 1993;2(3):106–12.
57. Magro CM, Crowson AN, Kovatich AJ, et al. Drug-induced reversible lymphoid dyscrasia: a clonal lymphomatoid dermatitis of memory and activated T cells. Hum Pathol 2003;34:119–29.
58. Diehl KJ, Lappin MR, Jones RL, et al. Monoclonal gammopathy in a dog with plasmacytic gastroenterocolitis. J Am Vet Med Assoc 1992;201(8):1233–6.
59. Posnett DN, Sinha R, Kabak S, et al. Clonal populations of T cells in normal elderly humans: the T cell equivalent to "benign monoclonal gammapathy". J Exp Med 1994;179:609–18.
60. Kokovic I, Novakovic BJ, Cerkovnik P, et al. Clonality analysis of lymphoid proliferations using the BIOMED-2 clonality assays: a single institution experience. Radiol Oncol 2014;48:155–62.
61. Marsilio S, Newman SJ, Estep JS, et al. Differentiation of lymphocytic-plasmacytic enteropathy and small cell lymphoma in cats using histology-guided mass spectrometry. J Vet Intern Med 2020. https://doi.org/10.1111/jvim.15742.
62. Pope KV, Tun AE, McNeill CJ, et al. Outcome and toxicity assessment of feline small cell lymphoma: 56 cases (2000-2010). Vet Med Sci 2015;1:51–62.
63. Sabattini S, Bottero E, Turba ME, et al. Differentiating feline inflammatory bowel disease from alimentary lymphoma in duodenal endoscopic biopsies. J Small Anim Pract 2016;57:396–401.

Canine Protein Losing Enteropathies and Systemic Complications

Karin Allenspach, Dr med vet, PhD, FVH, FHEA*,
Chelsea Iennarella-Servantez, BS, MS

KEYWORDS

- PLE • Protein loss • Hypercoagulability • Lymphangiectasia • Vitamin D3
- Tryptophan

KEY POINTS

- Hypercoagulability has been documented in 10% of dogs with protein-losing enteropathy but is likely to be more common. Prophylactic treatment of prevention of thromboembolism is performed with low-dose aspirin or clopidogrel.
- Vitamin D3 deficiency is common in dogs with protein-losing enteropathy (PLE) and should be investigated in all cases. Supplementation with vitamin D2 or D3 may improve survival.
- Serum tryptophan concentrations are decreased in many dogs with PLE and are critical to counteract the inflammation in the intestine. Supplementation with amino acids may be indicated in select cases.

INTRODUCTION

Protein-losing enteropathy (PLE) is not a disease but rather a syndrome characterized by an abnormal loss of serum proteins into the gastrointestinal lumen. Clinical signs include small intestinal diarrhea, vomiting, anorexia, and weight loss, with systemic manifestations such as pleural effusion, ascites, and/or peripheral edema developing secondary to severe hypoalbuminemia.[1-3] In addition, some cases may present without clinically significant diarrhea. Most commonly, PLE is considered to occur secondary to severe inflammatory bowel disease (IBD).[4] The outcome in dogs with PLE is poor with only about 50% of cases surviving longer than 4 months. It is therefore critical to detect and possibly correct individual risk factors for poor outcome in order to improve the odds for survival.

Veterinary Clinical Sciences, College of Veterinary Medicine, Iowa State University, 1809 South Riverside Drive, Ames, IA 50010, USA
* Corresponding author.
E-mail address: allek@iastate.edu

Vet Clin Small Anim 51 (2021) 111–122
https://doi.org/10.1016/j.cvsm.2020.09.010
0195-5616/21/Published by Elsevier Inc.

BREED PREDISPOSITIONS FOR PROTEIN-LOSING ENTEROPATHY

Longitudinal data spanning over 30 years have identified breed predispositions for PLE secondary to IBD in Yorkshire terriers, Border collies, German shepherds, and Rottweilers.[3] Among these, some Yorkshire terriers seem to respond favorably to dietary treatment alone, which is associated with a better prognosis.[5] To the contrary, Rottweilers with PLE have been reported to generally have poor survival rates.[6]

DIAGNOSTIC APPROACH

The workup of dogs suspected to have PLE is similar to that for dogs with chronic small intestinal diarrhea and therefore generally includes a complete blood count, serum biochemistry profile, urinalysis, serum cobalamin measurements, canine pancreatic lipase, and trypsin-like immunoreactivity if chronic pancreatitis or exocrine pancreatic insufficiency is clinically suspected, abdominal ultrasound, as well as biopsies from the small intestinal mucosa to confirm the diagnosis.[7] An adrenocorticotropic hormone stimulation test or basal serum cortisol level is also useful in many of these cases, as mild to moderate hypoalbuminemia has been reported in dogs with Addison's disease.[8] In addition, it may be important to rule out protein-losing nephropathy by confirming that there is no substantial proteinuria as confirmed by urine protein:creatine ratio less than 0.5 in an inactive urine sediment, and exclude liver dysfunction as a cause of the hypoalbuminemia (ie, a normal bile acid stimulation test). Furthermore, it is important to realize that in many PLE cases, the dogs are clinically severely debilitated and anorexic at the time of diagnosis; it is therefore important to prioritize intestinal biopsies over treatment trials in these cases. When obtaining intestinal biopsies, endoscopy is the preferred method in order to avoid complications such as dehiscence, which may be aggravated by hypoalbuminemia.[9] Duodenal and ileal biopsies are indicated in all cases of IBD, because it has been shown in several studies that lesions such as intestinal lymphoma and lymphangiectasia may only be found in the ileum.[10,11] Additional clinical pathologic tests that have prognostic value and may be important for individualized treatment plans are ionized calcium serum concentrations, serum vitamin D3 concentrations, and possibly tests to identify hypercoagulability, such as thromboelastography (TEG).[12,13]

Hypoalbuminemia

PLE is often suspected in the presence of panhypoproteinemia. Hypoalbuminemia is associated with a worse prognosis overall among dogs with chronic enteropathy.[1,14] A recent review reported hypoalbuminemia in 21/23 studies of dogs with PLE, with cumulative median serum albumin levels of 1.49 g/dL.[3]

Ultrasound Evaluation

Ultrasound examination of the abdomen has diagnostic value in identifying intestinal changes associated with PLE.[15–17] Unspecific findings such as mild thickening of the duodenal and jejunal wall can be seen 70% to 90% of cases.[15] More specific is the detection of hyperechoic mucosal striations that were associated with clinical PLE in 18/23 (78%) dogs and with histologic confirmation of lacteal dilation in 22/23 (95%) dogs.[15,18]

Endoscopy

Gross lesions associated with intestinal lymphangiectasia in dogs may be visible during endoscopic examination of the intestinal tract. Common lesions include white patchy appearance to the small intestinal mucosa, multifocal white granular mucosal foci[19](**Fig. 1**), white tipped intestinal villi, and occasionally lymphatic fluid in the intestinal lumen. However, gross endoscopic appearance of duodenal mucosa for diagnosis of intestinal lymphangiectasia still only has a sensitivity and specificity of 68% (confidence interval [CI] 46, 84%) and 42% (CI: 24, 63%), respectively, suggesting limited diagnostic value.[4,20,21] Histologic evaluation of intestinal biopsies is therefore still necessary for definitive diagnosis.

Intestinal Biopsies and Histologic Evaluation

As stated earlier, histologic evaluation of intestinal biopsies is required for a definitive diagnosis of the causes of PLE.[22] There is a risk of complications associated with full-thickness biopsies, which implies that endoscopic biopsies are the current gold standard.[23] However, endoscopic biopsies may be nondiagnostic in some cases as some areas, particularly the jejunum, are not accessible via endoscopy. Further, deeper lesions located within the intestinal submucosal and muscularis layers cannot be sampled via endoscopy.[7] Intestinal lymphoma, and especially small cell intestinal lymphoma, is in some cases easier to diagnose on full-thickness biopsies[24,25] and can be missed when endoscopic biopsies are obtained. Therefore, comprehensive owner information regarding the possibility of a missed diagnosis (for example for intestinal lymphoma) is important when obtaining endoscopic (mucosal) biopsies only.

Expression of tight junction markers in dogs with protein-losing enteropathy
Significant loss of serum proteins into the intestinal lumen with resulting panhypoproteinemia is the hallmark of PLE in dogs. In children diagnosed with primary lymphangiectasia, it has been shown that tight junction proteins are dysregulated, resulting in a "leaky" epithelial membrane, which may cause the leakage into the intestinal lumen. Recent research emphasized that cellular and architectural changes of the epithelium were the most important determinants of disease pathogenesis in canine PLE.[22,26] It is therefore reasonable to assume that changes in the structure of the epithelial cell layer, in addition to the well-described lymphangiectasia, contribute to the leakage of proteins in these dogs. Recent work in the author's laboratory using biopsies and

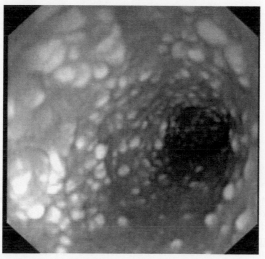

Fig. 1. Duodenal endoscopic appearance in a dog with PLE. Typical white patchy infiltrates of the mucosa can be seen.

organoids from dogs with PLE has demonstrated similar findings.[27] Canine organoids are 3-dimensional cultures derived from the epithelial cell layer and faithfully reproduce structural and functional changes of the epithelium of the individual dog.[28] The authors found that the percentage of intestinal stem cells in dogs with IBD or PLE is increased in the epithelium of affected dogs as compared with healthy dogs. This in turn leads to a lesser percentage of absorptive enterocytes, which may be one of the factors that ultimately causes diarrhea in these dogs. Furthermore, tight junctional expression of zonulin-1 was also increased in dogs with PLE compared with healthy dog epithelium.[27,29,30] Zonulin-1 protein loosens interepithelial cell junctions and therefore results in leakage of fluid into the intestinal lumen[31,32] (**Fig. 2**).These findings are promising as organoids from dogs with PLE could be used to investigate novel drugs that affect tight junctional regulation ex vivo, before using them in clinical trials. However, at this point, more research needs to be performed in order to better define the epithelial changes in dogs with PLE.

CAUSES OF PROTEIN-LOSING ENTEROPATHY
Intestinal Lymphangiectasia

A recent review paper reported 214/469 (58%) of dogs with PLE were diagnosed with intestinal lymphangiectasia, further supporting the association between histologically confirmed lymphatic dilation and PLE.[3] Most often, canine PLE is associated with secondary lymphangiectasia resulting from lymphoplasmacytic enteritis (314 of 469 dogs; 68%).[3] As a result, secondary intestinal lymphangiectasia is thought to result in an obstruction of lymphatic outflow with loss of lymphatic fluid into the intestinal lumen.[33]

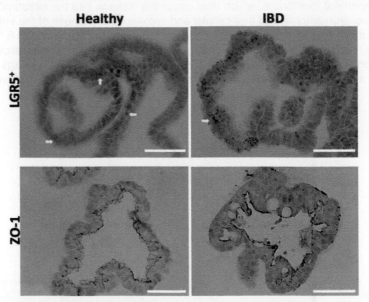

Fig. 2. Staining of stem cells and tight junctional proteins in organoids from dogs with PLE. RNA in situ hybridization (RNA-ISH) or immunohistochemistry for zonulin-1 was performed to stain for mRNA of intestinal stem cells (LGR5+) and tight junctional zonulin protein (Zo-1) in tissues and organoids from dogs with PLE and healthy dogs. Expression of stem cell markers (LGR5+) is increased in dogs with PLE, therefore decreasing the ratio of absorptive enterocytes/stem cells. Zonulin-1 was also upregulated in dogs with PLE versus healthy dogs, indicating "leaky" tight junctions in dogs with PLE.

Interestingly, some reports found lymphangiectasia in only about 50% (12/24) of dogs with PLE.[33] However, if intestinal lymphangiectasia was present in the histologic lesions, it was associated with hypoalbuminemia in most cases (76%).[33] However, when immunolabeling for lymphatic endothelial cells was performed, lymphangiectasia was identified in almost all PLE cases in which routine histopathology had missed the lesions[33] (**Fig. 3**). This seemed to be particularly important for ileal biopsies, again emphasizing the need to obtain ileal biopsies in PLE cases whenever possible.[10,33]

Crypt Disease

On histology, crypt lesions seem as dilated, cystic crypts packed with sloughed epithelial cells, mucus, leukocytes, and other proteinaceous and cellular debris with collapsed villous structures.[34] Yorkshire Terrier dogs specifically have been reported to be susceptible to crypt disease associated with PLE.[5,14] Crypt lesions can be found in as many as 90% to 100% percent of Yorkshire Terriers with PLE.[5] In one study, 20% of Yorkshire Terries even lacked any evidence of lymphatic dilation on histologic biopsies, which seemed to suggest that lymphangiectasia in this breed might be secondary to crypt pathology and/or inflammation.[5] The underlying pathogenesis of the crypt lesions is unclear; however, it is unlikely that a bacterial infection is at the origin of the lesions as evidenced by negative fluorescent in situ hybridization for bacterial DNA within the crypt lesions.[35]

TREATMENT
Immunosuppressive Therapy

Traditional therapy for PLE in dogs consists of dietary intervention in combination with immunosuppressant and/or antiinflammatory therapies.[1] In a recent review on dogs with PLE,[3] 15/16 studies with treatment information indicated use of immunosuppressive medication in PLE.

Immunosuppressive doses of prednisolone
The authors recommend to use 2 mg/kg PO daily for 2 weeks, then slowly tapering over 6 weeks, followed by azathioprine, cyclosporine, chlorambucil, and methotrexate. Because prednisolone can worsen hypercoagulability, cyclosporine (5 mg/kg po sid for 6–8 weeks) can be considered instead of steroid treatment.[13,36] Cyclosporine has been shown to act as a rescue treatment in steroid-resistant dogs (9/12

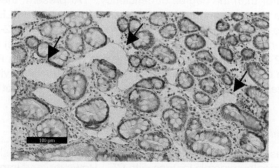

Fig. 3. Immunohistochemistry staining of ileal biopsies from a dog with PLE using antibodies against lymphatic vascular endothelial hyaluronic acid receptor (LYVE-1). The staining reveals dilated lymphatic vessels in the lower areas of the lamina propria that had been missed by routine histopathology. The arrow indicates positive staining for LYVE-1 in endothelial cells. (*Courtesy of* S. Wennogle, DVM, PhD, East Lansing, MI.)

dogs).[2] Furthermore, a recent study comparing the efficacy of prednisolone-chlorambucil combination treatment in dogs with PLE showed better treatment response and survival for this regimen in comparison to prednisolone combined with azathioprine.[37]

Dietary Therapy

Reports on dogs with PLE responding favorably to dietary treatment alone have increased in recent years.[12,38] Clinical efficacy of dietary intervention has been demonstrated across a wide variety of diet types (eg, homemade, commercial) and nutrient inclusion ratios (eg, fat-restricted, limited antigen).[18] In a study of Yorkshire Terrier dogs with PLE, dietary interventions, when prescribed, were categorized as either limited antigen (in 20/30 dogs; 66%) or low fat diet (in 7/30 dogs; 23%), respectively.[5] The clinical efficacy of dietary fat restriction in the treatment of dogs with PLE-associated intestinal lymphangiectasia has also been reported, and in one study up to 80% of dogs responded to low-fat diet alone.[38] At present, it is unclear whether low-fat (fat content 1.7–2.5 g/100 kcal or 15%–22.5% ME) or ultralow-fat (0.35 g/100 kcal or 3.1% ME) diet is more effective in PLE cases.[38,39] Importantly, dogs responding to diet alone had significantly lower clinical activity scores (Canine Chronic Enteropathy Clinical Activity Index [CCECAI][1]) at the time of diagnosis.[12,39]

SYSTEMIC COMPLICATIONS IN PROTEIN-LOSING ENTEROPATHY
Ionized Hypocalcemia and Vitamin D Deficiency

A decrease in ionized serum calcium concentrations has frequently been reported in dogs with PLE[40,41]. Across 23 canine PLE studies, ionized hypocalcemia was reported in approximately 10% of all cases.[3] In a case series of 5 Yorkshire Terriers with PLE, twitching episodes were reported in 3/5 dogs diagnosed.[40] The dogs were found to have profound hypocalcemia and hypomagnesemia, with an accompanying increase in serum concentration of parathyroid hormone.[40] A newer study found significantly higher mean 25(OH) vitamin D concentration in dogs with PLE with favorable outcome (37.0; range = 6–81 nmol/L) as compared with dogs that had to be euthanized due to intractable disease (16.5; range = 0–66 nmol/L),[12] which was not associated with serum albumin concentration. Further, incidence of hypovitaminosis D did not differ significantly between groups, indicating that presence of deficiency is a less valuable prognostic indicator than the degree of deficiency.[12] At present, there is no specific protocol available for supplementation of vitamin D in dogs with PLE. However, current practice is to supplement using either dihydrotachysterol (0.02–0.03 mg/kg PO q24 h initially, then 0.01–0.02 mg/kg PO q24–48 h for maintenance) or calcitriol (10–15 ng/kg PO q12 h for 3–4 days, then decrease to 2.5–7.5 ng/kg PO q12 h for 2–3 days, then give q24 h). However, whether supplementation with vitamin D in dogs with PLE is clinically useful and results in improved survival has not been evaluated yet.

Cobalamin (Vitamin B12) Deficiency

In previous studies, hypocobalaminemia has been identified to be of similar prognostic importance as hypoalbuminemia in dogs with CE.[1] However, and importantly, the risk associated with hypocobalaminemia can be reversed if the dogs are supplemented with cobalamin.[1] Cobalamin can be administered by weekly subcutaneous injections (see dosing protocol at https://vetmed.tamu.edu/gilab/research/cobalamin-information) or orally (0.25–1.0 mg cyanocobalamin daily according to body weight).[42]

If choosing oral cobalamin supplementation, much higher doses must be given to achieve similar serum concentrations than with subcutaneous administration, and no long-term effect can be expected. Therefore, oral supplementation necessitates long-term daily administration of cobalamin[42]

Hypercoagulability

Thromboembolic complications resulting from underlying hypercoagulability have been documented in dogs with PLE and occur in at least 10% of cases.[13,36] In Yorkshire Terriers with PLE, sudden death due to possible pulmonary thromboembolism (TE) occurred in 10% of cases in one study and was confirmed to be the cause of death in one of these cases.[5] Furthermore, in another study, 14/14 dogs with PLE were hypercoagulable based on TEG measurements.[13] The actual incidence of TE in PLE is therefore likely to be much higher, because our ability to clinically diagnose TE is often limited to severe disease resulting in death of the dog.

In humans with IBD, TE is also a fairly common complication and usually manifests in venous thrombosis.[43] The pathogenesis of TE in people with IBD has been attributed to a combination of factors, such as thrombocytosis, platelet hyperaggregation, hyperfibrinogenemia, endothelial lesions due to inflammation and immune-complex deposition, increased concentrations of plasminogen activator inhibitor, fibrin degradation products, factor XIII, and tissue plasminogen activator.[44] In the study by Goodwin and colleagues,[13] an attempt was made to investigate the reason for the hypercoagulability found in dogs with PLE when using TEG. TEG gives a global assessment of coagulation but does not generally help to distinguish between specific causes of hypercoagulability.[45] In this case series, serum antithrombin (AT) concentrations were therefore also measured and found to be normal in all dogs, which makes intestinal loss of AT less likely as a causative factor.[13] Other factors that are likely to contribute to hypercoagulability in dogs with PLE are thrombocytosis and increased WBC,[13,46] which also commonly occur in dogs with PLE.[13] Factors such as systemic inflammation and treatment with immunosuppressive drugs, such as prednisolone, are other possible causes that warrant further investigation. Current practice for dogs with PLE and hypercoagulability is to prescribe an antithrombotic agent such as low-dose aspirin (0.5 mg/kg PO q12 h) or clopidogrel (2-4 mg/kg PO q24 h). It is possible that prophylactic treatment against venous TE with heparin, as is done in people with IBD, may be more effective. However, the effect of thromboprophylactic measures on the risk of TE in dogs with PLE has not been investigated so far.

Tryptophan deficiency

Amino acid deficiencies, and in particular, decreased serum concentrations of tryptophan, have been identified in people with Crohn's disease.[47] Tryptophan is an essential amino acid in dogs and in people and is absorbed to a large degree in the small intestine. Tryptophan plays an important role in energy metabolism by being a precursor for kynurenine, which comprises at least 90% of tryptophan catabolism. About 5% of the absorbed tryptophan is metabolized in the host to serotonin and melatonin. Importantly, a small proportion of tryptophan reaches the colon and is metabolized by luminal bacteria to metabolites such as indole, skatole indicant, and tryptamine. These microbial metabolites play an essential role in counteracting intestinal inflammation, as they are essential for the induction of antiinflammatory cytokines such as interleukin-22 (IL-22)[48] (**Fig. 4**). Recently, it was shown that serum amino acids are frequently decreased in the serum of dogs with chronic enteropathies.[49] In dogs with PLE, tryptophan seems to be the only amino acid to be decreased in the serum.[50] Furthermore, lower serum tryptophan concentrations were also correlated with lower

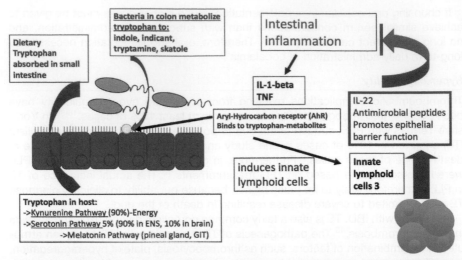

Fig. 4. Tryptophan acts as antiinflammatory mediator in the intestine. Most of the dietary tryptophan is metabolized in the small intestine; however, a small but important part is metabolized in the colon by resident commensal bacteria. The bacteria produce metabolites such as indole, tryptamine, and skatole from tryptophan, which bind to Aryl-hydrocarbon receptors (AhR) on the epithelial cells. Epithelial cells then release signals to innate lymphoid cells 3 in the lamina propria, which produce antiinflammatory cytokines such as IL-22 in the mucosa. IL-22 also induces the secretion of antimicrobial peptides and therefore improves the overall intestinal barrier function.

serum albumin and poor outcome in dogs with PLE.[50] Consistent with the notion that there is a severe intestinal dysbiosis in dogs with IBD, and therefore reduced production of tryptophan metabolites, other studies have shown that several indole compounds were significantly decreased in fecal samples.[51] It is therefore conceivable that tryptophan supplementation could have a positive therapeutic impact on some PLE cases, but further research is necessary to confirm this hypothesis.

PROGNOSIS

Median survival times for dogs with PLE reported across 8 different studies were highly variable and ranged from 1 to 28 months.[3] This is likely because overall survival is about 50% in dogs with PLE.[3,12]

The most commonly reported negative prognostic indicator is hypoalbuminemia.[1,14,52] Other negative prognostic factors reported include a CCECAI score greater than 5 at 1 month after diagnosis,[53] increased blood urea nitrogen at diagnosis,[54,55] intestinal villus blunting on histology,[33] and treatment with immunosuppressive drugs.[12,56] Other important negative prognostic factors in dogs with PLE are serum vitamin D concentrations[12] and serum tryptophan concentrations.[50] Overall, clinical activity measured with CCECAI, which includes serum albumin concentration[1] at the time of diagnosis and again after initiating treatment (2–4 weeks after diagnosis),[53] seems to be a reliable and easily obtainable prognostic indicator for dogs with PLE.[1,39]

In summary, treatment of dogs with PLE may therefore need to become more personalized, possibly correcting individual deficiencies of vitamins and essential amino acids and counteracting possible hypercoagulability in some dogs. In the future, such measure could lead to improved survival in severely affected dogs.

CLINICS CARE POINTS

- Canine PLE is associated with a unacceptably high rate of fatality.
- Some PLE cases die from complications that can be managed appropriately if identified early on.
- Individualized treatment is likely to improve overall outcome for PLE cases.

DISCLOSURE

K. Allenspach is a cofounder of 3D Health Solutions, Inc., a start-up company developing drug testing assays based on canine organoid technology.

REFERENCES

1. Allenspach K, Wieland B, Grone A, et al. Chronic enteropathies in dogs: evaluation of risk factors for negative outcome. J Vet Intern Med 2007;21:700–8.
2. Allenspach K, Rufenacht S, Sauter S, et al. Pharmacokinetics and clinical efficacy of cyclosporine treatment of dogs with steroid-refractory inflammatory bowel disease. J Vet Intern Med 2006;20:239–44.
3. Craven MD, Washabau RJ. Comparative pathophysiology and management of protein-losing enteropathy. J Vet Intern Med 2019;33(2):383–402.
4. Dossin O, Lavoue R. Protein-losing enteropathies in dogs. Vet Clin North Am Small Anim Pract 2011;41:399–418.
5. Simmerson SM, Armstrong PJ, Wunschmann A, et al. Clinical features, intestinal histopathology, and outcome in protein losing enteropathy in Yorkshire Terrier dogs. J Vet Intern Med 2014;28:331–7.
6. Dijkstra M, Kraus JS, Bosje JT, et al. [Protein-losing enteropathy in Rottweilers]. Tijdschrift voor diergeneeskunde 2010;135:406–12.
7. Washabau RJ, Day MJ, Willard MD, et al. Endoscopic, biopsy, and histopathologic guidelines for the evaluation of gastrointestinal inflammation in companion animals. J Vet Intern Med 2010;24:10–26.
8. Lyngby JG, Sellon RK. Hypoadrenocorticism mimicking protein-losing enteropathy in 4 dogs. Can Vet J 2016;57(7):757–60.
9. Shales CJ, Warren J, Anderson DM, et al. Complications following full-thickness small intestinal biopsy in 66 dogs: a retrospective study. J Small Anim Pract 2005; 46(7):317–21.
10. Procoli F, Motskula PF, Keyte SV, et al. Comparison of histopathologic findings in duodenal and ileal endoscopic biopsies in dogs with chronic small intestinal enteropathies. J Vet Intern Med 2013;27:268–74.
11. Casamian-Sorrosal D, Willard MD, Murray JK, et al. Comparison of Histopathologic Findings in Biopsies from the Duodenum and Ileum of Dogs with Enteropathy. J Vet Intern Med 2010;24(1):80–3.
12. Allenspach K, Rizzo J, Jergens AE, et al. Hypovitaminosis D is associated with negative outcome in dogs with protein losing enteropathy: a retrospective study of 43 cases. BMC Vet Res 2017;13(1):96.
13. Goodwin LV, Goggs R, Chan DL, et al. Hypercoagulability in dogs with protein-losing enteropathy. J Vet Intern Med 2011;25(2):273–7.

14. Craven M, Simpson JW, Ridyard AE, et al. Canine inflammatory bowel disease: retrospective analysis of diagnosis and outcome in 80 cases (1995-2002). J Small Anim Pract 2004;45(7):336–42.

15. Sutherland-Smith J, Penninck DG, Keating JH, et al. Ultrasonographic intestinal hyperechoic mucosal striations in dogs are associated with lacteal dilation. Vet Radiol Ultrasound 2007;48(1):51–7.

16. Gaschen L, Kircher P, Lang J, et al. Pattern recognition and feature extraction of canine celiac and cranial mesenteric arterial waveforms: normal versus chronic enteropathy–a pilot study. Vet J 2005;169:242–50.

17. Lecoindre P, Chevallier M, Guerret S. [Protein-losing enteropathy of non neoplastic origin in the dog: a retrospective study of 34 cases]. Schweiz Arch Tierheilkd 2010;152(3):141–6.

18. Rudinsky AJ, Howard JP, Bishop MA, et al. Dietary management of presumptive protein-losing enteropathy in Yorkshire terriers. J Small Anim Pract 2017;58(2): 103–8.

19. Tams TR, Rawlings CA. Small animal endoscopy. 3rd edition. Amsterdam (Netherlands): Elsevier; 2011.

20. Garcia-Sancho M, Rodriguez-Franco F, Sainz A, et al. Evaluation of clinical, macroscopic, and histopathologic response to treatment in nonhypoproteinemic dogs with lymphocytic-plasmacytic enteritis. J Vet Intern Med 2007;21:11–7.

21. Larson RN, Ginn JA, Bell CM, et al. Duodenal endoscopic findings and histopathologic confirmation of intestinal lymphangiectasia in dogs. J Vet Intern Med 2012; 26(5):1087–92.

22. Day MJ, Bilzer T, Mansell J, et al. Histopathological standards for the diagnosis of gastrointestinal inflammation in endoscopic biopsy samples from the dog and cat: a report from the World Small Animal Veterinary Association Gastrointestinal Standardization Group. J Comp Pathol 2008;138(Suppl 1):S1–43.

23. Snowdon KA, Smeak DD, Chiang S. Risk Factors for Dehiscence of Stapled Functional End-to-End Intestinal Anastomoses in Dogs: 53 Cases (2001-2012). Vet Surg 2016;45(1):91–9.

24. Lane J, Price J, Moore A, et al. Low-grade gastrointestinal lymphoma in dogs: 20 cases (2010 to 2016). J Small Anim Pract 2018;59(3):147–53.

25. Couto KM, Moore PF, Zwingenberger AL, et al. Clinical characteristics and outcome in dogs with small cell T-cell intestinal lymphoma. Vet Comp Oncol 2018;16(3):337–43.

26. Allenspach KA, Mochel JP, Du Y, et al. Correlating gastrointestinal histopathologic changes to clinical disease activity in dogs with idiopathic inflammatory bowel disease. Vet Pathol 2019;56(3):435–43.

27. Mao S, Atherly T, Borcherding D, et al. Phenotypic and functional characterizationof adult intestinal organoids from dogs with inflammatory bowel disease. Iowa State Research Day, August 2019, Ames, IA.

28. Chandra L, Borcherding DC, Kingsbury D, et al. Derivation of adult canine intestinal organoids for translational research in gastroenterology. BMC Biol 2019 11; 17(1):33.

29. Rossi G, Pengo G, Caldin M, et al. Comparison of Microbiological, Histological, and Immunomodulatory Parameters in Response to Treatment with Either Combination Therapy with Prednisone and Metronidazole or Probiotic VSL#3 Strains in Dogs with Idiopathic Inflammatory Bowel Disease. PLoS One 2014;9(4):e94699.

30. White R, Atherly T, Guard B, et al. Randomized, controlled trial evaluating the effect of multi-strain probiotic on the mucosal microbiota in canine idiopathic inflammatory bowel disease. Gut Microbes 2017;8(5):451–66.

31. Sturgeon C, Fasano A. Zonulin, a regulator of epithelial and endothelial barrier functions, and its involvement in chronic inflammatory diseases. Tissue Barriers 2016;4(4):e1251384.
32. Tripathi A, Lammers KM, Goldblum S, et al. Identification of human zonulin, a physiological modulator of tight junctions, as prehaptoglobin-2. Proc Natl Acad Sci U S A 2009;106(39):16799–804.
33. Wennogle SA, Priestnall SL, Suárez-Bonnet A, et al. Lymphatic endothelial cell immunohistochemical markers for evaluation of the intestinal lymphatic vasculature in dogs with chronic inflammatory enteropathy. J Vet Intern Med 2019; 33(4):1669–76.
34. Stroda K, Wakamatsu N, Gaschen L, et al. Histopathological , clinical, clinical, endoscopic and ultrasound features of dogs with chronic enteropathies and small intestinal crypt lesions. J Vet Intern Med 2012;26:767–8.
35. Craven MD, Duhamel GE, Sutter NB, et al. Absence of bacterial association in Yorkshire terriers with protein-losing enteropathy and cystic intestinal crypts. J Vet Intern Med 2009;757:23.
36. Jacinto AML, Ridyard AE, Aroch I, et al. Thromboembolism in dogs with protein-losing enteropathy with non-neoplastic chronic small intestinal disease. J Am Anim Hosp Assoc 2017;53(3):185–92.
37. Dandrieux JR, Noble PJ, Scase TJ, et al. Comparison of a chlorambucil-prednisolone combination with an azathioprine-prednisolone combination for treatment of chronic enteropathy with concurrent protein-losing enteropathy in dogs: 27 cases (2007-2010). J Am Vet Med Assoc 2013;242:1705–14.
38. Okanishi H, Yoshioka R, Kagawa Y, et al. The clinical efficacy of dietary fat restriction in treatment of dogs with intestinal lymphangiectasia. J Vet Intern Med 2014; 28:809–17.
39. Nagata N, Ohta H, Yokoyama N, et al. Clinical characteristics of dogs with food-responsive protein-losing enteropathy. J Vet Intern Med 2020;34(2):659–68.
40. Kimmel SE, Waddell LS, Michel KE. Hypomagnesemia and hypocalcemia associated with protein-losing enteropathy in Yorkshire terriers: five cases (1992-1998). J Am Vet Med Assoc 2000;217:703–6.
41. Gow AG, Else R, Evans H, et al. Hypovitaminosis D in dogs with inflammatory bowel disease and hypoalbuminaemia. J Small Anim Pract 2011;52:411–8.
42. Toresson L, Steiner JM, Suchodolski JS, et al. Oral Cobalamin Supplementation in Dogs with Chronic Enteropathies and Hypocobalaminemia. J Vet Intern Med 2016;30(1):101–7.
43. McCurdy JD, Kuenzig ME, Smith G, et al. Risk of venous thromboembolism after hospital discharge in patients with inflammatory bowel disease: a population-based study. Inflamm Bowel Dis 2020 ;izaa002.
44. Lagrange J, Lacolley P, Wahl D, et al. Shedding Light on Hemostasis in Patients With Inflammatory Bowel Diseases. Clin Gastroenterol Hepatol 2020 ;S1542-3565(20)30056-2.
45. Kol A, Borjesson DL. Application of thrombelastography/thromboelastometry to veterinary medicine. Vet Clin Pathol 2010;39(4):405–16.
46. Marschner CB, Wiinberg B, Tarnow I, et al. The influence of inflammation and hematocrit on clot strength in canine thromboelastographic hypercoagulability. J Vet Emerg Crit Care (San Antonio) 2018;28(1):20–30.
47. He F, Wu C, Li P, et al. Functions and Signaling Pathways of Amino Acids in Intestinal Inflammation. Biomed Res Int 2018;2018:9171905.
48. Kathrani A, Lezcano V, Hall EJ, et al. Indoleamine-pyrrole 2,3-dioxygenase-1 (IDO-1) mRNA is over-expressed in the duodenal mucosa and is negatively

correlated with serum tryptophan concentrations in dogs with protein-losing enteropathy. PLoS One 2019;14(6):e0218218.

49. Tamura Y, Ohta H, Kagawa Y, et al. Plasma amino acid profiles in dogs with inflammatory bowel disease. J Vet Intern Med 2019;33(4):1602–7.

50. Kathrani A, Allenspach K, Fascetti AJ, et al. Alterations in serum amino acid concentrations in dogs with protein-losing enteropathy. J Vet Intern Med 2018;32(3): 1026–32.

51. Agus A, Denizot J, Thévenot J, et al. Western diet induces a shift in microbiota composition enhancing susceptibility to Adherent-Invasive E. coli infection and intestinal inflammation. Sci Rep 2016;6:19032.

52. Allenspach K, Culverwell C, Chan D. Long-term outcome in dogs with chronic enteropathies: 203 cases. Vet Rec 2016;178:368.

53. Gianella P, Lotti U, Bellino C, et al. Clinicopathologic and prognostic factors in short- and long-term surviving dogs with protein-losing enteropathy. Schweiz Arch Tierheilkd 2017;159(3):163–9.

54. Equilino M, Theodoloz V, Gorgas D, et al. Evaluation of serum biochemical marker concentrations and survival time in dogs with protein-losing enteropathy. J Am Vet Med Assoc 2015;246:91–9.

55. Kathrani A, Sánchez-Vizcaíno F, Hall EJ. Association of chronic enteropathy activity index, blood urea concentration, and risk of death in dogs with protein-losing enteropathy. J Vet Intern Med 2019;33(2):536–43.

56. Nakashima K, Hiyoshi S, Ohno K, et al. Prognostic factors in dogs with protein-losing enteropathy. Vet J 2015;205(1):28–32.

Dietary and Nutritional Approaches to the Management of Chronic Enteropathy in Dogs and Cats

Aarti Kathrani, BVetMed (Hons), PhD, FHEA, MRCVS

KEYWORDS

- Nutrition • Hydrolyzed diet • Limited-ingredient novel protein diet
- Gastrointestinal diet • Malnutrition • Fat • Tryptophan • Magnesium

KEY POINTS

- Nutrition can influence those components and functions of the gastrointestinal tract that can be adversely affected in chronic enteropathy, such as microbiota, mucosal immune system, intestinal permeability, and motility.
- Malnutrition adversely affects outcome in people with inflammatory bowel disease. Approximately two-thirds of dogs with protein-losing enteropathy due to chronic enteropathy or lymphangiectasia are underweight.
- Some nutrients of concern in chronic enteropathy include fat; fiber; amino acids, such as tryptophan; vitamins, in particular cobalamin and vitamin D; and minerals, such as magnesium.
- Commercial therapeutic hydrolyzed, limited-ingredient novel protein, and gastrointestinal diets and home-prepared diets have all been used successfully in the management of chronic enteropathy.
- Fat restriction is the main dietary strategy for intestinal lymphangiectasia. Supplementation of medium-chain triglycerides, vitamin D, tryptophan, and magnesium warrants further investigation in intestinal lymphangiectasia.

INTRODUCTION

Nutrition has many direct effects on the gastrointestinal tract, including modulation of the microbiota, influencing the immune system, regulating gene expression and epigenetics, enhancing epithelial barrier function, and effecting motility. Therefore, in chronic enteropathy (CE), diet plays a central role in both disease pathogenesis, by serving as a risk factor, and as a therapeutic intervention.

Royal Veterinary College, Hawkshead Lane, Hatfield, Hertfordshire, AL9 7TA, UK
E-mail address: akathrani@rvc.ac.uk

Vet Clin Small Anim 51 (2021) 123–136
https://doi.org/10.1016/j.cvsm.2020.09.005
0195-5616/21/© 2020 Elsevier Inc. All rights reserved.
vetsmall.theclinics.com

INTESTINAL MICROBIOTA

Studies in dogs and cats have shown that diet can promote changes in the intestinal microbiota. An extruded animal protein–free diet was able to significantly increase fecal microbiota richness, which was significantly closer to a healthy microbiota in dogs with food-responsive enteropathy, but no changes were detected in the fecal microbiota of healthy dogs fed the same diet.[1] This suggests that diet is able to beneficially alter intestinal dysfunctions present in dogs with CE, but because these functional changes likely are absent in healthy dogs, similar effects are not seen. A separate study performed in dogs with CE showed that remission induced by a hydrolyzed diet was accompanied by alterations in microbial community structure marked by decreased abundance of pathobionts and reduced severity of dysbiosis.[2] Changes in the microbiota also have been documented in cats with naturally occurring chronic diarrhea following commercial gastrointestinal diets; however, this study could not conclude whether the changes were a consequence of the improvement in the diarrhea or the cause.[3]

MUCOSAL IMMUNE SYSTEM

Several nutrients, such as fat, amino acids, vitamin D, and vitamin A, have a direct effect on the gastrointestinal mucosal immune system. Unfortunately, there have been few studies assessing the effect of therapeutic diets, specifically on the intestinal mucosal immune response in dogs and cats with CE. One study was able to document that the mean duodenal lamina propria mononuclear cell score and duodenal lamina propria densities of eosinophils and mononuclear cells decreased in dogs with CE following a 6-week trial with a hydrolyzed soy protein diet.[4]

EPIGENETIC MODIFICATION

Epigenetics is the study of inheritable and reversible changes that modulate the function of genes without affecting their sequence.[5] DNA methylation and histone modification are 2 examples of epigenetic modification. Various dietary substrates necessary for DNA methylation, such as methionine, folate, choline, vitamin B_6, and vitamin B_{12}, have been suggested to influence DNA methylation.[6] In rats, a selenium-deficient diet resulted in markedly hypomethylated colonic DNA.[7] One study showed that a diet poor in fiber led to the suppression of microbiota-driven short-chain fatty acid (SCFA) production and disturbed chromatin effects.[8] Other dietary components, such as curcumin, also have been shown to have epigenetic effects.[9] To the author's knowledge, there have been no studies assessing the effect of diet on epigenetic modification in dogs and cats with CE.

ROLE OF DIET IN THE PATHOGENESIS OF CHRONIC ENTEROPATHY

To the author's knowledge, no epidemiologic studies have been performed assessing preillness dietary risk factors in dogs and cats with CE. A study with 1212 cats however, showed that those not exclusively fed commercial diet(s) meeting the World Small Animal Veterinary Association (WSAVA) Global Nutrition Committee (GNC) recommendations before 16 weeks of age were more likely to visit veterinary practices specifically for gastrointestinal signs on at least 2 occasions between 6 months and 30 months of age.[10] Feeding a diet that does not comply with the WSAVA GNC recommendations may raise concerns regarding quality control, source of ingredients, and nutritional composition of the diet, factors that may have an impact on the gastrointestinal mucosal immune system, microbiota, and intestinal permeability.

Longitudinal studies are required, however, to determine if and which specific dietary components serve as risk factors for the development of CE in dogs and cats.

ASSESSMENT OF NUTRITIONAL STATUS IN CHRONIC ENTEROPATHY

The World Health Organization refers to malnutrition as a deficiency, excess, or imbalance in a person's intake of energy and/or nutrients (https://www.who.int/features/qa/malnutrition/en/). Malnutrition is an important comorbidity in humans with inflammatory bowel disease (IBD), with a prevalence as high as 70% in patients with active disease and up to 38% in patients in remission.[11–13] Similarly, the prevalence of decreased body condition score (BCS) in canine protein-losing enteropathy (PLE) due to CE or lymphangiectasia was 47 of 71 dogs (66%), with 6 of 71 dogs (8%) being over-conditioned.[14] Malnutrition is linked to adverse outcomes in humans with IBD[15,16] and is associated with in-hospital death and increased hospital stay in these patients[17] as well as increased risk for infection, venous thromboembolism, and nonelective surgery.[18,19] Interestingly, 2 studies performed in dogs with PLE documented that BCS was not associated with treatment outcome.[14,20] BCS is informative of peripheral fat status in dogs, however, and this score does not take into account intra-abdominal fat, muscle condition, or bone density, all of which can be affected by malnutrition and, therefore, likely are important in the assessment of this. Unfortunately, to the author's knowledge, no studies have assessed muscle condition score or bone density in dogs and cats with CE and the effect of this on treatment outcome.

In human IBD, earlier identification of malnourished patients may allow for earlier intervention and impact on clinical outcomes.[21] One review study in human IBD suggests that nutrition screening tools hold promise in the prediction of clinical outcomes.[21] Unfortunately, no studies have been performed utilizing nutrition scores in canine or feline CE.

NUTRIENTS OF CONCERN IN CHRONIC ENTEROPATHY
Fat

High-fat diets have been shown to increase mRNA expression of the pattern recognition receptors, nucleotide oligomerization domain (NOD) 2, and Toll-like receptor (TLR) 5 in an experimental model of IBD,[22] whereas 21 days of fish oil supplementation down-regulated mRNA levels of NOD2 and TLR4 in lipopolysaccharide-treated pigs.[23] The innate immune receptors NOD2, TLR4, and TLR5 have all been implicated in the pathogenesis of canine CE.[24–28] Taken together, these results might support the benefit of a reduced fat diet or supplementation with omega-3 fatty acids in those dogs with a dysregulated mucosal innate immune response due to these receptors; however, studies are needed to assess this definitively.

Gastrointestinal disease can result in increased passage of fat into the colon due to reduced fat digestion and absorption in the small intestine. Increased fat in the colon potentially can result in dysbiosis as well as induce epithelial cell damage and fluid secretion into the colon.[29] Therefore, fat may be a nutrient of concern in some dogs with CE and trialing a low-fat diet may be beneficial in these cases. Dietary fat did not seem to affect the outcome of cats with chronic diarrhea.[30] Therefore, dietary fat may be less of a concern in cats with CE.

Amino Acids

Cats with chronic gastrointestinal disease have decreased plasma concentrations of the essential amino acids arginine, histidine, lysine, methionine, phenylalanine, taurine, and tryptophan.[31] Also, plasma histidine and tryptophan concentrations were inversely correlated with severity of signs in this study. Whole-blood taurine concentrations were not decreased significantly in cats with intestinal disease.[32] Dogs with CE and PLE have decreased plasma and serum concentrations of tryptophan, respectively.[33,34] Studies in murine and porcine models of colitis have shown an anti-inflammatory effect of dietary intervention with tryptophan or tryptophan metabolites, with supplementation ameliorating clinical signs, improving weight gain and histologic scores, and decreasing gut permeability and expression of proinflammatory cytokines.[35–37] Further studies are needed in canine CE and PLE and feline CE to determine if supplementation with tryptophan or other amino acids helps to improve clinical signs and disease outcome.

Fiber

Dietary fibers are plant-based carbohydrates, which cannot be digested by mammalian enzymes. Fiber is regarded as having numerous health benefits and is hypothesized as exerting an anti-inflammatory effect via fermentation by intestinal microbiota to SCFAs and playing a role in maintaining intestinal barrier function.[38] There have been few studies assessing the efficacy of dietary fiber in canine and feline CE. One retrospective study showed that treatment with a commercial therapeutic highly digestible diet supplemented with soluble fiber resulted in a very good to excellent response in most dogs with chronic idiopathic large bowel diarrhea.[39] In another study, 19 dogs with chronic colitis that had failed a low-fat diet responded to a fiber-supplemented diet, and maintenance could be achieved without the concurrent need for other medications.[40] In cats with colitis, 1 study showed response to diets high in fiber or supplemented with fiber.[41]

Fiber also can serve as a prebiotic, which is defined as a nondigestible food ingredient that is able to promote the growth of beneficial intestinal microorganisms. One study assessing the effects of chondroitin sulfate and several prebiotics, including resistant starch, beta-glucan and mannan-oligosaccharides in 27 dogs with IBD showed that the histologic score of dogs that received the supplement together with a hydrolyzed diet decreased by 1.53-fold.[42]

Vitamins

Several studies have documented low vitamin B_{12} in canine and feline CE[43,44] and this also has been shown to be a negative prognostic indicator in canine CE.[43] Studies showing the effects of oral cobalamin supplementation at normalizing serum vitamin B_{12} in dogs and cats have been reported.[45,46] Vitamin D concentrations are reduced in canine CE and PLE and are associated with outcome.[20,47] Currently, a consensus regarding vitamin D supplementation in dogs with CE and documented low concentrations has not been established.

Minerals and Other Micronutrients

Low blood magnesium concentrations requiring supplementation may be seen in some dogs with PLE. Magnesium can be supplemented orally with a dose of 1 mEq/kg/d to 2 mEq/kg/d using magnesium oxide, magnesium citrate, or magnesium sulfate. Supplementation also should be considered in those cases of refractory hypokalemia or hypocalcemia. The most frequent side effect of oral magnesium supplementation is diarrhea. Other micronutrient deficiencies, such as zinc, selenium, and iron, have not been investigated to date in canine or feline CE but are known to be of concern in human IBD.[48,49]

Emulsifiers

A majority of research on the negative effects of emulsifiers on the intestinal tract has been performed in experimental animal models. These studies have shown that various emulsifiers are able to promote proinflammatory microbiota and induce histopathologic changes in the intestinal tract.[50–52] Dogs and cats may be exposed to different emulsifiers through commercial pet foods and treats. The ingredients listed on a pet food label can be consulted to determine which specific additives are present in the food. To the author's knowledge, no studies have been performed assessing the effect of emulsifiers in dogs and cats with CE.

ASSESSMENT OF DIET IN DOGS AND CATS WITH CHRONIC ENTEROPATHY

Assessment of the diet just prior to or at the onset of gastrointestinal signs may help identify dietary triggers. The diet should be complete and balanced and should meet the recommendations outlined by the WSAVA GNC (https://wsava.org/wp-content/uploads/2020/01/Selecting-the-Best-Food-for-your-Pet.pdf). This ensures that a reputable and knowledgeable manufacturer has produced the diet. Collecting a full diet history of currently and historically fed diets, including snacks, treats, table foods, and foods used to administer medication, also is important to allow a full antigen exposure list to be compiled, which then can be used to determine ingredients that would be novel for the animal. Determining which ingredients are tolerated or help to improve gastrointestinal signs can help with selection of ingredients for home-prepared diets or commercial therapeutic diets. The dietary antigens identified most commonly in dogs are beef, dairy products, and wheat and those most commonly identified in cats are beef, dairy products, and fish.[53,54]

Dietary fiber can be estimated using total dietary fiber (TDF). Unfortunately, the regulations in the United States require that the maximum amount of crude fiber instead of TDF be listed on the pet food label. Crude fiber measures most of the insoluble fiber but none of the soluble fiber. One study demonstrated that crude fiber concentration was not a reliable indicator of TDF concentration or dietary fiber composition.[55] Unfortunately, TDF often is unavailable from the manufacturers of over-the-counter diets but may be found in the product guides for therapeutic diets. Determining the fiber content of the current diet helps to determine which strategy should be trialed next. For example, if a dog with colitis already is consuming a high-fiber diet with minimal improvement in signs, a diet with lower fiber and, therefore, higher digestibility should be trialed.

The fat content of the diet also should be assessed to determine which levels already have been trialed and their effects on the gastrointestinal signs. The fat content should be compared on an energy basis to remove any differences in energy density between diets; this can be done on a percentage or gram per 1000-kcal basis. Although there currently is no consensus on the definition of low fat, diets below 20% fat on a calorie basis are considered to be suitably low in fat.

DIETARY INTERVENTIONS IN CHRONIC ENTEROPATHY

A beneficial response to specific dietary strategies in animals with CE is variable and likely dependent on the underlying genetic susceptibility as well as environmental risk factor; therefore, nutrition should be applied as an individualized therapeutic intervention. Unfortunately, at this time, dietary therapy remains trial and error to determine which strategy is most effective in a dog or cat with CE. Although this may be frustrating for owners, studies have shown a clinical response to diet in dogs and cats with CE within or at 2 weeks of feeding.[4,43,56–58]

Enteral Nutrition

Hydrolyzed diets have been used successfully in the management of CE in dogs and cats.[2,4,59–62] These diets use several different dietary strategies that may be beneficial for CE. The hydrolyzed strategy may help influence the immune system, which is known to be dysregulated in this disease. Two studies assessing the ex vivo whole-blood cytokine response to commercial hydrolyzed diets showed that these diets elicit no to minimal response in dogs and cats.[63,64] However, 1 study showed that hydrolyzed diets might stimulate food-reactive lymphocytes in dogs.[65] Therefore, further studies are needed to ascertain the immunologic effect of hydrolyzed diets, especially at the intestinal mucosal surface. The hydrolyzed approach also helps increase digestibility, which may be beneficial for gastrointestinal disease. Digestibility alone, however, may be unlikely to maintain remission, because 1 study demonstrated that although a highly digestible therapeutic gastrointestinal diet was able to induce remission in dogs with CE, they were less likely to remain asymptomatic at subsequent rechecks compared with dogs managed with a hydrolyzed diet.[60] Although studies have demonstrated that highly digestible gastrointestinal diets can help with clinical signs of CE in cats, further studies assessing these diets are needed in dogs.[66,67] Some hydrolyzed formulas have a lower fat content, which may be beneficial, and some hydrolyzed diets contain omega-3 fatty acids and soy, which are known to be immunomodulatory. Some formulas are vegetarian and a study in humans showed that a semivegetarian diet was highly effective for maintaining remission in IBD patients.[68] Gluten-free diets have been shown to improve clinical symptoms in people with IBD.[69] Therefore, because some hydrolyzed formulas are gluten-free, this strategy may explain the improvement in clinical signs associated with these diets in some dogs and cats with CE. Randomized controlled trials are needed, however, to determine the effect of gluten-free diets on clinical signs in dogs and cats with CE. Given the anecdotal success of hydrolyzed diets in CE and that in 1 study, 2 of 6 dogs that failed an elimination diet trial with a novel protein diet responded to a hydrolyzed diet,[59] the author elects to try this category of diets first. If the animal does not consume the diet, then a commercial therapeutic novel protein diet can be tried.

Approximately 50% of cats and 60% of dogs with chronic gastrointestinal signs responded to a novel protein diet.[69,70] Interestingly, 1 study showed no difference in response rate between hydrolyzed and limited ingredient novel protein diets when used in dogs with CE.[62] A study demonstrated the presence of other common food antigens in over-the-counter novel protein diets, and, therefore, these diets should be avoided for the treatment of suspected CE.[71] Some therapeutic novel protein formulas have the advantage of having a higher TDF content and, therefore, may be beneficial in those cases with large intestinal signs, especially if a highly digestible diet failed to improve clinical signs.

Certain emulsifiers and preservatives have been shown to have negative effects on the intestinal microbiota and gastrointestinal mucosal immune system in experimental gene knockout models of IBD. Thus, there may be a subset of canine and feline CE cases that, due to their underlying genetic susceptibility, may not be able to tolerate commercial foods and may need a home-prepared diet for resolution of their signs. Home-prepared diets should be formulated with the guidance of a board-certified veterinary nutritionist. The pros and cons of different categories of diets for treatment of CE are listed in **Table 1**.

Table 1
Pros and cons of different categories of diet used in the management of chronic enteropathy in dogs and cats.

Diet Category	Pros	Cons
Commercial therapeutic gastrointestinal diet	• Generally higher digestibility than over-the-counter diets • Possibly less expensive than hydrolyzed diets • Likely higher palatability compared with hydrolyzed diets • Some formulas are low in fat • Studies have shown efficacy for chronic gastrointestinal signs in cats.[66,67]	• One study suggests less able to maintain remission compared with hydrolyzed diet in dogs with CE[60]
Commercial therapeutic, limited-ingredient, novel protein diet	• Likely higher palatability • Some formulas have higher TDF to help with large intestinal signs. • Studies have shown efficacy for canine and feline CE.[43,57,62,69,70,79]	• Thorough diet history needed • Generally higher fat content • Possible relapse due to reaction to new antigens over time • Contamination concerns with over-the-counter diets[71]
Commercial therapeutic hydrolyzed diet	• Thorough diet history not needed • Anecdotally less relapse seen compared with novel protein diets • Some formulas contain less fat than commercial novel protein diets. • Studies have shown efficacy for canine and feline CE.[2,4,59–62]	• Possibly lower palatability compared with other categories of diets • Possibly more expensive than other categories of commercial diets
Home-prepared diet	• Generally higher digestibility • Likely higher palatability • Ability to precisely set macronutrient profile, such as fat content • Avoids antigens from processing and certain emulsifiers • Studies have shown efficacy in canine IL and feline colitis[57,75]	• More expensive compared with other categories of diet • More labor intensive • Guidance from board-certified veterinary nutritionist required • Possible relapse due to reaction to new antigens over time • Novel protein may be difficult to source if case has extensive antigen exposure list. • May be difficult to transition to in cats that have developed fixed preferences for certain ingredients, flavors or textures • Closer monitoring with regular blood work may be required if bioavailability of diet is unknown.

(*Data from* Refs.[2,4,43,57,59–62,66,67,69–71,75,79]).

Fortunately, most dogs and cats with CE can be transitioned back to their original diet without showing any relapse. In 1 study, 21% of dogs, and in another study, 29% of cats with gastrointestinal signs relapsed on challenge[43,69]; these cases likely were food allergic or had a significant dietary risk factor that may have triggered a relapse. Unfortunately, at this time, it is not possible to distinguish food allergy, intolerance, or CE that is responsive to diet alone. Therefore, these studies assessing diet in dogs and cats with CE may have included animals with food allergy or intolerance (**Fig. 1**). Further studies are needed to help distinguish between these 3 gastrointestinal conditions in dogs and cats to help guide optimal dietary treatment.

Parenteral Nutrition

Parenteral nutrition (PN) allows for bowel rest, correction of nutritional deficiency, and removal of dietary antigen that may stimulate the gastrointestinal mucosal immune system.[72] PN, however, is expensive, needs to be carried out in a specialized facility, requires closer monitoring, and may predispose to infection and thromboembolism. Based on the studies in human medicine, it can be concluded that PN is less advantageous than enteral nutrition, which is considered a more physiologic modality with regard to mucosal healing and, therefore, should be prioritized. However, in certain cases PN may be indicated, such as supplementary therapy with enteral nutrition to ensure that the daily requirement of calories are met, if enteral nutrition is not possible in the absence of access, for example, when the patient is comatose, debilitated or unable to swallow, has intractable regurgitation, vomiting or diarrhea or is coagulopathic. There has been 1 case report of the use of PN in the management of a dog with CE and severe PLE.[73]

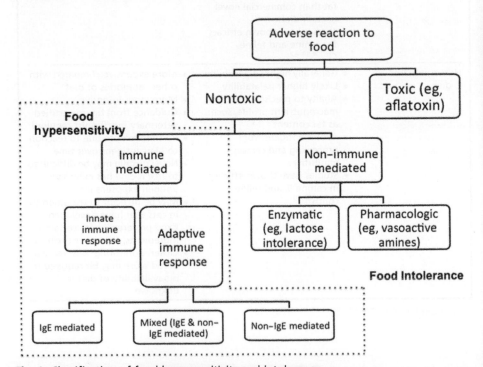

Fig. 1. Classification of food hypersensitivity and intolerance.

DIETARY MANAGEMENT OF CANINE PROTEIN-LOSING ENTEROPATHY DUE TO INTESTINAL LYMPHANGIECTASIA

The main therapeutic strategies for intestinal lymphangiectasia (IL) are treatment of the underlying cause if identified, decreased fat intake, and, therefore, decreased fat absorption and reduction of intestinal inflammation. Low-fat diets are hypothesized to decrease lymphatic flow and pressure due to decreased chylomicron production. This reduced flow and pressure prevent lacteal dilation and lymph leakage resulting from lacteal rupture. Also, long-chain triglycerides have proinflammatory properties and are hypothesized to cause lipogranulomas. Therefore, a low-fat diet is prioritized in the management of IL. Although there is no consensus for the definition of low fat, nutritionists generally consider less than 20% fat on a metabolizable energy (ME) basis to be suitably low. Ultra–low-fat diets are considered by the author to be generally less than 15% fat on an ME basis. Therefore, a home-cooked diet using low-fat ingredients is the ideal way to achieve an ultra–low-fat diet as well as increased digestibility. Consultation with a board-certified veterinary nutritionist should be sought to ensure ultra–low-fat diets still contain the minimum requirement of essential fatty acids as well as being balanced. The amount of dietary fat chosen depends on the level the dog currently is consuming. Therefore, between 15% and 20% fat on an ME basis (ie, low-fat) may be chosen if a dog currently is consuming at least 30%. Whereas, if the dog is consuming less than 30% fat on an ME basis and still is showing clinical signs and abnormal biochemical parameters, an ultra–low-fat diet (less than 15% fat on an ME basis) can be trialed. An ultra–low-fat diet also can be chosen if the dog's clinical signs and laboratory parameters fail to respond to a commercial therapeutic low-fat diet in the first instance. In addition to dogs with primary lymphangiectasia, the author also attempts a trial with a low-fat or ultra–low-fat diet in dogs with inflammatory PLE with secondary lymphangiectasia. Although 1 study demonstrated an optimal canine CE clinical activity index cutoff value of 8 as being able to distinguish ultra–low-fat food-responsive PLE group (less than 8) from immunosuppressant-responsive or nonresponsive PLE, additional studies are needed to further define which population of dogs with PLE are most likely to benefit solely from these diets. Although glucocorticoids also are used in canine IL to decrease intestinal inflammation, 1 small retrospective study in Yorkshire terriers with IL documented that some dogs could respond satisfactorily in the short term to a low-fat diet alone.[74] In addition, another study documented that dietary fat restriction could be used as an effective treatment in dogs with IL that were unresponsive to prednisolone or experienced a relapse with dose reduction.[75] If clinical signs or biochemical abnormalities persist with an appropriate low fat commercial therapeutic diet, then a home-prepared diet should be considered for further dietary fat reduction. Supplementation with medium-chain triglycerides (MCTs) is used in human IL due to their direct absorption into the portal vein. In dogs, however, MCTs still are absorbed into the lymphatic system and, therefore, may not help reduce lymph flow.[76] MCTs have been shown to modulate intestinal inflammation and cause less damage than long-chain triglycerides in an animal model of ileitis[77] and, therefore, might help reduce inflammation in canine IL. In addition to dietary fat and cobalamin, other nutrients of concern include vitamin D, tryptophan, and magnesium.[20,33,78] Further studies are needed, however, to definitively ascertain the effects of supplementation of these specific nutrients in canine PLE due to IL.

SUMMARY

In conclusion, nutrition plays a central role in the management of canine and feline CE. An understanding of the different dietary strategies available for canine and feline CE helps ensure the most appropriate diet is selected, although at this time trial and error of these different dietary strategies is needed to ensure optimization for each case. Future studies should focus on additional dietary strategies that may be efficacious in canine and feline CE and defining which specific subpopulations within this condition are most likely to benefit from these.

DISCLOSURE

The author has nothing to disclose.

REFERENCES

1. Bresciani F, Minamoto Y, Suchodolski JS, et al. Effect of an extruded animal protein-free diet on fecal microbiota of dogs with food-responsive enteropathy. J Vet Intern Med 2018;32:1903–10.
2. Wang S, Martins R, Sullivan MC, et al. Diet-induced remission in chronic enteropathy is associated with altered microbial community structure and synthesis of secondary bile acids. Microbiome 2019;7:126.
3. Ramadan Z, Xu H, Laflamme D, et al. Fecal microbiota of cats with naturally occurring chronic diarrhea assessed using 16S rRNA gene 454-pyrosequencing before and after dietary treatment. J Vet Intern Med 2014;28:59–65.
4. Walker D, Knuchel-Takano A, McCutchan A, et al. A comprehensive pathological survey of duodenal biopsies from dogs with diet-responsive chronic enteropathy. J Vet Intern Med 2013;27:862–74.
5. Desiderio A, Spinelli R, Ciccarelli M, et al. Epigenetics: spotlight on type 2 diabetes and obesity. J Endocrinol Invest 2016;39:1095–103.
6. Anderson OS, Sant KE, Dolinoy DC. Nutrition and epigenetics: an interplay of dietary methyl donors, one-carbon metabolism and DNA methylation. J Nutr Biochem 2012;23:853–9.
7. Davis CD, Uthus EO, Finley JW. Dietary selenium and arsenic affect DNA methylation in vitro in Caco-2 cells and in vivo in rat liver and colon. J Nutr 2000;130: 2903–9.
8. Krautkramer KA, Kreznar JH, Romano KA, et al. Diet-microbiota interactions mediate global epigenetic programming in multiple host tissues. Mol Cell 2016; 64:982–92.
9. Reuter S, Gupta SC, Park B, et al. Epigenetic changes induced by curcumin and other natural compounds. Genes Nutr 2011;6:93–108.
10. Kathrani A, Blackwell EJ, Williams JL, et al. Exploring early life events including diet in cats presenting for gastrointestinal signs in later life. Vet Rec 2019; 185:144.
11. Mijac DD, Jankovic GL, Jorga J, et al. Nutritional status in patients with active inflammatory bowel disease: prevalence of malnutrition and methods for routine nutritional assessment. Eur J Intern Med 2010;21:315–9.
12. Vadan R, Gheorghe LS, Constantinescu A, et al. The prevalence of malnutrition and the evolution of nutritional status in patients with moderate to severe forms of Crohn's disease treated with Infliximab. Clin Nutr 2011;30:86–91.
13. Benjamin J, Makharia GK, Kalaivani M, et al. Nutritional status of patients with Crohn's disease. Indian J Gastroenterol 2008;27:195–200.
14. Kathrani A, Sanchez-Vizcaino F, Hall EJ. Association of chronic enteropathy activity index, blood urea concentration, and risk of death in dogs with protein-losing enteropathy. J Vet Intern Med 2019;33:536–43.

15. Pirlich M, Schutz T, Kemps M, et al. Prevalence of malnutrition in hospitalized medical patients: impact of underlying disease. Dig Dis 2003;21:245–51.
16. Gassull MA. Nutrition and inflammatory bowel disease: its relation to pathophysiology, outcome and therapy. Dig Dis 2003;21:220–7.
17. Nguyen GC, Munsell M, Harris ML. Nationwide prevalence and prognostic significance of clinically diagnosable protein-calorie malnutrition in hospitalized inflammatory bowel disease patients. Inflamm Bowel Dis 2008;14:1105–11.
18. Ananthakrishnan AN, McGinley EL. Infection-related hospitalizations are associated with increased mortality in patients with inflammatory bowel diseases. J Crohns Colitis 2013;7:107–12.
19. Ananthakrishnan AN, McGinley EL, Binion DG, et al. A novel risk score to stratify severity of Crohn's disease hospitalizations. Am J Gastroenterol 2010;105:1799–807.
20. Allenspach K, Rizzo J, Jergens AE, et al. Hypovitaminosis D is associated with negative outcome in dogs with protein losing enteropathy: a retrospective study of 43 cases. BMC Vet Res 2017;13:96.
21. Li S, Ney M, Eslamparast T, et al. Systematic review of nutrition screening and assessment in inflammatory bowel disease. World J Gastroenterol 2019;25:3823–37.
22. Martinez-Medina M, Denizot J, Dreux N, et al. Western diet induces dysbiosis with increased E coli in CEABAC10 mice, alters host barrier function favouring AIEC colonisation. Gut 2014;63:116–24.
23. Liu Y, Chen F, Odle J, et al. Fish oil enhances intestinal integrity and inhibits TLR4 and NOD2 signaling pathways in weaned pigs after LPS challenge. J Nutr 2012;142:2017–24.
24. Kathrani A, Lee II, White C, et al. Association between nucleotide oligomerisation domain two (Nod2) gene polymorphisms and canine inflammatory bowel disease. Vet Immunol Immunopathol 2014;161.32–41.
25. Kathrani A, House A, Catchpole B, et al. Polymorphisms in the TLR4 and TLR5 gene are significantly associated with inflammatory bowel disease in German shepherd dogs. PLoS One 2010;5:e15740.
26. Kathrani A, Holder A, Catchpole B, et al. TLR5 risk-associated haplotype for canine inflammatory bowel disease confers hyper-responsiveness to flagellin. PLoS One 2012;7:e30117.
27. Swerdlow MP, Kennedy DR, Kennedy JS, et al. Expression and function of TLR2, TLR4, and Nod2 in primary canine colonic epithelial cells. Vet Immunol Immunopathol 2006;114:313–9.
28. Allenspach K, House A, Smith K, et al. Evaluation of mucosal bacteria and histopathology, clinical disease activity and expression of Toll-like receptors in German shepherd dogs with chronic enteropathies. Vet Microbiol 2010;146:326–35.
29. Ramakrishna BS, Mathan M, Mathan VI. Alteration of colonic absorption by long-chain unsaturated fatty acids. Influence of hydroxylation and degree of unsaturation. Scand J Gastroenterol 1994;29:54–8.
30. Laflamme DP, Xu H, Long GM. Effect of diets differing in fat content on chronic diarrhea in cats. J Vet Intern Med 2011;25:230–5.
31. Sakai K, Maeda S, Yonezawa T, et al. Decreased plasma amino acid concentrations in cats with chronic gastrointestinal diseases and their possible contribution in the inflammatory response. Vet Immunol Immunopathol 2018;195:1–6.
32. Kathrani A, Fascetti AJ, Larsen JA, et al. Whole-blood taurine concentrations in cats with intestinal disease. J Vet Intern Med 2017;31:1067–73.

33. Kathrani A, Allenspach K, Fascetti AJ, et al. Alterations in serum amino acid concentrations in dogs with protein-losing enteropathy. J Vet Intern Med 2018;32: 1026–32.
34. Tamura Y, Ohta H, Kagawa Y, et al. Plasma amino acid profiles in dogs with inflammatory bowel disease. J Vet Intern Med 2019;33:1602–7.
35. Kim CJ, Kovacs-Nolan JA, Yang C, et al. l-Tryptophan exhibits therapeutic function in a porcine model of dextran sodium sulfate (DSS)-induced colitis. J Nutr Biochem 2010;21:468–75.
36. Shizuma T, Mori H, Fukuyama N. Protective effect of tryptophan against dextran sulfate sodium- induced experimental colitis. Turk J Gastroenterol 2013;24:30–5.
37. Islam J, Sato S, Watanabe K, et al. Dietary tryptophan alleviates dextran sodium sulfate-induced colitis through aryl hydrocarbon receptor in mice. J Nutr Biochem 2017;42:43–50.
38. Gu P, Feagins LA. Dining with inflammatory bowel disease: a review of the literature on diet in the pathogenesis and management of IBD. Inflamm Bowel Dis 2019;26(2):181–91.
39. Leib MS. Treatment of chronic idiopathic large-bowel diarrhea in dogs with a highly digestible diet and soluble fiber: a retrospective review of 37 cases. J Vet Intern Med 2000;14:27–32.
40. Lecoindre P, Gaschen FP. Chronic idiopathic large bowel diarrhea in the dog. Vet Clin North Am Small Anim Pract 2011;41:447–56.
41. Dennis JS, Kruger JM, Mullaney TP. Lymphocytic/plasmacytic colitis in cats: 14 cases (1985-1990). J Am Vet Med Assoc 1993;202:313–8.
42. Segarra S, Martinez-Subiela S, Cerda-Cuellar M, et al. Oral chondroitin sulfate and prebiotics for the treatment of canine inflammatory bowel disease: a randomized, controlled clinical trial. BMC Vet Res 2016;12:49.
43. Allenspach K, Wieland B, Grone A, et al. Chronic enteropathies in dogs: evaluation of risk factors for negative outcome. J Vet Intern Med 2007;21:700–8.
44. Simpson KW, Fyfe J, Cornetta A, et al. Subnormal concentrations of serum cobalamin (vitamin B12) in cats with gastrointestinal disease. J Vet Intern Med 2001;15: 26–32.
45. Toresson L, Steiner JM, Suchodolski JS, et al. Oral cobalamin supplementation in dogs with chronic enteropathies and hypocobalaminemia. J Vet Intern Med 2016; 30:101–7.
46. Toresson L, Steiner JM, Olmedal G, et al. Oral cobalamin supplementation in cats with hypocobalaminaemia: a retrospective study. J Feline Med Surg 2017;19: 1302–6.
47. Titmarsh H, Gow AG, Kilpatrick S, et al. Association of vitamin D status and clinical outcome in dogs with a chronic enteropathy. J Vet Intern Med 2015;29: 1473–8.
48. Massironi S, Rossi RE, Cavalcoli FA, et al. Nutritional deficiencies in inflammatory bowel disease: therapeutic approaches. Clin Nutr 2013;32:904–10.
49. Castro Aguilar-Tablada T, Navarro-Alarcon M, Quesada Granados J, et al. Ulcerative colitis and crohn's disease are associated with decreased serum selenium concentrations and increased cardiovascular risk. Nutrients 2016;8:780.
50. Chassaing B, Koren O, Goodrich JK, et al. Dietary emulsifiers impact the mouse gut microbiota promoting colitis and metabolic syndrome. Nature 2015;519:92–6.
51. Shang Q, Sun W, Shan X, et al. Carrageenan-induced colitis is associated with decreased population of anti-inflammatory bacterium, Akkermansia muciniphila, in the gut microbiota of C57BL/6J mice. Toxicol Lett 2017;279:87–95.

52. Watt J, Marcus R. Carrageenan-induced ulceration of the large intestine in the guinea pig. Gut 1971;12:164–71.

53. White SD. Food hypersensitivity in 30 dogs. J Am Vet Med Assoc 1986;188: 695–8.

54. Jeffers JG, Meyer EK, Sosis EJ. Responses of dogs with food allergies to single-ingredient dietary provocation. J Am Vet Med Assoc 1996;209:608–11.

55. Owens TJ, Larsen JA, Farcas AK, et al. Total dietary fiber composition of diets used for management of obesity and diabetes mellitus in cats. J Am Vet Med Assoc 2014;245:99–105.

56. Schmitz S, Glanemann B, Garden OA, et al. A prospective, randomized, blinded, placebo-controlled pilot study on the effect of Enterococcus faecium on clinical activity and intestinal gene expression in canine food-responsive chronic enteropathy. J Vet Intern Med 2015;29:533–43.

57. Nelson RW, Dimperio ME, Long GG. Lymphocytic-plasmacytic colitis in the cat. J Am Vet Med Assoc 1984;184:1133–5.

58. Guilford WG, Jones BR, Markwell PJ, et al. Food sensitivity in cats with chronic idiopathic gastrointestinal problems. J Vet Intern Med 2001;15:7–13.

59. Marks SL, Laflamme DP, McAloose D. Dietary trial using a commercial hypoallergenic diet containing hydrolyzed protein for dogs with inflammatory bowel disease. Vet Ther 2002;3:109–18.

60. Mandigers PJ, Biourge V, van den Ingh TS, et al. A randomized, open-label, positively-controlled field trial of a hydrolyzed protein diet in dogs with chronic small bowel enteropathy. J Vet Intern Med 2010;24:1350–7.

61. Mandigers PJ, Biourge V, German AJ. Efficacy of a commercial hydrolysate diet in eight cats suffering from inflammatory bowel disease or adverse reaction to food. Tijdschr Diergeneeskd 2010;135:668–72.

62. Allenspach K, Culverwell C, Chan D. Long-term outcome in dogs with chronic enteropathies: 203 cases. Vet Rec 2016;178:368.

63. Kathrani A, Hall E. A preliminary study assessing cytokine production following ex vivo stimulation of whole blood with diet in dogs with chronic enteropathy. BMC Vet Res 2019;15:185.

64. Kathrani A, Larsen JA, Cortopassi G, et al. A descriptive pilot study of cytokine production following stimulation of ex-vivo whole blood with commercial therapeutic feline hydrolyzed diets in individual healthy immunotolerant cats. BMC Vet Res 2017;13:297.

65. Masuda K, Sato A, Tanaka A, et al. Hydrolyzed diets may stimulate food-reactive lymphocytes in dogs. J Vet Med Sci 2019;82:177–83.

66. Laflamme DP, Xu H, Cupp CJ, et al. Evaluation of canned therapeutic diets for the management of cats with naturally occurring chronic diarrhea. J Feline Med Surg 2012;14:669–77.

67. Perea SC, Marks SL, Daristotle L, et al. Evaluation of Two Dry Commercial Therapeutic Diets for the Management of Feline Chronic Gastroenteropathy. Front Vet Sci 2017;4:69.

68. Chiba M, Abe T, Tsuda H, et al. Lifestyle-related disease in Crohn's disease: relapse prevention by a semi-vegetarian diet. World J Gastroenterol 2010;16: 2484–95.

69. Herfarth HH, Martin CF, Sandler RS, et al. Prevalence of a gluten-free diet and improvement of clinical symptoms in patients with inflammatory bowel diseases. Inflamm Bowel Dis 2014;20:1194–7.

70. Luckschander N, Allenspach K, Hall J, et al. Perinuclear antineutrophilic cytoplasmic antibody and response to treatment in diarrheic dogs with food responsive disease or inflammatory bowel disease. J Vet Intern Med 2006;20:221–7.
71. Raditic DM, Remillard RL, Tater KC. ELISA testing for common food antigens in four dry dog foods used in dietary elimination trials. J Anim Physiol Anim Nutr (Berl) 2011;95:90–7.
72. Scolapio JS. The role of total parenteral nutrition in the management of patients with acute attacks of inflammatory bowel disease. J Clin Gastroenterol 1999;29: 223–4.
73. Lane IF, Miller E, Twedt DC. Parenteral nutrition in the management of a dog with lymphocytic-plasmacytic enteritis and severe protein-losing enteropathy. Can Vet J 1999;40:721–4.
74. Rudinsky AJ, Howard JP, Bishop MA, et al. Dietary management of presumptive protein-losing enteropathy in Yorkshire terriers. J Small Anim Pract 2017;58: 103–8.
75. Okanishi H, Yoshioka R, Kagawa Y, et al. The clinical efficacy of dietary fat restriction in treatment of dogs with intestinal lymphangiectasia. J Vet Intern Med 2014; 28:809–17.
76. Jensen GL, McGarvey N, Taraszewski R, et al. Lymphatic absorption of enterally fed structured triacylglycerol vs physical mix in a canine model. Am J Clin Nutr 1994;60:518–24.
77. Tsujikawa T, Ohta N, Nakamura T, et al. Medium-chain triglycerides modulate ileitis induced by trinitrobenzene sulfonic acid. J Gastroenterol Hepatol 1999; 14:1166–72.
78. Kathrani A, Lezcano V, Hall EJ, et al. Indoleamine-pyrrole 2,3-dioxygenase-1 (IDO-1) mRNA is over-expressed in the duodenal mucosa and is negatively correlated with serum tryptophan concentrations in dogs with protein-losing enteropathy. PLoS One 2019;14:e0218218.
79. Sauter SN, Benyacoub J, Allenspach K, et al. Effects of probiotic bacteria in dogs with food responsive diarrhoea treated with an elimination diet. J Anim Physiol Anim Nutr (Berl) 2006;90:269–77.

From Bench Top to Clinics
How New Tests Can Be Helpful in Diagnosis and Management of Dogs with Chronic Enteropathies

Juan Hernandez, Dr med vet, PhD[a,b],
Julien Rodolphe Samuel Dandrieux, BSc, Dr med vet, PhD[c,*]

KEYWORDS

- Chronic enteropathy • Inflammatory bowel disease • Biomarker • Cytokine • Dogs

KEY POINTS

- There are currently only a few tests that have been validated and are offered commercially for dogs with chronic enteropathies.
- In dogs with suggestive histologic changes, polymerase chain reaction for antigen receptor gene rearrangements and fluorescence in situ hybridization testing have the potential to change the treatment plan.
- Several promising biomarkers such as calprotectin and calgranulin C are currently not available commercially.
- It is likely that a panel of biomarkers will be needed to increase the yield for diagnostic and prognostic purposes in the future.

INTRODUCTION

Chronic enteropathies (CE) are a group of primary intestinal diseases characterized by persistent or recurrent gastrointestinal signs and are a common presentation in dogs.[1] CE is often further classified upon treatment response in food-responsive enteropathy (FRE), antibiotic-responsive enteropathy (ARE), steroid-responsive or immunosuppressant-responsive therapy (IRE), and nonresponsive enteropathy. CE is a common presentation in the canine population and there is active research on

[a] Université Paris-Saclay, INRAE, AgroParisTech, UMR 1319 Micalis, Microbiota Interactions with Human and Animal Team (MIHA), F-78350, Jouy-en Josas, France; [b] Department of Clinical Sciences, Nantes-Atlantic College of Veterinary Medicine and Food Sciences (Oniris), University of Nantes, 101 route de Gachet, Nantes 44300, France; [c] Department of Veterinary Clinical Sciences, Melbourne Veterinary School, Faculty of Veterinary and Agricultural Sciences, University of Melbourne, U-Vet, 250 Princes Highway, Werribee, Victoria 3030, Australia
* Corresponding author.
E-mail address: julien.dandrieux@unimelb.edu.au

Vet Clin Small Anim 51 (2021) 137–153
https://doi.org/10.1016/j.cvsm.2020.09.008
0195-5616/21/© 2020 Elsevier Inc. All rights reserved.

vetsmall.theclinics.com

the subject. Despite this activity, our ability to differentiate among the different types of enteropathies before treatment trials remains elusive. The requirements of sequential treatment trials can be frustrating and costly for the owners and their pets. For this reason, there is a strong interest in finding tests and biomarkers that can help in diagnostic evaluation, prognostication, and clinical monitoring of dogs with CE. A biomarker is defined as "a characteristic that is objectively measured and evaluated as an indicator of normal biological processes, pathogenic processes, or pharmacologic responses to a therapeutic intervention."[2]

Biomarkers can be used in a clinical setting for different goals such as:

1. Identifying animals with a specific disease.
2. Disease staging.
3. Prognostic indicator.
4. Surrogate for monitoring the effects of a therapeutic intervention.

A biomarker that could help predicting the probability that a dog with CE would respond to a particular treatment would be especially desirable. Several biomarkers have been evaluated in canine CE during the last decade, and some are now translated from basic science into commercially available tests.

The present review is limited to tests that are commercially available or tests that have been used clinically and hold promise for future commercialization. The commercially available blood tests include concentrations of C-reactive protein (CRP), cobalamin or vitamin B_{12}, methylmalonic acid (MMA), and folate. The commercially available fecal tests include concentration of alpha$_1$-proteinase inhibitor (α_1PI) and the fecal dysbiosis index (DI). Two tests performed on tissue biopsies are also commercially available: fluorescence in situ hybridization and polymerase chain reaction for antigen receptor gene rearrangements (PARR). Although the latter two are not biomarkers, their results can drastically change the treatment plan and outcome in some instances. We have focused our review of tests that are not commercially available on those that do not require tissue biopsies and can be used by the clinicians before a histologic diagnosis is made or for monitoring purposes. We refer the readers to a recent publication for an extensive list of clinically relevant biomarkers.[3]

COMMERCIALLY AVAILABLE BIOMARKERS
Cobalamin, Folate, and Methylmalonic Acid

Disorders of cobalamin (vitamin B_{12}) metabolism were reviewed recently and the reader is directed to this publication for in depth information.[4] Folate and cobalamin are both water-soluble vitamins. Folate is absorbed in the duodenum, whereas cobalamin is absorbed in the ileum; hence, hypofolatemia suggests duodenal disease and hypocobalaminemia ileal disease. Exocrine pancreatic insufficiency needs to be ruled out in the presence of hypocobalaminemia because lack of intrinsic factor, predominantly produced by the pancreas in dogs, is a cause for cobalamin malabsorption. Other causes for hypocobalaminemia include dysbiosis, small cell intestinal lymphoma, and Imerslund–Grasbeck syndrome, described in Beagles, Border Collies, Giant Schnauzers, and Australian Shepherds.[5–9]

Accumulation of MMA develops secondary to cobalamin deficiency at the cellular level (**Fig. 1**). Because serum hypocobalaminemia does not indicate cellular cobalamin deficiency, an increase in MMA supports significant hypocobalaminemia. MMA concentration can be determined in serum and urine samples and is useful to further assess the stores of cobalamin.[10] Other causes of increased MMA include renal disease and intestinal dysbiosis.[4]

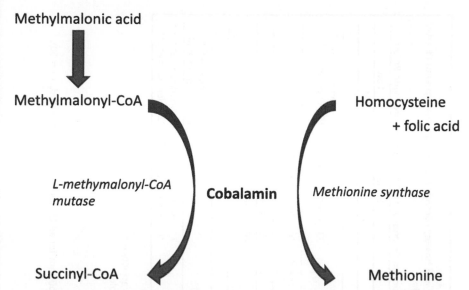

Fig. 1. Vitamin B_{12} is required for MMA to be converted to succinyl-coenzyme A (CoA), and in combination with folic acid, for homocysteine to be converted to methionine.

Hence, measurements of serum cobalamin and folate can be useful to assess which part of the intestinal tract is most affected, and ileal biopsies should be considered in dogs with hypocobalaminemia. Furthermore, hypocobalaminemia has been reported as a negative prognostic factor for dogs with exocrine pancreatic insufficiency and CE, whereas there is no evidence that hypofolatemia is.[11–14] The usefulness of MMA as a prognostic factor has not yet been studied.

C-Reactive Protein

CRP is a positive acute phase protein produced by the liver and a very sensitive marker of inflammation.[15] However, CRP is increased with a number of inflammatory diseases and for this reason is a nonspecific biological marker of inflammation.[16]

Quantification of canine CRP in serum can be done with several assays, including heterologous and homologous immunoassays with typical values of less than 10 mg/L in healthy dogs.[17] CRP is offered by most large commercial laboratories. Because of large intraindividual variability, the serum concentration of CRP must increase or decrease at least 2.7-fold for this change to be considered clinically relevant. For this reason, CRP might have more of a role to monitor treatment response rather than as a disease biomarker CE.[18] CRP has been shown to be useful to monitor treatment response in dogs with steroid-responsive meningitis arteritis, idiopathic polyarthritis, and in dogs treated for bacterial pneumonia.[19–21]

Documented differences in serum biomarkers between healthy dogs and dogs with CE as well as changes after treatment are summarized in **Table 1**. Serum CRP has been shown to be increased in dogs with CE compared with normal dogs and to decrease after treatment in some studies, but not in others.[11,22,23] Correlation between serum biomarkers and clinical or histologic scoring is summarized in **Table 2**. Serum CRP showed a significant moderate correlation with clinical scoring in some studies, but not in others.[11,23–26] No correlation was found between histologic score and serum CRP.[23,26] One study reported significantly higher CRP concentrations in

Table 1
Summary of the studies assessing differences in biomarkers concentration between dogs with CE and healthy controls and changes in dogs with CE after treatment

	Concentration in CE Compared with Healthy Dogs						Concentration in CE Dogs After Therapy Compared with Before					
	Higher		Same		Lower		Higher		Same		Lower	
	n	Ref	n	Ref	n	Ref	n	Ref	n	Ref	n	Ref
Serum												
CRP	28†	Jergens et al[22,a]	58g	Jergens et al[22,a]					33	Allenspach et al[11]	58	Jergens et al[22,a]
	16	Otoni et al[23,b]									15	Otoni et al[23,b]
	16	Heilmann et al[d]										
Calprotectin	34	Heilmann et al[24,c]	16	Otoni et al[23,b]			34	Heilmann et al[24,c]	16	Otoni et al[23,b]		
			16	Heilmann et al[47,d]								
S100A12									20	Heilmann et al[47,d]		
sRAGE					20	Heilmann et al[67,e]			20	Heilmann et al[67,e]		
Fecal												
Calprotectin	16	Otoni et al[23,b]							16	Otoni et al[23,b]	12	Heilmann et al[25,f]
S100A12	26	Heilmann et al[47,d]							7	Heilman et al[48,h]	20	Heilmann et al[67,e]
									9	Heilman et al[48,h]	22	Heilmann et al[48,h]

Abbreviation: NRE, nonresponsive enteropathy.
a IRE (n = 58) versus healthy (n = 9). CRP was significantly increased only in dogs with canine IBD activity index scores of ≥ 5 (n = 28).
b IRE/NRE (n = 16) versus healthy (n = 13). One CE dog did not have a post-treatment serum sample.
c IRE (n = 34) versus healthy dogs (n = 139).
d IRE (n = 26) versus healthy dogs (n = 90).
e CE (n = 20) versus healthy dogs (n = 15).
f CE (n = 127). Follow-up in 12 dogs with IRE.
g Significant difference for dogs with canine IBD activity index scores of greater than 5 (n = 28), but not for all CE dogs included in the study (n = 58).
h CE classification: ARE (n = 7), FRE (n = 9), and IRE (N = 22).
Data from Refs. 6,17–19,25,41,59 .

Table 2
Difference in biomarkers concentration between dogs with different subgroups of CE

| Group 1 | vs | Group 2 | Ref | Serum | | | Fecal | |
				CRP	Calprotectin	S100A12	Calprotectin	S100A12
IRE (n = 14)		PLE (n = 12)	Heilmann[47,a]					Same
FRE (n = 18)		PLE (n = 18)	Equilino[27,b]	Lower	Same	Same		
ARE/FRE (n = 13)		IRE (n = 19)	Heilmann[25,c]	Lower	Same	Same	Same	Same
IRE (n = 12)		NRE (n = 5)	Heilmann[25,c]	Same			Same	
PLE-FRE (n = 23)		PLE-IRE/NRE (n = 10)	Nagata[31,d]	Lower				
ARE/FRE (n = 39)		IRE (n = 25)	Heilmann[48]					Lower
FRE/ARE/IRE (n = 51)		PLE (n = 13)	Heilmann[48]					Lower
IRE (n = 12)		NRE (n = 4)	Heilmann[48]					Lower

Abbreviations: NRE, nonresponsive enteropathy; PLE, protein-losing enteropathy.
[a] Groups comparison: IRE (n = 14) versus PLE (n = 12).
[b] Groups comparison PLE (n = 18) versus FRE (n = 18).
[c] CE (n = 127). Groups comparison: ARE/FRE (n = 13) versus IRE (n = 19) and IRE (n = 12) versus NRE (n = 5).
[d] Groups comparison: PLE-FRE (n = 23) versus PLE-IRE/NRE (n = 10).
Data from Refs. [25, 27, 47, 81].

dogs with IRE compared with dogs with FRE or ARE, and another study between dogs with protein-losing enteropathy (PLE) and FRE.[25,27] A serum CRP concentration of 9.1 mg/L or greater distinguished dogs with IRE from dogs with FRE or ARE with a sensitivity of 72% (95% confidence interval [CI]: 47–90) and a specificity of 100% (95% CI, 74–100).[25] With the current body of knowledge, CRP use to distinguish IRE dogs would be clinically very relevant, but further studies are required to confirm this result. There is limited support for the use of CRP as a biomarker for clinical outcome or histologic severity.

Alpha$_1$-Proteinase Inhibitor

α_1PI is a major proteinase inhibitor that is, primarily synthesized in the liver.[28] Canine α_1PI has a molecular weight similar to that of albumin and is expected to be lost into the intestinal lumen at approximately the same rate in dogs with PLE. Increased fecal canine α_1PI concentration is a useful clinical marker for gastrointestinal protein loss and histologic lesions seen with PLE in dogs.[29,30]

Because of relatively large day-to-day variation in fecal α_1PI concentrations, fecal samples should be collected over 3 consecutive days, and a 3-day mean fecal α_1PI concentration of 13.9 µg/g or greater or a 3-day maximum fecal α_1PI concentration of 21.0 µg/g or greater are interpreted as abnormal.[25,31] A 3-day mean fecal α_1PI concentration of 19.0 µg/g or greater is a good confirmatory test for histologic lesions of lacteal dilatation, crypt abscesses, or both.[29] Fecal α_1PI concentrations in dogs less than 1 year of age are significantly higher and should be verified at 1 year of age or older.[31] Fecal canine α_1PI seems to be particularly useful for early detection of gastrointestinal protein loss in Soft Coated Wheaten Terriers because it can precede the onset of clinical signs or hypoalbuminemia.[32]

Fecal Dysbiosis Index

AlShawaqfeh et al[33] have developed a fecal DI based on a mathematical model using quantitative polymerase chain reaction of 8 bacterial groups (ie, Blautia, Clostridium hiranonis, Escherichia coli, Faecalibacterium, Fusobacterium, Streptococcus, Turicibacter, and total bacteria) that are commonly altered in canine CE. DI with a threshold value of greater than 0 distinguishes dogs with CE from healthy dogs with 74% sensitivity (95% CI, 0.65–0.82) and 95% specificity (95% CI, 0.89–0.98).[33] This tool enables detection of fecal dysbiosis and return to eubiosis after treatment. An abnormal DI supports the presence of dysbiosis either as the primary cause for CE or as a consequence of CE; however, it does not imply the need for a specific treatment (eg, antibiotics). The reader is referred to the Anna-Lena Ziese and Jan. S. Suchodolski's article, "Impact of Changes in GI Microbiota in Canine and Feline Digestive Diseases," in this issue for more information about DI.

TESTS COMMERCIALLY AVAILABLE ON TISSUE BIOPSIES
Polymerase Chain Reaction for Antigen Receptor Rearrangement

PARR is a molecular diagnostic tool used to differentiate lymphoid malignancies from benign processes. As discussed in the Sina Marsilio's article, "Differentiating IBD from Alimentary Lymphoma in Cats: Does it Matter?," in this issue, the accuracy of this test to differentiate feline inflammatory bowel disease (IBD) from small cell intestinal lymphoma (SCIL) is currently subject to controversy. A recent study assessing PARR testing on canine formalin-fixed paraffin-embedded tissue suggested a 92% accuracy (95% CI, 81–98) to differentiate lymphoma from other causes of enteropathy among 89% of dogs passing the quality control testing.[34] However, false-positive results have also been reported in 4 of 35 dogs with CE.[35] Care needs to be taken in the interpretation of this study as cases of SCIL cannot be fully excluded in view of the short follow-up (10 weeks). Overall, this suggest that PARR testing may be more reliable in dogs than in cats, although more data are required to further support this finding.

Canine SCIL is reported with increased frequency, often in association with PLE.[5,36] Therefore, it is likely that PARR testing will be used more widely in dogs. As discussed for cats, this test should only be considered in cases where histology and immunohistochemistry are suggestive for SCIL to account for the risk of false-positive results until more studies are available. Diagnosing SCIL has therapeutic and prognostic implications, as demonstrated in dogs with PLE.[37] Dogs of different breeds diagnosed with SCIL are reported to have a median survival time of more than 1 year with appropriate chemotherapy in 2 retrospective studies, although a much shorter median survival time of 48 days has been reported in Shiba Inus with clonality.[5,36,38]

Fluorescence In Situ Hybridization

Fluorescence in situ hybridization is a very sensitive method to detect, identify and localize bacteria and other micro-organisms in formalin-fixed tissue. This technique has been very useful to study the role of *E coli* in granulomatous colitis of Boxer dogs.[39] This method can be useful in dogs and cats with neutrophilic or granulomatous enteritis. These inflammatory patterns raise concern for an underlying infectious etiology that might benefit from antibiotic treatment, whereas other treatments, especially immunosuppressants, would be contraindicated.

PROMISING BIOMARKERS CURRENTLY AVAILABLE ON A RESEARCH BASIS

The following tests have been validated in dogs and have been used in peer-reviewed clinical studies. However, they are not currently available commercially: calprotectin (CAL; serum and feces) and calgranulin C (serum and feces).

Calprotectin (Serum and Feces)

The S100 protein family belongs to the calcium-binding EF-hand protein superfamily; these proteins are mainly restricted to granulocytes and monocytes and include S100A8, S100A9, and S100A12.[40] Once released in the extracellular compartment, S100 proteins act as damage-associated molecular pattern molecules and promote innate immune response via Toll-like receptor 4. CAL is a heterodimer of S100A8 and S100A9 proteins and a nonspecific marker of acute or chronic inflammation mainly expressed by activated neutrophils, monocytes, and some epithelial cells.[41]

In dogs, CAL increases are not specific to intestinal diseases (similar to CRP) and have also been reported in dogs with sepsis and atopic dermatitis.[3,42] A radioimmunoassay has been validated and is available for research purposes to measure CAL both in serum and feces.[43]

Serum CAL was increased in dogs with IRE compared with healthy dogs in 1 study, but not in another one.[23,24] Serum CAL must be interpreted with caution in corticosteroid-treated dogs because the CAL concentration significantly increased in 1 study after treatment with prednisolone or combination of prednisolone and metronidazole despite clinical improvement.[24] CAL has not been shown to be useful in differentiating ARE from FRE or IRE dogs. As mentioned for serum CRP, the literature for serum CAL in dogs with CE is currently limited and serum CAL does not seem to correlate with clinical or histologic scores (**Table 3**).

Fecal CAL concentration is a good surrogate marker of disease severity in canine CE, with a cut-off value of about 50 μg/g of wet feces to identify dogs with severe

Table 3
Correlation of serum and fecal biomarkers with clinical score or histology score in dogs with CE

Correlation	With Clinical Score		With Histologic Score	
	Yes	No	Yes	No
CRP	Heilmann et al[25,a] (n = 127)	Allenspach et al[11] (n = 33) Otoni et al[23,b] (n = 16) McCann et al[26,c] (n = 16) Heilmann et al[24,d] (n = 34)		Allenspach et al[11] (n = 33) McCann et al[26,c] (n = 16) Otoni et al[23,b] (n = 16) Heilmann et al[25,a] (n = 127)
S-CAL		Heilmann et al[24,d] (n = 34) Otoni et al[23,b] (n = 16) Heilmann et al[25] (n = 127)		Otoni et al[23,b] (n = 16) Heilmann et al[24,d] (n = 34) Heilmann et al[48] (n = 16)
F-CAL	Otoni et al[23,b] (n = 16) Heilmann et al[25,a] (n = 127)			Otoni et al[23,b] (n = 16) Heilmann et al[25,a] (n = 127)
S-S100A12		Heilmann et al[25,a] (n = 127)		
F-S100A12	Heilmann et al[47,e] (n = 26)	Heilmann et al[25,a] (n = 127)		Heilmann et al[47,e] (n = 26) Heilmann et al[24,a] (n = 127)
sRAGE		Heilmann et al[67,f] (n = 20)		Heilmann et al[67,f] (n = 20)

Abbreviations: F-CAL, fecal calprotectin; F-S100A12, fecal S100A12; S-CAL, serum calprotectin; S-S100A12, serum S100A12.

a CE (n = 127). Follow-up in 32 dogs (steroid-responsive therapy/IRE n = 19, FRE/ARE n = 13). Low to moderate correlation between F-CAL or CRP and Canine Chronic Enteropathy Activity Index Score (rho = 0.27, P = .039 and rho = 0.42, P < .001). High correlation between overall cumulative inflammatory lesion score and F-CAL (rho = 0.52, P = .018).
b Correlation fecal CAL with pretreatment canine IBD activity index score rho = 0.60, P = .1.
c 2007; CE (n = 16).
d IRE (n = 34) versus healthy dogs (n = 139). Moderate correlation between F-S100A12 and CCECAI (rho = 0.48, P = .0408).
e IBD (n = 26) versus healthy dogs (n = 90).
f RAGE. CE (n = 20) versus healthy dogs (n = 15).
Data from Refs. 11, 23–26, 47, 48, 67.

clinical disease (Canine Chronic Enteropathy Activity Index Score of $\geq$12).[44] Fecal CAL concentration also seems to have usefulness in predicting the response to immunosuppressant in dogs with CE: a cut-off of 15.2 μg/g or greater distinguish partial responders or nonresponders from dogs that achieve complete clinical remission with a sensitivity of 80% (95% CI, 28–100) and a specificity of 75% (95% CI, 43–95).[25] Because fecal CAL has been shown to be an indicator of overall gastrointestinal health and can also be increased in acute gastrointestinal inflammatory conditions, the population of dogs tested with fecal CAL must be carefully selected to gain relevant information. The possibility of an effect of gastrointestinal neoplasia on fecal CAL concentrations remains to be determined.

Calgranulin C (Serum and Feces)

Calgranulin C (S100A12) is another damage-associated molecular pattern molecule that belongs also to the S100 protein family and has a cellular expression and distribution similar to CAL.[45(p12)] S100A12 seems to be mainly expressed by neutrophils in dogs as reported in humans. The S100A12 protein is a ligand of the pattern recognition receptors RAGE and Toll-like receptor 4 and plays a central role in the innate and acquired immune response.

No difference in serum S100A12 concentration has been reported between dogs with FRE or ARE versus IRE or between dogs with FRE and PLE. Furthermore, the serum S100A12 concentration in dogs with CE is very similar to the reference interval reported in healthy dogs: 206 μg/L (interquartile range, 144–328) with a reported reference interval of 49 to 320 μg/L. Finally, there was no correlation between S100A12 and clinical score or histology score in dogs with CE. In view of these results, serum S100A12 seems to be of little use in canine CE. In contrast with CAL, the serum S100A12 concentration is not affected by corticosteroid treatment.[46]

Fecal S100A12 concentration seems more useful as a biomarker of gastrointestinal inflammation. It is correlated with the severity of clinical signs and endoscopic lesions, but not with the severity of histopathologic changes.[47] A fecal S100A12 concentration of 490 ng/g or greater can differentiate dogs requiring anti-inflammatory or immunosuppressive treatment from dogs with FRE or ARE with a sensitivity of 64% (95% CI, 43%–81%) and a specificity of 77% (95% CI, 60%–88%).[48] Fecal S100A12 concentrations at the time of diagnosis 2700 ng/g or greater distinguished nonresponsive enteropathy dogs from dogs with partial or full response with a sensitivity of 100% (95% CI, 40%–100%) and a specificity of 76% (95% CI, 53%–91%).[48] The fecal S100A12 concentration can also increase with acute gastrointestinal inflammation; thus, patient selection for the use of this marker is important. The effect of gastrointestinal neoplasia on fecal S100A12 concentrations has not been investigated.

BIOMARKERS WITH LIMITED INFORMATION SUPPORTING CLINICAL USE
Perinuclear Antineutrophilic Cytoplasmic and Anti-Saccharomyces cerevisiae Antibodies

Useful serologic tests in dogs with CE include perinuclear antineutrophilic cytoplasmic antibodies (pANCA) and anti-Saccharomyces cerevisiae antibody titers. The percentage of pANCA seropositive dogs was significantly higher in FRE dogs than in IBD dogs (62% vs 23%) before treatment in 1 study.[49] The median titer was also higher in FRE dogs (1:100 in the FRE group vs <1:10 in the IBD group). Soft Coated Wheaten Terriers with PLE or protein-losing nephropathy also produce pANCA that can be detected more than 2 years prior hypoalbuminemia.[50] However, specificity is limited because pANCA seropositivity occurs with other immune-mediated, infectious or neoplastic diseases.[51,52] Reported sensitivity and specificity of pANCA to detect IRE dogs was 0.51 (95% CI, 0.35–0.67) and 0.83 (95% CI, 0.85–0.96), respectively.[53] In the same study, the sensitivity of anti-*Saccharomyces cerevisiae* antibody to detect IBD dogs was 0.44 (95% CI, 0.22–0.69).

Recently, Estruch and colleagues[54] detected IgA seropositivity (defined as serum level of IgA antibodies exceeding 2 standard deviations above the mean for the normal control serum level) to canine polymorphonuclear leukocytes, canine-isolated bacterial outer membrane porin, and flagellin, food-derived gliadins, and canine CAL in 70 dogs diagnosed with chronic inflammatory enteropathy. The results indicated that dogs were seropositive for polymorphonuclear leukocytes (77%), canine-isolated bacterial outer membrane porin (76%), gliadins (54%), canine CAL (43%), and flagellin (39%). For non-IBD control dogs, 52% displayed positive titers against gliadins, 13% of the cohort members tested positive for polymorphonuclear leukocytes, canine-isolated bacterial outer membrane porin, and ACNA, and none displayed seropositivity for flagellin. Furthermore, the overall mean levels of these selected markers in the patient cohort were higher than in the control cohorts.

Also, Hernandez's group evaluated serum anti-flagellin- and anti-lipopolysaccharide immunoglobulin levels (IgA and IgG) using an enzyme-linked immunosorbent assay adapted from the method described in humans and found significantly higher concentrations of anti-flagellin and anti-lipopolysaccharide IgGs in IBD dogs compared with control dogs[55] (J. Hernandez, personal communication, May 2020).

The clinical relevance of these antibodies as new serologic markers needs to be further assessed.

Serum Citrulline

Citrulline is a nondietary amino acid involved in intermediary metabolism produced almost exclusively by the enterocytes of the small intestinal mucosa. For this reason, plasma or serum citrulline concentrations have been proposed as a biomarker of small bowel mass and function.[56] In human medicine, a decreased plasma citrulline concentration correlates with a decreased enterocyte mass in short bowel syndrome, villous atrophy states, and during follow-up of patients after small bowel transplantation.[56] In veterinary medicine, variation of postprandial plasma citrulline concentration has been showed in healthy Beagles leading to the recommendation to withhold food for 8 to 12 hours before blood collection.[57] Parvovirus enteritis is associated with a severe decrease in plasma citrulline concentrations (median concentration of 2.8 μmol/L [range, 0.3–49.0 μmol/L] for survivors, of 2.1 μmol/L [range, 0.5–6.4 μmol/L] for nonsurvivors, and 38.6 μmol/L [range, 11.4–96.1 μmol/L] for healthy control dogs), but is of no prognostic value.[58]

Rossi and colleagues[59] observed increased plasma citrulline concentrations in IRE dogs treated with the probiotic VSL#3, suggesting an increase of global enterocyte functional mass.

Serum citrulline concentration failed to distinguish healthy dogs and dogs with CE or to stratify the different subtypes of CE including dogs with PLE. There is no correlation with the canine IBD activity index and no prognostic value reported.[60] Therefore, the use of serum citrulline cannot currently be recommended in canine CE.

3-Bromotyrosine

Serum 3-bromotyrosine (3-BrY) is a stable metabolite used as surrogate marker of eosinophils activation.[61] It is produced by eosinophil peroxidase that is released during eosinophils activation.

Significant increases in serum 3-BrY concentrations have been reported in dogs with pancreatitis, lymphoplasmacytic enteritis, and eosinophilic enteritis compared with healthy dogs.[61] However, there is a marked overlap between these groups, precluding the use of 3-BrY for differentiation. The serum concentration of 3-BrY has also been reported to be significantly increased in IRE dogs compared with FRE dogs or healthy dogs and in FRE dogs compared with healthy dogs.[62] It was neither correlated with the peripheral eosinophil count nor the Canine Chronic Enteropathy Activity Index Score.[61,62] The current information does not suggest that serum 3-BrY will be a good biomarker to differentiate between different CE etiologies in view of the marked overlap between dogs with different diseases. There is currently no information about its use as a prognostic marker.

An assay to measure 3-BrY concentrations in canine fecal samples was recently validated.[63] The 3-day mean and the 3-day maximum fecal 3-BrY concentration for the dogs with CE was significantly higher than that for the healthy control dogs. Further investigations with more precise disease subclassification (FRE, ARE, and IRE) are needed to determine the clinical relevance of fecal 3-BrY concentration.

Soluble Advanced Glycation End Product Receptor

Advanced glycation end products (AGEs) are reactive derivatives from protein, lipids, and nucleic acids formed after they exposure to reducing sugars (nonenzymatic reaction). Oxidative stress is produced by AGEs binding to their receptor (RAGE) that in turn promotes inflammation and thrombogenic reactions.[64] Soluble RAGE (sRAGE) consists of the extracellular portion of RAGE and acts as a decoy protein that can bind to AGE and prevent RAGE activation. Another ligand of sRAGE is S100A12. Variations of serum concentrations of sRAGE are subject to controversy in people with ulcerative.[65,66]

Only 1 study has evaluated sRAGE in dogs with IRE.[67] The authors found a lower sRAGE concentrations in IRE dogs than control dogs, but no correlation between sRAGE and canine IBD activity index or histologic score. Further studies are needed to better assess the use of sRAGE in canine CE.

Cytokine Concentrations

Cytokines are glycoproteins that are released by immune cells and activated cells in various tissues. They are often divided into T-helper 1 cytokines (such as tumor necrosis factor [TNF]α and IL-2), and (IFNγ), or T-helper 2 cytokines (such as IL-4 and IL-6) and anti-inflammatory cytokines (such as IL-10 and TNFβ).[68] No clear polarization into T-helper 1 or T-helper 2 response has been shown in canine CE compared with IBD in people.[69] Although several studies have looked at cytokine production in the intestinal mucosa, as reviewed elsewhere, there is little information of the role of serum cytokines as biomarkers in dogs with CE.[70]

The IL-6 concentration was increased in serum from people with ulcerative colitis (UC) or Crohn's disease compared with healthy controls.[71,72] Furthermore, IL-6 correlated with the clinical activity index in patients with UC. More recently, IL-9 has been shown to be increased in patients with UC or Crohn's disease with a strong correlation between IL-9 and endoscopic mucosal healing in UC.[73] Contradictory findings are available for TNFα, with some studies reporting a correlation with disease activity, whereas other report no TNFα detectable.[72,74,75]

Little information is available on basal cytokine serum concentrations in canine CE. In 1 study, no TNFα was detected in 12 dogs with IRE.[26] More recently, a significant increase in IL-2, IL-6, and TNFα, but not IL-8 was reported in dogs with CE at diagnosis (n = 68) compared with healthy dogs (n = 25).[76]

Similar to people, a decrease in the IL-6 concentration and an increase in IL-10 has been reported after treatment of dogs with IRE with immunomodulators (beta-1,3/1,6-D-glucan, beta-hydroxy-beta-methyl butyrate or levamisole) for 6 weeks.[77] A significant reduction in IL-6 with successful treatment in 8 dogs with CE (4 dogs with FRE, 3 with ARE, and 1 with IRE) was also noted in a pilot study in one of the authors' institution, whereas the reduction was not significant for IL-2 and TNFα.[78]

Recently, an assay was validated to measure serum-soluble CD25 as a marker of T-cell activation.[79] The study included 15 dogs diagnosed with CE and histologic evidence of intestinal inflammation. Fourteen dogs had normal CD25 concentration, which suggests limited use of CD25 in canine CE, although more work is required to further assess the usefulness of the assay.

Basal cytokine concentrations can be markedly elevated in healthy people and we have found similar results in our pilot study with concentrations of up to 8000 pg/mL in healthy dogs.[80] For this reason, cytokine concentrations should be interpreted in conjunction with the clinical signs and not used a sole diagnostic or therapeutic test. Cytokines might be more useful for monitoring a disease over time rather than at single time points.

There is currently not enough information to assess the usefulness of serum cytokine concentrations as biomarkers for canine CE. Larger cohorts of healthy dogs and dogs with CE assessed before treatment and after remission are necessary to further evaluate the biological variability of serum cytokines.

SUMMARY

In current practice, several laboratory tests can be useful during the diagnostic process to confirm the origin of the disease (intestinal protein loss with α_1PI, involvement of different part of the small intestine with cobalamin, folate) or to point to the underlying etiology (fluorescence in situ hybridization and PARR). Distinction between different subtypes of CE remains elusive with contradictory results between different studies (CRP, α_1PI, fecal S100A12, and pANCA). Other tests are of prognostic interest and might play a role in predicting response to treatment (CRP, cobalamin, fecal CAL, and fecal S100A12). Finally, some tests might be useful to monitor therapeutic response (CRP and MMA after cobalamin supplementation).

Overall, fecal tests seem to be more powerful in distinguishing the different subtypes of CE and guiding therapeutic choices, but studies on larger cohorts of dogs are required to obtain more meaningful data. Both in veterinary and human medicine, the evaluation and development of markers remain a real challenge. It is likely that panels of biomarkers will be required to increase the yield of each test.

DISCLOSURE

The authors have nothing to disclose.

CLINICS CARE POINTS

- If a dog is deficient in cobalamin, measurements of methylmalonic acid can be useful to confirm cobalamin deficiency at the cellular level.
- Oral or parenteral cobalamin supplementation is recommended in dogs diagnosed with hypocobalaminaemia.
- There are currently no validated biomarkers to predict treatment response in dogs with CE.

REFERENCES

1. Dandrieux JRS. Inflammatory bowel disease versus chronic enteropathy in dogs: are they one and the same? J Small Anim Pract 2016;57(11):589–99.
2. Biomarkers Definitions Working G. Biomarkers and surrogate endpoints: preferred definitions and conceptual framework. Clin Pharmacol Ther 2001;69: 89–95.
3. Heilmann RM, Steiner JM. Clinical utility of currently available biomarkers in inflammatory enteropathies of dogs. J Vet Intern Med 2018;32(5):1495–508.
4. Kather S, Grützner N, Kook PH, et al. Review of cobalamin status and disorders of cobalamin metabolism in dogs. J Vet Intern Med 2020;34(1):13–28.
5. Lane J, Price J, Moore A, et al. Low-grade gastrointestinal lymphoma in dogs: 20 cases (2010 to 2016). J Small Anim Pr 2017;59(3):147–53.
6. Fyfe JC, Hemker SL, Venta PJ, et al. Selective intestinal cobalamin malabsorption with proteinuria (Imerslund-Gräsbeck Syndrome) in juvenile beagles. J Vet Intern Med 2014;28(2):356–62.
7. Owczarek-Lipska M, Jagannathan V, Drögemüller C, et al. A Frameshift Mutation in the Cubilin Gene (CUBN) in border collies with Imerslund-Gräsbeck Syndrome (Selective Cobalamin Malabsorption). PLoS One 2013;8(4):e61144.
8. He Q, Madsen M, Kilkenney A, et al. Amnionless function is required for cubilin brush-border expression and intrinsic factor-cobalamin (vitamin B12) absorption in vivo. Blood 2005;106:1447–53.
9. Gold AJ, Scott MA, Fyfe JC. Failure to thrive and life-threatening complications due to inherited selective cobalamin malabsorption effectively managed in a juvenile Australian shepherd dog. Can Vet J 2015;56(10):1029–34.
10. Berghoff N, Parnell NK, Hill SL, et al. Serum cobalamin and methylmalonic acid concentrations in dogs with chronic gastrointestinal disease. Am J Vet Res 2013;74(1):84–9.
11. Allenspach K, Wieland B, Grone A, et al. Chronic enteropathies in dogs: evaluation of risk factors for negative outcome. J Vet Intern Med 2007;21:700–8.
12. Batchelor DJ, Noble PJ, Taylor RH, et al. Prognostic factors in canine exocrine pancreatic insufficiency: prolonged survival is likely if clinical remission is achieved. J Vet Intern Med 2007;21:54–60.
13. Soetart N, Rochel D, Drut A, et al. Serum cobalamin and folate as prognostic factors in canine exocrine pancreatic insufficiency: an observational cohort study of 299 dogs. Vet J 2019;243:15–20.
14. Volkmann M, Steiner JM, Fosgate GT, et al. Chronic diarrhea in Dogs – retrospective study in 136 cases. J Vet Intern Med 2017;31(4):1043–55.
15. Rhodes B, Fürnrohr BG, Vyse TJ. C-reactive protein in rheumatology: biology and genetics. Nat Rev Rheumatol 2011;7(5):282–9.
16. Nakamura M, Takahashi M, Ohno K, et al. C-reactive protein concentration in dogs with various diseases. J Vet Med Sci 2008;70(2):127–31.
17. Muñoz-Prieto A, Tvarijonaviciute A, Escribano D, et al. Use of heterologous immunoassays for quantification of serum proteins: the case of canine C-reactive protein. PLoS ONE 2017;12(2).
18. Carney PC, Ruaux CG, Suchodolski JS, et al. Biological variability of c-reactive protein and specific canine pancreatic lipase immunoreactivity in apparently healthy dogs: variability of CRP and spec cPL. J Vet Intern Med 2011;25(4): 825–30.

19. Lowrie M, Penderis J, Eckersall PD, et al. The role of acute phase proteins in diagnosis and management of steroid-responsive meningitis arteritis in dogs. Vet J 2009;182(1):125–30.

20. Ohno K, Yokoyama Y, Nakashima K, et al. C-Reactive Protein Concentration in Canine Idiopathic Polyarthritis. J Vet Med Sci 2006;68(12):1275–9.

21. Viitanen SJ, Lappalainen AK, Christensen MB, et al. The utility of acute-phase proteins in the assessment of treatment response in dogs with bacterial pneumonia. J Vet Intern Med 2017;31(1):124–33.

22. Jergens AE, Schreiner CA, Frank DE, et al. A scoring index for disease activity in canine inflammatory bowel disease. J Vet Intern Med 2003;17:291–7.

23. Otoni CC, Heilmann RM, García-Sancho M, et al. Serologic and fecal markers to predict response to induction therapy in dogs with idiopathic inflammatory bowel disease. J Vet Intern Med 2018;32(3):999–1008.

24. Heilmann RM, Jergens AE, Ackermann MR, et al. Serum calprotectin concentrations in dogs with idiopathic inflammatory bowel disease. Am J Vet Res 2012;73: 1900–7.

25. Heilmann RM, Berghoff N, Mansell J, et al. Association of fecal calprotectin concentrations with disease severity, response to treatment, and other biomarkers in dogs with chronic inflammatory enteropathies. J Vet Intern Med 2018;32(2): 679–92.

26. McCann TM, Ridyard AE, Else RW, et al. Evaluation of disease activity markers in dogs with idiopathic inflammatory bowel disease. J Small Anim Pract 2007; 48(11):620–5.

27. Equilino M, Theodoloz V, Gorgas D, et al. Evaluation of serum biochemical marker concentrations and survival time in dogs with protein-losing enteropathy. J Am Vet Med Assoc 2015;246:91–9.

28. Travis J. Structure, function, and control of neutrophil proteinases. Am J Med 1988;84(6):37–42.

29. Heilmann RM, Parnell NK, Grützner N, et al. Serum and fecal canine α1-proteinase inhibitor concentrations reflect the severity of intestinal crypt abscesses and/ or lacteal dilation in dogs. Vet J 2016;207:131–9.

30. Murphy KF, German AJ, Ruaux CG, et al. Fecal alpha1-proteinase inhibitor concentration in dogs with chronic gastrointestinal disease. Vet Clin Pathol 2003; 32(2):67–72.

31. Heilmann RM, Paddock CG, Ruhnke I, et al. Development and analytical validation of a radioimmunoassay for the measurement of alpha1-proteinase inhibitor concentrations in feces from healthy puppies and adult dogs. J Vet Diagn Invest 2011;23(3):476–85.

32. Vaden SL, Vidaurri A, Levine JF, et al. Fecal alpha1-proteinase inhibitor activity in soft coated wheaten Terriers. J Vet Intern Med 2002;16(3):382.

33. AlShawaqfeh MK, Wajid B, Minamoto Y, et al. A dysbiosis index to assess microbial changes in fecal samples of dogs with chronic inflammatory enteropathy. FEMS Microbiol Ecol 2017;93(11).

34. Ehrhart EJ, Wong S, Richter K, et al. Polymerase chain reaction for antigen receptor rearrangement: benchmarking performance of a lymphoid clonality assay in diverse canine sample types. J Vet Intern Med 2019;33(3):1392–402.

35. Luckschander-Zeller N, Hammer SE, Ruetgen BC, et al. Clonality testing as complementary tool in the assessment of different patient groups with canine chronic enteropathy. Vet Immunol Immunopathol 2019;214:109893.

36. Couto KM, Moore PF, Zwingenberger AL, et al. Clinical characteristics and outcome in dogs with small cell T-cell intestinal lymphoma. Vet Comp Oncol 2018;16(3):337–43.

37. Nakashima K, Hiyoshi S, Ohno K, et al. Prognostic factors in dogs with protein-losing enteropathy. Vet J 2015;205:28–32.

38. Ohmi A, Ohno K, Uchida K, et al. Significance of clonal rearrangements of lymphocyte antigen receptor genes on the prognosis of chronic enteropathy in 22 Shiba dogs. J Vet Med Sci 2017;79(9):1578–84.

39. Mansfield CS, James FE, Craven M, et al. Remission of histiocytic ulcerative colitis in boxer dogs correlates with eradication of invasive intramucosal Escherichia coli. J Vet Intern Med 2009;23(5):964–9.

40. Holzinger D, Foell D, Kessel C. The role of S100 proteins in the pathogenesis and monitoring of autoinflammatory diseases. Mol Cell Pediatr 2018;5:7.

41. Striz I, Trebichavsky I. Calprotectin - a pleiotropic molecule in acute and chronic inflammation. Physiol Res 2004;53:245–53.

42. Chung T-H, Oh J-S, Lee Y-S, et al. Elevated serum levels of S100 calcium binding protein A8 (S100A8) reflect disease severity in canine atopic dermatitis. J Vet Med Sci 2010;72(6):693–700.

43. Heilmann RM, Suchodolski JS, Steiner JM. Development and analytic validation of a radioimmunoassay for the quantification of canine calprotectin in serum and feces from dogs. Am J Vet Res 2008;69(7):845–53.

44. Grellet A, Heilmann RM, Lecoindre P, et al. Fecal calprotectin concentrations in adult dogs with chronic diarrhea. Am J Vet Res 2013;74(5):706–11.

45. Heilmann RM, Suchodolski JS, Steiner JM. Purification and partial characterization of canine S100A12. Biochimie 2010;92(12):1914–22.

46. Heilmann RM, Cranford SM, Ambrus A, et al. Validation of an enzyme-linked immunosorbent assay (ELISA) for the measurement of canine S100A12. Vet Clin Pathol 2016;45(1):135–47.

47. Heilmann RM, Grellet A, Allenspach K, et al. Association between fecal S100A12 concentration and histologic, endoscopic, and clinical disease severity in dogs with idiopathic inflammatory bowel disease. Vet Immunol Immunopathol 2014; 158(3–4):156–66.

48. Heilmann RM, Volkmann M, Otoni CC, et al. Fecal S100A12 concentration predicts a lack of response to treatment in dogs affected with chronic enteropathy. Vet J 2016;215:96–100.

49. Luckschander N, Allenspach K, Hall J, et al. Perinuclear antineutrophilic cytoplasmic antibody and response to treatment in diarrheic dogs with food responsive disease or inflammatory bowel disease. J Vet Intern Med 2006;20(2):221.

50. Allenspach K, Lomas B, Wieland B, et al. Evaluation of perinuclear antineutrophilic cytoplasmic autoantibodies as an early marker of protein-losing enteropathy and protein-losing nephropathy in Soft Coated Wheaten Terriers. Am J Vet Res 2008;69(10):1301–4.

51. Mancho C, Sainz A, Garcia-Sancho M, et al. Evaluation of perinuclear antineutrophilic cytoplasmic antibodies in sera from dogs with inflammatory bowel disease or intestinal lymphoma. Am J Vet Res 2011;72:1333–7.

52. Karagianni AE, Solano-Gallego L, Breitschwerdt EB, et al. Perinuclear antineutrophil cytoplasmic autoantibodies in dogs infected with various vector-borne pathogens and in dogs with immune-mediated hemolytic anemia. Am J Vet Res 2012; 73(9):1403–9.

53. Allenspach K, Luckschander N, Styner M, et al. Evaluation of assays for perinuclear antineutrophilic cytoplasmic antibodies and antibodies to Saccharomyces

cerevisiae in dogs with inflammatory bowel disease. Am J Vet Res 2004;65(9): 1279–83.

54. Estruch JJ, Barken D, Bennett N, et al. Evaluation of novel serological markers and autoantibodies in dogs with inflammatory bowel disease. J Vet Intern Med 2020;34(3):1177–86.

55. Ziegler TR, Luo M, Estívariz CF, et al. Detectable serum flagellin and lipopolysaccharide and upregulated anti-flagellin and lipopolysaccharide immunoglobulins in human short bowel syndrome. Am J Physiol Regul Integr Comp Physiol 2008;294(2):R402–10.

56. Crenn P, Messing B, Cynober L. Citrulline as a biomarker of intestinal failure due to enterocyte mass reduction. Clin Nutr 2008;27(3):328–39.

57. Dahan JM, Giron C, Concordet D, et al. Circadian and postprandial variation in plasma citrulline concentration in healthy dogs. Am J Vet Res 2016;77(3):288–93.

58. Dossin O, Rupassara SI, Weng H-Y, et al. Effect of parvoviral enteritis on plasma citrulline concentration in dogs: plasma citrulline and enteritis. J Vet Intern Med 2011;25(2):215–21.

59. Rossi G, Pengo G, Caldin M, et al. Comparison of microbiological, histological, and immunomodulatory parameters in response to treatment with either combination therapy with prednisone and metronidazole or probiotic VSL#3 strains in dogs with idiopathic inflammatory bowel disease. PLoS One 2014;9(4):e94699.

60. Gerou-Ferriani M, Allen R, Noble P-JM, et al. Determining optimal therapy of dogs with chronic enteropathy by measurement of serum citrulline. J Vet Intern Med 2018;32(3):993–8.

61. Sattasathuchana P, Grützner N, Lopes R, et al. Stability of 3-bromotyrosine in serum and serum 3-bromotyrosine concentrations in dogs with gastrointestinal diseases. BMC Vet Res 2015;11:5.

62. Sattasathuchana P, Allenspach K, Lopes R, et al. Evaluation of serum 3-bromotyrosine concentrations in dogs with steroid-responsive diarrhea and food-responsive diarrhea. J Vet Intern Med 2017;31(4):1056–61.

63. Sattasathuchana P, Thengchaisri N, Suchodolski JS, et al. Analytical validation of fecal 3-bromotyrosine concentrations in healthy dogs and dogs with chronic enteropathy. J Vet Diagn Invest 2019;31(3):434–9.

64. Yamagishi S. Soluble form of a receptor for advanced glycation end products sRAGE as a biomarker. Front Biosci 2010;E2(4):1184–95.

65. Malíčková K, Kalousová M, Fučíková T, et al. Anti-inflammatory effect of biological treatment in patients with inflammatory bowel diseases: calprotectin and IL-6 changes do not correspond to sRAGE changes. Scand J Clin Lab Invest 2010; 70(4):294–9.

66. Ciccocioppo R, Imbesi V, Betti E, et al. The circulating level of soluble receptor for advanced glycation end products displays different patterns in ulcerative colitis and Crohn's disease: a cross-sectional study. Dig Dis Sci 2015;60(8):2327–37.

67. Heilmann RM, Otoni CC, Jergens AE, et al. Systemic levels of the anti-inflammatory decoy receptor soluble RAGE (receptor for advanced glycation end products) are decreased in dogs with inflammatory bowel disease. Vet Immunol Immunopathol 2014;161(3–4):184–92.

68. Pucheu-Haston CM, Bizikova P, Marsella R, et al. Review: lymphocytes, cytokines, chemokines and the T-helper 1-T-helper 2 balance in canine atopic dermatitis. Vet Dermatol 2015;26. 124-e32.

69. Heilmann RM, Suchodolski JS. Is inflammatory bowel disease in dogs and cats associated with a Th1 or Th2 polarization? Vet Immunol Immunopathol 2015; 168(3–4):131–4.

70. Kołodziejska-Sawerska A, Rychlik A, Depta A, et al. Cytokines in canine inflammatory bowel disease. Pol J Vet Sci 2013;16(1):165–71.
71. Aleksandra Nielsen A, Nederby Nielsen J, Schmedes A, et al. Saliva Interleukin-6 in patients with inflammatory bowel disease. Scand J Gastroenterol 2005;40(12): 1444–8.
72. Gustot T, Lemmers A, Louis E, et al. Profile of soluble cytokine receptors in Crohn's disease. Gut 2005;54(4):488–95.
73. Matusiewicz M, Neubauer K, Bednarz-Misa I, et al. Systemic interleukin-9 in inflammatory bowel disease: association with mucosal healing in ulcerative colitis. World J Gastroenterol 2017;23(22):4039–46.
74. Gardiner KR, Halliday MI, Barclay GR, et al. Significance of systemic endotoxaemia in inflammatory bowel disease. Gut 1995;36(6):897–901.
75. Nielsen O. Established and emerging biological activity markers of inflammatory bowel disease. Am J Gastroenterol 2000;95(2):359–67.
76. Buono A, Minamoto T, Minamoto Y, et al. Serum IL-2, IL-6, IL-8, and TNF-α concentrations in dogs with chronic enteropathies. J Vet Intern Med 2018;32(6): 2144–309.
77. Rychlik A, Nieradka R, Kander M, et al. The effectiveness of natural and synthetic immunomodulators in the treatment of inflammatory bowel disease in dogs. Acta Vet Hung 2013;61:297–308.
78. Dandrieux JRS, Santos L, Martinez Lopez LM, et al. Serum cytokines before and after treatment in a cohort of dogs with chronic enteropathy. J Vet Intern Med 2019;33(5):2375–547.
79. Buono A, Lidbury JA, Wood C, et al. Development, analytical validation, and initial clinical evaluation of a radioimmunoassay for the measurement of soluble CD25 concentrations in canine serum. Vet Immunol Immunopathol 2019;215:109901.
80. Karlsson I, Hagman R, Johannisson A, et al. Multiplex cytokine analyses in dogs with pyometra suggest involvement of KC-like chemokine in canine bacterial sepsis. Vet Immunol Immunopathol 2016;170:41–6.
81. Nagata N, et al. Clinical characteristics of dogs with food-responsive protein-losing enteropathy. J. Vet. Intern. Med 2020 Mar;34(2):659–68. https://doi.org/10.1111/jvim.15720.

Impact of Changes in Gastrointestinal Microbiota in Canine and Feline Digestive Diseases

Anna-Lena Ziese, Dr med vet[a], Jan S. Suchodolski, Dr med vet, PhD[b],*

KEYWORDS

- Microbiome • Dysbiosis • Dysbiosis index • Bile acids • SCFA
- Chronic enteropathy • AHDS • *Clostridium hiranonis*

KEY POINTS

- The microbiome is a complex immune and metabolic organ that protects the host against pathogens, promotes the intestinal barrier, and provides nutrients to the host.
- Depending on the type of dysbiosis, luminal versus mucosa-adherent, different therapeutic approaches should be considered, with dietary modulation as the primary step.
- Although antibiotics may improve clinical signs in a subset of patients with gastrointestinal disease, they may cause long-term negative alterations of the intestinal microbiota and should not be used as first-line treatment.

INTRODUCTION

The intestinal microbiota is the collection of all microorganisms in the gastrointestinal tract (GIT) (ie, bacteria, viruses, fungi, and protozoa), whereas the intestinal microbiome is the collective genome of these microorganisms. More than 100 trillion microbial cells inhabit the GIT, outnumbering the host cells approximately 10-fold.[1]

Microbiome in Health

Bacteria make up most microbial cells and show increasing abundance from the stomach to the colon.[2] Culture-based studies showed concentrations of 10^1 to 10^6 colony forming units (CFU) per gram in the stomach, 10^2 to 10^6 CFU/g in the small intestine, and 10^{11} CFU/g in the colon.[3] The small intestine harbors aerobic and facultative anaerobes, whereas the colonic microbiome consists mainly of anaerobes.[4]

[a] Clinic of Small Animal Medicine, Ludwig Maximilian University of Munich, Veterinärstrasse 13, Munich 80539, Germany; [b] Gastrointestinal Laboratory, College of Veterinary Medicine, Texas A&M University, 4474 TAMU, College Station, TX 77845, USA
* Corresponding author.
E-mail address: jsuchodolski@cvm.tamu.edu

Vet Clin Small Anim 51 (2021) 155–169
https://doi.org/10.1016/j.cvsm.2020.09.004
0195-5616/21/© 2020 The Authors. Published by Elsevier Inc. This is an open access article under the CC BY-NC-ND license (http://creativecommons.org/licenses/by-nc-nd/4.0/).

The predominant phyla in the GIT of healthy cats and dogs are Firmicutes, Bacteroidetes, Actinobacteria, and Fusobacteria.[4,5] Every animal shows an individual microbial profile, characterized by individual proportions of bacterial species and strains.[4,5] Nevertheless, the microbial gene content is conserved, resulting in comparable microbial function across individuals.[6] The intestinal epithelium is covered by a mucus layer that acts as an important barrier between the luminal content and the epithelial wall. Bacteria can be found in the intestinal lumen or be mucosa adherent on the surface or crypts and, therefore, have direct contact to intestinal cells.[7]

The intestinal microbiome is a metabolic organ and participates in a variety of different pathways. A balanced microbiome promotes host health; however, imbalances in some of these pathways may lead to deleterious effects (**Table 1**). The microbiome plays a role in the development of the GIT, modulates the immune system, protects the host from pathogens, helps in intestinal barrier function, and provides beneficial metabolites.[8] Examples for important microbial pathways are bile acid (BA), short-chain fatty acid (SCFA), and indole metabolism.

Recent research has shown that particularly intestinal BAs and the BA 7α-dehydroxylating bacterium *Clostridium hiranonis* seem to play a major role in host health and maintaining a normal microbiota in dogs.[9–11] Primary BAs, cholic acid and chenodeoxycholic acid, are synthetized in the liver from cholesterol and conjugated with either taurine or glycine. They are stored in the gallbladder until released into the small intestine after a meal to enable lipid digestion. Reabsorption of BA through the apical sodium-BA transporter takes place in the terminal ileum, where BA enter enterohepatic cycle.[12] The small amount of primary BAs that subsequently reach the colon is converted by 7α-dehydroxylation to secondary BAs, such as deoxycholic acid and lithocholic acid, which is why secondary BAs occur physiologically at a higher concentrations in the colon than primary BAs.[13] In dogs, *C hiranonis* is the main BA-converting bacterial species.[13,14] Secondary BAs have different effects on the host. They bind to the transmembrane G protein-coupled bile acid receptor GPBAR-1, also known as TGR5 as signaling molecules, and have antiinflammatory properties.[15] They have a glucose level–lowering effect by binding to the farnesoid X receptor. Because the abundance of *C hiranonis* is often depleted in dogs with, chronic enteropathies, and with antibiotic-induced dysbiosis, these dogs have a decreased proportion of secondary BAs in the colon.[14,16,17] Fecal microbiota transplant (FMT) can restore *C hiranonis*, leading to proper conversion of primary to secondary BAs and normalization of the microbiota.[14] In contrast, broad-spectrum antibiotics such as tylosin or metronidazole lead to reduction of *C hiranonis* and therefore reduction in secondary BA conversion, and lack of these leads to long-lasting subclinical dysbiosis in some dogs[11,14,17] (**Fig. 1**).

Other important metabolic pathways involve SCFA and indoles. Some bacteria, such as *Ruminococcus*, *Faecalibacterium*, and *Turicibacter*, ferment dietary carbohydrates to SCFAs.[18] Those SCFAs, mainly butyrate, acetate, and propionate, act as nutrients, regulate satiety, have antiinflammatory properties, regulate intestinal motility, and downregulate the intestinal pH to create an environment that is not suitable for pH-sensitive enteropathogens.[8,19] Indole compounds, metabolized by intestinal bacteria from the essential amino acid tryptophan, improve gut permeability and increase mucin production.[20] Other examples of microbial-derived metabolites are B vitamins and vitamin K.

A healthy microbiome contributes to an intact intestinal barrier, because it promotes tight junction formation, preventing translocation of pathogens, toxins, or dietary antigens.[21] Some bacteria produce antimicrobials that can directly kill enteropathogens.[22] Indirect mechanisms, such as competition for nutrients or receptor sites,

Table 1
Examples of beneficial and deleterious metabolic pathways carried out by the intestinal microbiome and their effects on the host

Source	Bacterial Groups Involved	Derived Metabolites	Consequence for Host	
			Beneficial (In Normal Concentrations)	Potentially Deleterious (In Abnormal Concentrations)
Dietary carbohydrates	Various (Faecalibacterium, Ruminococcus, Bacteroides, Blautia)	Fermentation to SCFAs such as butyrate, acetate, propionate	Antiinflammatory Maintain intestinal barrier function Regulate motility Energy source systemic and local for epithelial cells	Depending on the SCFA ratio and intestinal site, they activate virulence factors of enteropathogens (eg, type III secretion system of Salmonella)
Primary bile acids from liver	Mostly Clostridium hiranonis in dogs and cats	Transformation to secondary BAs in colon	Antiinflammatory in various organ systems Secondary BAs inhibit the growth of Clostridium difficile, Clostridium perfringens, Escherichia coli Modulate glucose/insulin secretion from pancreas	In chronic enteropathies, mostly increase in primary BAs, can lead to secretory BA diarrhea; dysbiosis is associated with decrease in secondary BAs (caused by lack of C hiranonis) In humans, fat-rich diets increase secondary BAs in colon, which is associated with colon cancer
Dietary fat	Various (eg, C perfringens, Bifidobacterium bifidum, Propionibacterium)	Conversion to hydroxystearic acids	—	In high concentration causes fatty acid diarrhea
Dietary amino acid tryptophan	Various	Various indole metabolites	Antiinflammatory Maintain intestinal barrier function	In increased concentrations cytotoxic, putrefactive Indoxyl sulfate acts as uremic toxin
Dietary amino acids tyrosine and phenylalanine	Various	P-cresol	—	Acts as uremic toxin and leads to progression of chronic kidney disease
Drug mycophenolate mofetil	Various	MPA acyl glucuronide	—	Produces proinflammatory cytokines and causes diarrhea

Abbreviations: BAs, bile acids; MPA, mycophenolic acid; SCFAs, short-chain fatty acids.

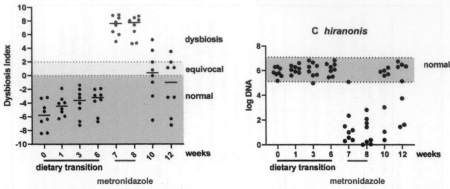

Fig. 1. Effect of diet and metronidazole on intestinal microbiome in healthy dogs. Diet (hydrolyzed protein diet) has only a minor effect on intestinal microbiota as assessed by the quantitative polymerase chain reaction–based dysbiosis index (*left*) and abundance of the primary to secondary BA-converting bacterium *C hiranonis* (*right*). In contrast, metronidazole treatment induces significant dysbiosis and reduction of *C hiranonis*, which is associated with improper BA conversion. One month after metronidazole cessation, some dogs did not recover their proper microbiome composition (week 12). This is 1 potential explanation for why a subset of clinically healthy dogs lack the important beneficial bacterium *C hiranonis*. Data based on Pilla and colleagues.[11]

modulating the immune system, or producing metabolites such as SCFAs, can also prevent growth of pathogens.[23] Modulation of the immune system occurs through contact between host cells (eg, dendritic cells or Toll-like receptors) and microbes or through microbial metabolites (eg, indole, SCFAs, and BAs).[23]

Microbiome in Disease

Table 2 summarizes the different types of dysbiosis, which often overlap in the same patients, especially those with chronic enteropathies. Understanding the

Table 2
Dysbiosis patterns and their consequences

Major Types of Dysbiosis	Possible Consequences
Abnormal substrate in intestinal lumen (eg, undigested nutrients, medications)	Increase in microbial metabolites causing osmotic/secretory diarrhea (eg, metabolites of mycophenolate mofetil, conversion of fatty acids to hydroxystearic acids)
Loss of microbiota function caused by loss of beneficial commensal bacteria (eg, *C hiranonis*)	No conversion from primary to secondary BAs leads to promotion of pathogenic invasion and increase in *C difficile*, *C perfringens*, *E coli* Lack of antiinflammatory microbial-derived metabolites
Increase in total bacterial load, especially in small intestine	Increased production of microbial metabolites causing osmotic/secretory diarrhea Increased inflammatory immune response
Increased mucosa-adherent and/or invasive bacteria	Increased attachment of bacteria to intestinal mucosa causes increased inflammatory immune response

pathophysiology of the various dysbiosis patterns can lead to a more rational treatment approach. Dysbiosis can appear as changes in luminal or mucosa-adherent bacterial species and/or amounts, and as impaired microbiota function, resulting in altered microbial metabolic pathways compared with a healthy state. There are various reasons why dysbiosis develops (**Box 1**), and the consequences of dysbiosis can be diverse. Alterations in the microbiota can cause a disruption of the intestinal barrier, leading to higher susceptibility for translocation of pathogens, toxins, or dietary antigens. Moreover, the immune system can be affected, which in turn promotes proinflammatory processes.[24] Levels of bacterial metabolites can either increase or decrease and, depending on their physiologic role, this may affect host health (see **Table 1**). Within BA metabolism, the inability of the dysbiotic microbiota (ie, decrease in *C hiranonis*) to convert primary into secondary BAs results in increased concentrations of primary BAs in the colon, which was shown to cause secretory diarrhea in humans.[25] In humans with *Clostridium difficile* infection, increased primary BA levels were shown to promote germination of *C difficile* spores.[26] Studies in humans also reported associations between dysbiosis-induced altered metabolic pathways and different systemic diseases, such as diabetes mellitus type 2, asthma, and obesity.[27,28]

Most cats and dogs with gastrointestinal (GI) disease have concurrent intestinal dysbiosis.[5,10] Although the patterns of dysbiosis generally differ between acute and chronic diseases, there are some similarities across all conditions. In most cases it remains unclear whether the dysbiosis is a cause or a secondary effect of the underlying

---

Box 1
Conditions that may lead to Intestinal dysbiosis

Anatomic abnormalities
  Blind loops
  Small bowel strictures or adhesions
  Surgical resection of the ileocolic valve
  Neoplasia
  Foreign bodies

Motility disorders
  Hypothyroidism
  Diabetic autonomic neuropathy
  Scleroderma
  Abnormal migrating motor complexes

Decreased gastric acid output
  Atrophic gastritis
  Administration of acid suppressing drugs (H_2-blockers, omeprazole)

Exocrine pancreatic insufficiency
  Decreased output of pancreatic antimicrobial factors
  Increase of undigested substrate in lumen leading to bacterial overgrowth

Chronic enteropathies
  Intestinal inflammation fosters aerobic conditions and changes in pH at mucosal site
  Reduction in mucus layer allows attachment of bacteria to mucosa

Miscellaneous
  Decreased mucosal immunity
  Antibiotic induced (eg, tylosin, metronidazole)
  Diets high in fat and protein and low in fiber (increase in *Escherichia coli* and *Clostridium perfringens*)

disease process. In the latter situation, it is also unclear to what extent the dysbiosis promotes the disease process and vice versa. Clinical signs caused by dysbiosis are also likely influenced by the localization and extent of microbial changes and can range from mild to severe acute or chronic GI signs.[29]

Microbiota in acute diarrhea

Dogs with acute uncomplicated diarrhea (AD) and acute hemorrhagic diarrhea syndrome (AHDS) have similar dysbiosis patterns, with dogs with AHDS showing the more profound alterations in their microbial profile.[30] In both types, a reduction in Actinobacteria and Firmicutes (eg, Ruminococcaceae, *Blautia*, *Faecalibacterium*, and *Turicibacter*) has been shown.[30] In addition, in dogs with AHDS, numbers of *Escherichia coli*, *Sutterella*, and *Clostridium perfringens* are increased.[30] *C perfringens* is a commensal of the intestinal tract and can therefore be detected in healthy individuals.[31] Although an overgrowth of *C perfringens* is observed in dogs with AD and chronic enteropathy (CE), toxin-producing *C perfringens* have been associated with AHDS.[31] Several studies showed that dogs with AHDS have an increase in *C perfringens* and enterotoxin-producing *C perfringens* (*cpe*).[32,33] Furthermore, the enterotoxin (CPE) measured by enzyme-linked immunosorbent assay can be detected more frequently in dogs with AHDS.[32] However, because patients either positive or negative for *cpe* or CPE do not show significant differences in clinical or laboratory parameters, enterotoxin is unlikely to be the main cause of AHDS.[32] A novel pore-forming toxin gene called *netF* was recently identified in a *C perfringens* type A strain isolated from a dog with AHDS.[34] The NetF toxin has high cytotoxic potential, causing severe intestinal necrosis by assembling transmembrane channels in enterocytes. Compared with other GI diseases, such as canine parvovirus infection, CE, AD, or exocrine pancreas insufficiency (EPI), the prevalence of *netF* is significantly higher in dogs with AHDS.[35,36] A prevalence from 45% up to 100% has been described in dogs with AHDS depending on the detection method, suggesting a significant association between the *netF* toxin gene and AHDS.[34–36]

Microbiota in chronic diarrhea

An important consideration to understand the full spectrum of dysbiosis patterns leading to GI signs is the localization of dysbiosis. Alterations in intestinal bacteria can occur either in lumenal and/or in mucosa-adherent microbiota. Disruption of the mucus layer (eg, caused by intestinal inflammation) is a key pathway in the pathogenesis of mucosa-adherent dysbiosis.[7] Dysbiosis that is mostly restricted to the intestinal lumen is found in patients with maldigestion (eg, EPI),[37] following antibiotic treatment,[11] or in individuals with a delay in the maturation of their microbiomes and immune systems.[38]

Studies on dysbiosis in chronic GI disease mainly focused on patients with inflammatory bowel disease (IBD). Duodenal mucosa-adherent genera within the Proteobacteria (*E coli*) are increased, whereas mucosa-adherent Fusobacteria, Bacteroidaceae, Prevotellaceae, and Clostridiales are decreased in IBD.[39] A study that used fluorescence in situ hybridization (FISH) investigated the distribution of the microbiota in colonic mucosal biopsies in dogs with chronic inflammatory enteropathy (CIE).[7] Dogs with CIE had decreased total bacterial counts in the colonic crypts, whereas there was no significant difference in total bacterial counts on the mucosal surface compared with healthy controls. *E coli/Shigella* were significantly increased. In contrast, *Helicobacter* and *Akkermansia* were significantly decreased in both crypts and on the mucosal surface in dogs with CIE, suggesting that those bacteria are beneficial commensals in the canine colon.[7] Especially in the pathogenesis of granulomatous colitis in boxer dogs and French bulldogs, the localization of intestinal bacteria plays a crucial role. Enteroinvasive *E coli* adhere to and invade the colonic mucosa, as shown via FISH.[40]

Other studies described luminal dysbiotic patterns in dogs with chronic GI signs. Dogs with IBD show reduced abundances of Firmicutes and Bacteroidetes and increased abundances of Proteobacteria and Actinobacteria.[9] Dogs with IBD have a significantly decreased fecal bacterial diversity and richness, reduced abundances of Firmicutes and Bacteroidetes, and increased abundances of Proteobacteria and Actinobacteria.[9,30] Numbers of *Blautia*, *Faecalibacterium*, and *Turicibacter* were decreased, whereas *E coli* und *Streptococcus* were increased in dogs with CE.[10,41] Dogs with EPI have significantly reduced bacterial diversity, with lactic acid bacteria Bifidobacteriaceae, Enterococcaceae, and Lactobacillaceae increased, likely because of overgrowth associated with maldigestion.[16,37]

There are only a few studies in cats with GI diseases.[5] Cats with IBD have increased numbers of Enterobacteriaceae adherent to the duodenal mucosa, and numbers of Enterobacteriaceae also correlate with changes in mucosal architecture.[42] *E coli* and *Clostridium* spp also correlate with intestinal inflammation, suggesting that alterations in intestinal bacteria contribute to the pathophysiology of IBD in cats.[42] Luminal microbiota in cats with IBD is characterized by significantly decreased *Bifidobacterium* and significantly increased *Desulfovibrio*.[43] In kittens with unspecific diarrhea, it was shown that increases in mucosa-adherent *E coli* in the ileum were significantly associated with mortality.[44]

Assessment of the Microbiome

Various approaches are necessary to describe the intestinal microbiome.[45] Bacterial culture focusses mainly on pathogenic bacteria. It is obvious now that the loss of beneficial bacteria leads to functional dysbiosis. Because most beneficial intestinal bacteria are strict anaerobes, they cannot be detected by standard culture.[46] Therefore, traditional bacterial culture is not useful for the assessment of the complex intestinal microbiome. Molecular methods have made it possible to detect as-yet unknown intestinal bacteria. Sequencing techniques using detection of the 16S ribosomal RNA gene provide information on the phylogenetic composition of a sample.[45] Using metagenomic shotgun sequencing, microbial DNA can be sequenced without prior amplification, and this provides information on the functional microbial genes from a sample.[45] Both methods are currently mostly available for research purposes, are expensive, and have long turnaround times. More rapid results with lower costs can be provided by polymerase chain reaction–based assays that detect specific bacterial groups. A novel approach, called the dysbiosis index (DI), has been developed to assess the canine fecal microbiota.[10] The DI measures the fecal abundance of 7 bacterial taxa (ie, *Faecalibacterium*, *Turicibacter*, *Streptococcus*, *E coli*, *Blautia*, *Fusobacterium*, and *C hiranonis*) as well as the total bacterial abundance. Therefore, it provides reference intervals for these 8 bacterial groups and additionally calculates a single number that expresses the extent of intestinal dysbiosis. A value greater than 2 indicates dysbiosis, a value less than 0 indicates a normal microbiota, and values between 0 and 2 are equivocal. The higher the DI, the less diverse the microbiome is.[11] The DI can be used to assess the normal versus abnormal microbiota and changes in microbiota over time or in response to treatment such as FMT (**Fig. 2**). Microbes can also be visualized via FISH directly in tissue samples using fluorescent probes that bind to bacterial DNA or RNA. Therefore, this method not only detects and quantifies microorganisms but also provides information on their localization; for example, whether bacteria are localized within the intestinal lumen or adhere to the mucosa. FISH is

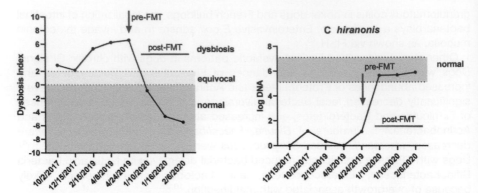

Fig. 2. Effect of FMT on the intestinal microbiome. The DI (*left*) and abundance of *C hirano-nis* (*right*) in a dog with long-lasting antibiotic-induced dysbiosis and intermittent episodes of diarrhea. After FMT, the microbiota and the abundance of the BA-converting bacterium *C hiranonis* normalize, also leading to proper conversion of primary to secondary BAs.

the method of choice in diagnosing dogs with granulomatous colitis caused by inva-sive *E coli*.[40]

Therapeutic Approaches to Dysbiosis

Dysbiosis plays a key role in GI and systemic diseases; hence, the normalization of microbiota composition and function is an important therapeutic target. The intestinal microbiome can be modulated by dietary approaches, antimicrobials, prebiotics and probiotics, and FMT. Each of these treatments has a different mechanism with advan-tages and possible drawbacks and side effects (**Table 3**). The underlying disease has to be taken into account because there is no treatment that addresses all kinds of dys-biosis (**Fig. 3**). Especially in chronic inflammatory GI diseases, such as CE in dogs, a treatment of the underlying inflammation is required for improvement of the disease process, and modulation of the microbiome should be considered as an adjunct treatment.

Dietary modulation should be always part of the treatment. A highly digestible diet reduces the potential for undigested substrate within the intestinal lumen that would allow bacterial overgrowth. In addition, in CE, a novel or hydrolyzed protein diet may reduce the host inflammatory response, a major driver of dysbiosis. In many cases of food-responsive enteropathy, this may be sufficient to achieve clinical response, with gradual improvement of mucosal inflammation and reduction of dys-biosis over several weeks or months.[47,48]

Prebiotics are indigestible carbohydrates that can be used selectively by microor-ganisms and therefore promote host health.[8] In general, prebiotics can be divided into soluble/nonsoluble and fermentable/nonfermentable (**Table 4**). The mechanism of fermentable prebiotics is their fermentation by colonic bacteria to SCFAs, with mul-tiple beneficial effects.[49] Because fermentable prebiotics serve as nutrients for micro-organisms, they are able to promote the growth of specific bacteria (eg, Bifidobacteria and Lactobacilli).[8] Psyllium, a soluble and fermentable dietary fiber, can also affect BA metabolism by binding BAs in the intestinal lumen.[50] A dose of 0.5 to 1 g/kg body weight is recommended, starting with a small amount to avoid possible side effects, such as flatulence and diarrhea. A prebiotic trial should be considered in patients with luminal and mucosa-adherent dysbiosis.

Table 3
Treatment approaches to dysbiosis differ in their mechanisms

Type of Treatment	Likely Mechanism	Potential Side Effects and Other Notes
Dietary modulation	Improved digestibility leads to less residual dietary substrate available for bacterial growth or conversion; can be hypoallergenic	None when highly digestible and no food sensitivity
Prebiotics/fibers	Promote growth of beneficial bacteria converted by bacteria to beneficial SCFA, some fibers bind deleterious bacterial metabolites (eg, psyllium has BA-binding properties)	Can initially cause flatulence, diarrhea in some patients, very individualized response in patients
Probiotics	Depending on the strains used, they can improve barrier function, be immunomodulatory, antimicrobial	In general, only rare side effects, but, because of strain-specific function, it is often unclear which patient would benefit best from which strain
Antibiotics	Reduction in total bacterial load and/or mucosa-adherent bacteria Leads to less antigenic stimulation and less conversion of toxic metabolites	Causes long-term changes in microbiota composition, when stopped, regrowth of bacterial load, concern for increased antimicrobial resistance
FMT	Alters luminal microbiota and also some microbial-derived metabolites	In general, no side effects expected, likely minor effect on mucosa-adherent bacteria, effect depends on underlying disease, recurrence of dysbiosis when concurrent intestinal inflammation still present

Probiotics are defined as live microorganisms that confer a health benefit to the host when administered in adequate amounts. The mechanism of probiotics is strain specific, which means that every bacterial strain has individual effects on the host. Examples are immune modulation, inhibition of pathogens, or improving the intestinal barrier.[51] Besides these strain-specific mechanisms, probiotic bacteria can also promote normalization of the normal microbiota and suppression of enterotoxigenic *C perfringens*, as shown in dogs with AHDS.[33] Probiotics have only a minor impact on the total microbiota composition in GI disease and are not able to prevent development of dysbiosis caused by antibiotic treatment.[52] When considering probiotic treatment, it is important to choose a probiotic product based on high quality and scientific evidence confirming its benefits for specific diseases.

Antibiotics (eg, tylosin or metronidazole) are often used in chronic GI diseases and can lead to improvement of clinical signs, but some patients tend to get worse during treatment and most patients that show improvement during treatment relapse after

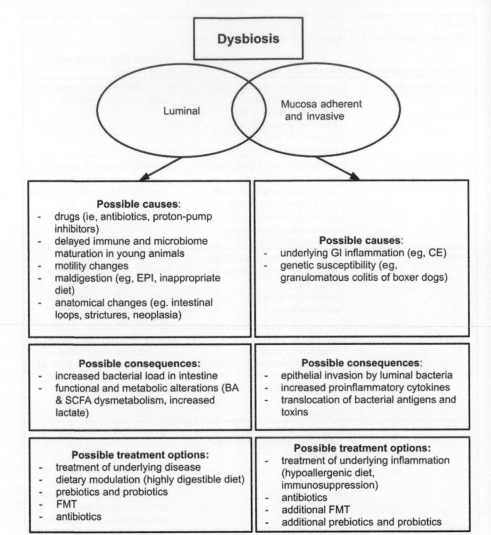

Fig. 3. Treatment approach to intestinal dysbiosis. Intestinal dysbiosis is associated with various disorders, and often it remains unclear whether the dysbiosis is the cause or effect of the disease. Intestinal dysbiosis can be localized in the intestinal lumen, be mucosa adherent and/or mucosa invasive, and there is likely an overlap between these patterns in some disorders. Detailed clinical history and assessment of underlying intestinal disorders may guide initial approaches to therapy.

cessation.[53] One possible explanation is that some of these animals have an increase in total bacterial load in the small intestine or increased mucosa-adherent bacteria,[7] with both causing a proinflammatory host response. Antibiotics lead to a reduction of bacterial load with improvement of clinical signs,[54] but, after antibiotic cessation, it is likely that bacteria will regrow,[55] leading to relapse of clinical signs. Antibiotics also promote the development of antimicrobial resistance and often cause alterations in intestinal microbiota that can last for months.[11,14,17] Examples of bacterial alterations following antibiotic treatment in companion animals are amoxicillin–clavulanic

Table 4
Overview of characteristics of commonly used prebiotics

Prebiotic	Soluble in Water	Can Be Metabolized by Colonic Bacteria	Source (Examples)	Mechanism	Notes
Cellulose	–	–	Cell wall component in plants	• Bind water Bulking effect • Increase fecal volume • Promote intestinal motility	Increase saturation
Lignin	–	–	Cell wall component in plants, especially wood	• Bind water Bulking effect • Increase fecal volume • Promote intestinal motility	• Consist of phenolic polymers • Increase saturation
Pectin	+++	+++	Berries, apples, pears	SCFA	Mainly fermented to acetate
Psyllium	++	+	Flea seeds	• Production of mucilage • SCFA	• Can bind BAs • Slow down carbohydrate resorption
Guar	+++	+++	Legume seeds	SCFA	Slow down carbohydrate resorption
Fructo-oligosaccharides	+++	+++	Asparagus, chicory, artichokes	SCFA	Increase in bifidobacteria

acid, which causes a decrease in abundance of bacterial species in cats, or tylosin and metronidazole, which lead to increases in *E coli* and reductions of beneficial bacteria in dogs.[11,14,52] In healthy dogs receiving metronidazole, microbial composition significantly differed after 2 weeks of administration compared with baseline (see **Fig. 1**).[11] Recent data in dogs with acute diarrhea show that metronidazole promotes lasting dysbiosis,[14] and amoxicillin–clavulanic acid promotes lasting increase in resistant *E coli*.[56] Because of these negative effects, antibiotics should not be used as a routine treatment in patients with GI diseases but should be considered in patients that failed dietary and antiinflammatory trials in chronic cases or with signs of systemic inflammation in acute cases.

Fecal microbiota transplant can aid in restoration of the normal microbiota[14] (see **Fig. 2**) and is discussed in more detail elsewhere in this issue.

In conclusion, the intestinal microbiome plays an important role in GI and systemic host health. Most animals with GI disease experience changes in their intestinal microbiota compositions, resulting in impaired microbial pathways. Because intestinal dysbiosis can have different underlying causes and therefore different pathophysiologies, multimodal therapeutic approaches are necessary to improve dysbiosis.

CLINICS CARE POINTS

- Intestinal dysbiosis can be a marker for the presence of underlying GI disease.
- Increased Dysbiosis Index and decreased abundance of Clostridium hiranonis together suggest the presence of chronic inflammatory enteropathy.
- Overgrowth of Clostridioides difficile or Clostridium perfringens can be secondary to intestinal dysbiosis (ie, lack of secondary bile acids) present in chronic enteropathy.
- In dogs with chronic enteropathy that respond clinically to novel or hydrolyzed protein diets, the microbiome dysbiosis will normalize over a few months without the need for additional antibiotic treatment.

DISCLOSURE

A.-L. Ziese has nothing to disclose; J.S. Suchodolski is an employee of the Gastrointestinal Laboratory, which offers microbiome testing on a fee-for-service basis.

REFERENCES

1. Human Microbiome Project Consortium. Structure, function and diversity of the healthy human microbiome. Nature 2012;486:207–14.

2. Swanson KS, Dowd SE, Suchodolski JS, et al. Phylogenetic and gene-centric metagenomics of the canine intestinal microbiome reveals similarities with humans and mice. ISME J 2011;5:639–49.

3. Mentula S, Harmoinen J, Heikkila M, et al. Comparison between cultured small-intestinal and fecal microbiotas in beagle dogs. Appl Environ Microbiol 2005; 71(8):4169–75.

4. Honneffer JB, Steiner JM, Lidbury JA, et al. Variation of the microbiota and metabolome along the canine gastrointestinal tract. Metabolomics 2017;13.3:26.

5. Marsilio S, Pilla R, Sarawichitr B, et al. Characterization of the fecal microbiome in cats with inflammatory bowel disease or alimentary small cell lymphoma. Sci Rep 2019;9:19208.

6. Guard BC, Suchodolski JS. HORSE SPECIES SYMPOSIUM: canine intestinal microbiology and metagenomics: from phylogeny to function. J Anim Sci 2016; 94:2247–61.

7. Giaretta PR, Suchodolski JS, Jergens AE, et al. Bacterial biogeography of the colon in dogs with chronic inflammatory enteropathy. Vet Pathol 2020;57:258–65.

8. Rowland I, Gibson G, Heinken A, et al. Gut microbiota functions: metabolism of nutrients and other food components. Eur J Nutr 2018;57:1–24.

9. Vazquez-Baeza Y, Hyde ER, Suchodolski JS, et al. Dog and human inflammatory bowel disease rely on overlapping yet distinct dysbiosis networks. Nat Microbiol 2016;1:16177.

10. AlShawaqfeh MK, Wajid B, Minamoto Y, et al. A dysbiosis index to assess microbial changes in fecal samples of dogs with chronic inflammatory enteropathy. FEMS Microbiol Ecol 2017;93(11).

11. Pilla R, Gaschen FP, Barr JW, et al. Effects of metronidazole on the fecal microbiome and metabolome in healthy dogs. J Vet Intern Med 2020;34(5):1853–66.

12. Giaretta PR, Suchodolski JS, Blick AK, et al. Distribution of bile acid receptor TGR5 in the gastrointestinal tract of dogs. Histol Histopathol 2019;34:69–79.

13. Giaretta PR, Rech RR, Guard BC, et al. Comparison of intestinal expression of the apical sodium-dependent bile acid transporter between dogs with and without chronic inflammatory enteropathy. J Vet Intern Med 2018;32:1918–26.

14. Chaitman J, Ziese AL, Pilla R, et al. Fecal microbial and metabolic profiles in dogs with acute diarrhea receiving either fecal microbiota transplantation or oral metronidazole. Front Vet Sci 2020;7:192.

15. Pavlidis P, Powell N, Vincent RP, et al. Systematic review: bile acids and intestinal inflammation-luminal aggressors or regulators of mucosal defence? Aliment Pharmacol Ther 2015;42:802–17.

16. Blake AB, Guard BC, Honneffer JB, et al. Altered microbiota, fecal lactate, and fecal bile acids in dogs with gastrointestinal disease. PLoS One 2019;14: e0224454.

17. Manchester AC, Webb CB, Blake AB, et al. Long-term impact of tylosin on fecal microbiota and fecal bile acids of healthy dogs. J Vet Intern Med 2019;33: 2605–17.

18. Arpaia N, Campbell C, Fan X, et al. Metabolites produced by commensal bacteria promote peripheral regulatory T-cell generation. Nature 2013;504:451–5.

19. Cherrington CA, Hinton M, Pearson GR, et al. Short-chain organic acids at ph 5.0 kill *Escherichia coli* and *Salmonella* spp. without causing membrane perturbation. J Appl Bacteriol 1991;70:161–5.

20. Whitfield-Cargile CM, Cohen ND, Chapkin RS, et al. The microbiota-derived metabolite indole decreases mucosal inflammation and injury in a murine model of NSAID enteropathy. Gut Microbes 2016;7:246–61.

21. Gasbarrini G, Montalto M. Structure and function of tight junctions. Role in intestinal barrier. Ital J Gastroenterol Hepatol 1999;31:481–8.

22. Dobson A, Cotter PD, Ross RP, et al. Bacteriocin production: a probiotic trait? Appl Environ Microbiol 2012;78:1–6.

23. Hooper LV, Gordon JI. Commensal host-bacterial relationships in the gut. Science 2001;292:1115–8.

24. Levy M, Kolodziejczyk AA, Thaiss CA, et al. Dysbiosis and the immune system. Nat Rev Immunol 2017;17:219–32.

25. Duboc H, Rajca S, Rainteau D, et al. Connecting dysbiosis, bile-acid dysmetabolism and gut inflammation in inflammatory bowel diseases. Gut 2013;62:531–9.

26. Weingarden AR, Chen C, Bobr A, et al. Microbiota transplantation restores normal fecal bile acid composition in recurrent *Clostridium difficile* infection. Am J Physiol Gastrointest Liver Physiol 2014;306:G310–9.
27. Saari A, Virta LJ, Sankilampi U, et al. Antibiotic exposure in infancy and risk of being overweight in the first 24 months of life. Pediatrics 2015;135:617–26.
28. Cox LM, Blaser MJ. Antibiotics in early life and obesity. Nat Rev Endocrinol 2015; 11:182–90.
29. Jalanka-Tuovinen J, Salonen A, Nikkila J, et al. Intestinal microbiota in healthy adults: temporal analysis reveals individual and common core and relation to intestinal symptoms. PLoS One 2011;6:e23035.
30. Suchodolski JS, Markel ME, Garcia-Mazcorro JF, et al. The fecal microbiome in dogs with acute diarrhea and idiopathic inflammatory bowel disease. PLoS One 2012;7:e51907.
31. Minamoto Y, Dhanani N, Markel ME, et al. Prevalence of *Clostridium perfringens, Clostridium perfringens* enterotoxin and dysbiosis in fecal samples of dogs with diarrhea. Vet Microbiol 2014;174:463–73.
32. Busch K, Suchodolski JS, Kuhner KA, et al. *Clostridium perfringens* enterotoxin and *Clostridium difficile* toxin A/B do not play a role in acute haemorrhagic diarrhoea syndrome in dogs. Vet Rec 2015;176:253.
33. Ziese AL, Suchodolski JS, Hartmann K, et al. Effect of probiotic treatment on the clinical course, intestinal microbiome, and toxigenic *Clostridium perfringens* in dogs with acute hemorrhagic diarrhea. PLoS One 2018;13:e0204691.
34. Mehdizadeh Gohari I, Parreira VR, Nowell VJ, et al. A novel pore-forming toxin in type A *Clostridium perfringens* is associated with both fatal canine hemorrhagic gastroenteritis and fatal foal necrotizing enterocolitis. PLoS One 2015;10: e0122684.
35. Sindern N, Suchodolski JS, Leutenegger CM, et al. Prevalence of *Clostridium perfringens* netE and netF toxin genes in the feces of dogs with acute hemorrhagic diarrhea syndrome. J Vet Intern Med 2019;33:100–5.
36. Sarwar F, Ziese AL, Werner M, et al. Prevalence of *Clostridium perfringens* encoding netF gene in dogs with acute and chronic gastrointestinal diseases. J Vet Intern Med 2018;32:2241 (abstract).
37. Isaiah A, Parambeth JC, Steiner JM, et al. The fecal microbiome of dogs with exocrine pancreatic insufficiency. Anaerobe 2017;45:50–8.
38. Aguilera M, Vergara P, Martinez V. Stress and antibiotics alter luminal and wall-adhered microbiota and enhance the local expression of visceral sensory-related systems in mice. Neurogastroenterol Motil 2013;25:e515–29.
39. Suchodolski JS, Dowd SE, Wilke V, et al. 16S rRNA gene pyrosequencing reveals bacterial dysbiosis in the duodenum of dogs with idiopathic inflammatory bowel disease. PLoS One 2012;7:e39333.
40. Simpson KW, Dogan B, Rishniw M, et al. Adherent and invasive *Escherichia coli* is associated with granulomatous colitis in boxer dogs. Infect Immun 2006;74: 4778–92.
41. Rossi G, Pengo G, Caldin M, et al. Comparison of microbiological, histological, and immunomodulatory parameters in response to treatment with either combination therapy with prednisone and metronidazole or probiotic VSL#3 strains in dogs with idiopathic inflammatory bowel disease. PLoS One 2014;9:e94699.
42. Janeczko S, Atwater D, Bogel E, et al. The relationship of mucosal bacteria to duodenal histopathology, cytokine mRNA, and clinical disease activity in cats with inflammatory bowel disease. Vet Microbiol 2008;128:178–93.

43. Inness VL, McCartney AL, Khoo C, et al. Molecular characterisation of the gut microflora of healthy and inflammatory bowel disease cats using fluorescence in situ hybridisation with special reference to Desulfovibrio spp. J Anim Physiol Anim Nutr 2007;91:48–53.

44. Ghosh A, Borst L, Stauffer SH, et al. Mortality in kittens is associated with a shift in ileum mucosa-associated enterococci from Enterococcus hirae to biofilm-forming Enterococcus faecalis and adherent Escherichia coli. J Clin Microbiol 2013;51: 3567–78.

45. Costa M, Weese JS. Methods and basic concepts for microbiota assessment. Vet J 2019;249:10–5.

46. Leser TD, Amenuvor JZ, Jensen TK, et al. Culture-independent analysis of gut bacteria: the pig gastrointestinal tract microbiota revisited. Appl Environ Microbiol 2002;68:673–90.

47. Bresciani F, Minamoto Y, Suchodolski JS, et al. Effect of an extruded animal protein-free diet on fecal microbiota of dogs with food-responsive enteropathy. J Vet Intern Med 2018;32:1903–10.

48. Wang S, Martins R, Sullivan MC, et al. Diet-induced remission in chronic enteropathy is associated with altered microbial community structure and synthesis of secondary bile acids. Microbiome 2019;7:126.

49. Patra AK. Responses of feeding prebiotics on nutrient digestibility, faecal microbiota composition and short-chain fatty acid concentrations in dogs: a meta-analysis. Animal 2011;5:1743–50.

50. Buhman KK, Furumoto EJ, Donkin SS, et al. Dietary psyllium increases fecal bile acid excretion, total steroid excretion and bile acid biosynthesis in rats. J Nutr 1998;128:1199–203.

51. White R, Atherly T, Guard B, et al. Randomized, controlled trial evaluating the effect of multi-strain probiotic on the mucosal microbiota in canine idiopathic inflammatory bowel disease. Gut Microbes 2017;0.

52. Torres-Henderson C, Summers S, Suchodolski J, et al. Effect of Enterococcus faecium strain SF68 on gastrointestinal signs and fecal microbiome in cats administered amoxicillin-clavulanate. Top Companion Anim Med 2017;32:104–8.

53. Westermarck E, Skrzypczak T, Harmoinen J, et al. Tylosin-responsive chronic diarrhea in dogs. J Vet Intern Med 2005;19:177–86.

54. Westermarck E, Myllys V, Aho M. Effect of treatment on the jejunal and colonic bacterial flora of dogs with exocrine pancreatic insufficiency. Pancreas 1993;8: 559–62.

55. Johnston KL, Lamport AI, BallŠvre OP, et al. Effects of oral administration of metronidazole on small intestinal bacteria and nutrients of cats. Am J Vet Res 2000;61:1106–12.

56. Werner M, Suchodolski JS, Straubinger RK, et al. Effect of amoxicillin-clavulanic acid on clinical scores, intestinal microbiome, and amoxicillin-resistant Escherichia coli in dogs with uncomplicated acute diarrhea. J Vet Intern Med 2020;34: 1166–76.

Value of Probiotics in Canine and Feline Gastroenterology

Silke Salavati Schmitz, Drmedvet, PhD, FHEA, MRCVS

KEYWORDS

- Synbiotics • Prebiotics • Probiotics • Gastrointestinal • Microbiota
- Mucosal immunity • Chronic enteropathy • Inflammatory bowel disease

KEY POINTS

- Probiotics are live microbial organisms with a proven health benefit to the host and can be regulated as food supplement, medical food, or drugs.
- Evidence of health promoting or disease preventing effects of probiotics or synbiotics in healthy dogs and cats is scarce.
- Probiotics or synbiotics are likely to be beneficial in some acute or infectious gastrointestinal conditions in dogs and cats (eg, acute hemorrhagic diarrhea syndrome or parvovirus infection).
- Probiotics or synbiotics add little benefit when treating food- or antibiotic-responsive canine chronic enteropathies, but could be promising adjunctive treatments in canine inflammatory bowel disease.
- Specific probiotics might be beneficial in feline *Tritrichomonas fetus* infection and feline chronic constipation.

INTRODUCTION

The current definition of probiotics was established by the Food and Agriculture Organization of the United Nations and the World Health Organization in 2001 and 2002[1] and amended by the International Scientific Association for Probiotics and Prebiotics in 2014,[2] and states that probiotics are "live microorganisms which when administered in adequate amounts confer a health benefit on the host". Unfortunately, the label "probiotic" is often misused as an umbrella term and applied to products that do not meet this strict definition.[3] In a further attempt to clarify what constitutes a probiotic, a newly created "probiotic framework"[2] separates live microbes used as processing aids or those in naturally fermented foods from those administered primarily for their health benefits (**Fig. 1**). It also dictates that, until any micro-organisms or gut commensals are isolated, characterized and their health effects are convincingly demonstrated, they are not truly probiotics.[2,3]

Hospital for Small Animals, Royal (Dick) School of Veterinary Studies, The Roslin Institute, College of Medicine and Veterinary Medicine, University of Edinburgh, Easter Bush, Midlothian EH25 9RG, UK
E-mail address: Silke.Salavati@ed.ac.uk

Vet Clin Small Anim 51 (2021) 171–217
https://doi.org/10.1016/j.cvsm.2020.09.011
vetsmall.theclinics.com

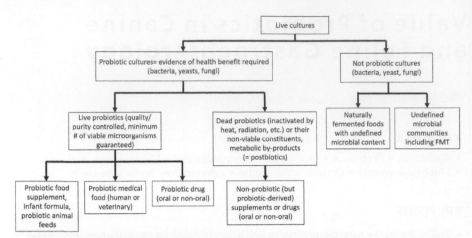

Fig. 1. The probiotic framework and its regulation. The definition of probiotics currently includes live cultures with a proven health benefit to the host (see also **Box 1**). FMT, fecal microbiota transplantation. (*Data from* Hill C, Guarner F, Reid G, et al. The International Scientific Association for Probiotics and Prebiotics consensus statement on the scope and appropriate use of the term probiotic. Nat Rev Gastroenterol Hepatol. 2014;11:506-514 and de Simone C. The Unregulated Probiotic Market. Clin Gastroenterol Hepatol. 2019;17(5):809-817.)

The main challenge seems to be the achievement of transparency for regulating specific products labeled as probiotics, because there is an increased interest in their use as novel or alternative treatments for a wide number of conditions. However, marketing is often based on their attractive theoretic modes of action and not matched by sufficient scientific evidence proving any claimed benefits. Worldwide, there is insufficient regulation of the probiotic market to scrutinize if a product can be defined as a probiotic, and legislation varies from including them as foods for human consumption, animal feeds, nutritional supplements or drugs (see **Fig. 1**). To uphold principles of evidence-based veterinary medicine in small animals, it seems prudent that sufficient scientific scrutiny is applied to assess if a presumptive probiotic achieves desired outcomes in the disease of interest and—crucially—in the target species.

So far, even though many studies examining probiotic effects are available, these investigations were mostly conducted in laboratory animals, cell cultures, or other "ex vivo" systems. Human clinical trials often examine small numbers of patients and are not controlled or do not include sufficiently specific information about the probiotics used. The number of high-quality probiotic trials in dogs and cats is even more limited. In smaller studies, the presumptive probiotic bacterial strains used were often isolated specifically for the study purpose, making it nearly impossible to reproduce any reported findings. This article aims to summarize legislation around the quality and safety of probiotic products used in small animals in the United States, their supposed or demonstrated mechanisms of action, and to examine the evidence for their use in clinical gastrointestinal (GI) diseases in dogs and cats.

DEFINITIONS OR PROBIOTICS, PREBIOTICS, SYNBIOTICS, AND POSTBIOTICS

The definition of *probiotics* as live micro-organisms benefiting the host (as described elsewhere in this article and in **Box 1**) is originally derived from the observation by Eli Metchnikoff at the beginning of the last century that specific bacteria and their

> **Box 1**
> **Key definitions**
>
> - *Probiotics* are supplements, foods, or drugs that contain viable micro-organisms with a proven benefit to the host
> - *Prebiotics* are supplements or foods (often dietary fibers or carbohydrates) that selectively stimulate the growth and/or activity of indigenous micro-organisms
> - *Postbiotics* are nonviable bacterial products that have a beneficial effect on the host
> - *Synbiotics* are products that contain both probiotics and prebiotics

metabolites could be harnessed to "replace" harmful microbes in the intestine.[4] At the same time, Henry Tissier, a French pediatrician, observed that children with diarrhea demonstrated a low number of peculiar, Y-shaped bacteria in their stools in comparison with healthy children.[5] He suggested that these "bifid" bacteria could be administered to diarrheic patients to restore their gut flora. The word "probiotic" was coined in 1960 to name substances that promoted the growth of other micro-organisms,[6] and later redefined to describe "a live microbial feed supplement that improves the host's intestinal balance."[7,8] This process eventually resulted in the more recent definition that is still used by the Food and Agriculture Organization of the United Nations and the World Health Organization today,[1] in turn based on the 1998 definition by Guarner and Schaafsma.[9]

In contrast, *prebiotics* are defined as "non-digestible food ingredients that beneficially affect the host by selectively stimulating the growth and/or activity of one or a limited number of bacterial species already established in the colon, and thus in effect improve host health," as outlined originally by Gibson and Roberfroid in 1995.[10]

In a report from 2001, the Food and Agriculture Organization of the United Nations and the World Health Organization claims that in some cases prebiotics may be directly beneficial for a probiotic, providing a synbiotic concept. *Synbiotics* are hence defined as "mixtures of probiotics and prebiotics that beneficially affect the host by improving the survival and implantation of live microbial dietary supplements in the gastrointestinal tract of the host."[1,11]

Postbiotics is a relatively new term that has been created to refer to the nonviable metabolic byproducts of (probiotic) micro-organisms that have biological activity in the host. Even though the field is still largely unexplored, some researchers believe that postbiotics are responsible for many of the beneficial effects of probiotics.[12]

REGULATION, QUALITY CONTROL, AND SAFETY OF PROBIOTIC PRODUCTS

Government regulation of probiotics in the Unites States is complex and depends on the probiotic product's intended use. The US Food and Drug Administration (FDA) might regulate it as a dietary supplement, a food ingredient or a drug or biological (see **Fig. 1**).[13]

Many probiotics are sold as a dietary supplements, which do not require FDA approval before they are marketed. Their labels may make claims about how the product affects the structure or function of the body without FDA approval, but health claims are not permitted without the FDA's consent. In 2016, the FDA issued a revised draft New Dietary Ingredient guidance, which raises questions regarding the regulatory status of innovative probiotic strains not isolated from food.[14] In addition, the FDA's interpretation of "chemical alteration" in the revised draft guidance could impact probiotics, because fermentation is mentioned as a process that results in chemical alteration, triggering the requirement for New Dietary Ingredient notification.

If a probiotic is marketed as a medical food, claims of the product being intended for the "dietary management of disease or medical condition" are also permitted without FDA approval. Only probiotics marketed as drugs for the prevention or treatment of a disease or disorder have to be proven safe and effective for their intended use through clinical trials and receive FDA approval before being sold.[13,15]

Assessing the safety of probiotic products (especially when marketed as drugs) necessitates the establishment of an adverse effect profile, with the principal theoretic risks including infection, ill effects from toxins of the probiotics or contaminants, and immunologic effects. In addition, marketed preparations need to meet stringent quality standards to make certain that the correct strain(s) are present in consistent amounts and the product is free of contamination. For this, self-regulatory initiatives have been put in place in the face of lack of governmental regulation. For example, in 2017, the Council for Responsible Nutrition and the International Probiotics Association developed scientifically based best practice guidelines for the labeling, storing, and stability testing of dietary supplements and functional foods containing probiotics.[16] A key element of the guidelines is the recommendation to label probiotic products in colony forming units, which has also been recommended in the 2018 draft guidance by the FDA.[17]

However, it is somewhat unclear how this translates into the pet food or pharmaceutical sectors. Studies investigating commercial pet foods or products claiming to contain probiotics showed worrisome results: none of the 19 commercial dog and cat foods tested contained all the probiotic organisms claimed, whereas 11 samples contained additional related micro-organisms and more than 25% of tested foods showed no relevant bacterial growth at all.[18] Of 25 commercial products claiming to consist of probiotics, only 4 met or exceeded their label claim, with overall viable growth ranging from 0 to 2×10^9 colony forming units per gram.[19]

When it comes to using probiotics in a clinical setting, the great majority of human clinical trials have not given rise to major safety concerns.[20,21] However, a few examples of serious adverse effects have been documented in people: sepsis, fungemia in critically ill patients treated with *Saccharomyces boulardii*,[22] death from mold contamination in a child,[23] and an increased risk of mortality in multistrain-probiotic treated patients with pancreatitis.[24] Therefore, careful safety evaluation is required before the use of probiotics in vulnerable patient groups, including patients with damaged intestinal mucosa or immune dysregulation. In people, this can include inflammatory bowel disease (IBD), liver diseases, and human immunodeficiency virus. In small animals, no specific contraindications for the use of probiotics have been identified so far.

THEORETIC MECHANISMS OF ACTION OF PROBIOTICS

Several mechanisms of action within the GI tract and the gut-associated immune system have been proposed for probiotics (**Fig. 2**), but very few of them have been confirmed specifically in small animals. These include displacement of intestinal pathogens,[25] for example, by interfering with their adherence to the intestinal epithelial cells or by induction of mucus or mucin production,[26] production of antimicrobial substances like organic acids[27] or defensins,[28,29] specific toxins aimed at pathogens[30] or proteases that in turn can deactivate toxins,[31] enhancement of innate and adaptive immune responses within intestinal epithelial cells[28] or in the lamina propria immune cells,[32] and/or upregulation of various nonspecific cellular defense mechanisms, for example, heat shock proteins or the inflammasome.[33]

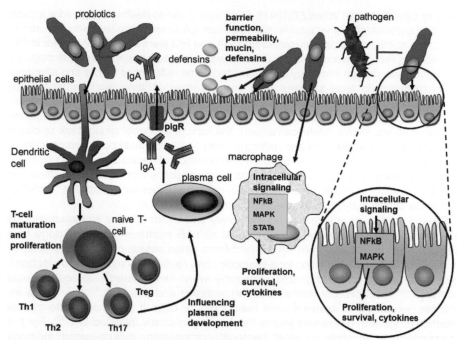

Fig. 2. Proposed mechanisms of action of probiotics on the intestinal mucosa (intestinal epithelial cells in green) and the associated local immune system. *Arrows* indicate direct promoting effects, red "T"-shaped bars indicate inhibitory effects. MAPK, mitogen-activated protein kinase; NFκB, nuclear factor kappa B; pIgR, polymeric immune globulin receptor; STAT, signal transducer and activator of transcription; Th, T-helper lymphocyte cell. (*Data from* Oelschlaeger TA. Mechanisms of probiotic actions - A review. *Int J Med Microbiol.* 2010;300(1):57-62.)

Many of these actions are strain specific; even bacterial strains of the same species can alter cellular responses in different ways. For example, *Lactobacillus reuteri* ATCC PTA 6475, can inhibit lipopolysaccharide-induced tumor necrosis factor alpha production from myeloid cells in vitro through suppression of the activator protein-1 pathway, whereas another *L reuteri* strain, DSM 17938, does not exhibit this behavior.[34] Details on the cellular interactions of specific probiotic strains have been summarized in several reviews,[28,29,35–37] but it is overall believed that key biological signaling pathways, for example, for the transcription of cytokines and other molecules involved in cell survival and apoptosis are common targets for probiotics or their products both in vitro and in vivo,[29] particularly in innate immune cells like macrophages and intestinal epithelial cells (see **Fig. 2**). Probiotics also regulate adaptive local immunity by influencing T-cell maturation and proliferation toward a more tolerogenic environment (shift to regulatory T cells), and plasma cell development/class switching to specific IgA production (see **Fig. 2**).[29]

THE EFFECT OF SELECTED PROBIOTICS ON PARAMETERS OF GUT HEALTH IN HEALTHY DOGS AND CATS

Enterococcus faecium (*EF*) is one of the most widely used presumed probiotic in small animals, but not many studies have focused on its effects when administered to healthy dogs or cats (**Table 1**). When *EF* 10415 SF68 was given to healthy puppies for a year, they had significantly higher total fecal and serum IgA levels compared with the control dogs.[38] In addition, vaccination-associated IgA and IgG were significantly higher in *EF*-treated puppies. In a second study, *EF* EE3 was orally administered to adult dogs for 1 week.[39] Even though this study demonstrated some differences before and after probiotic treatment in fecal samples (total concentration of lactic acid bacteria [LAB] increased, *Pseudomonas*-like bacteria and *Staphylococcus* spp. decreased) and serum biochemistry parameters (total serum lipids and protein decreased but were never outside their respective reference ranges), the lack of a control group, lack of clarity about the strain identification and methods used to assess fecal composition (culture vs next-generation sequencing), make the interpretation of results and clinical relevance difficult. Similarly, when EF 10415 SF68 was given to healthy kittens, it did not affect any developmental or immune parameters, even though the percentage of CD4$^+$ lymphocytes was significantly higher in the treatment group.[40]

Several studies have investigated the safety and effect of other single-strain LAB preparations (eg, lactobacilli, bifidobacteria) or LAB mixtures in healthy dogs (see **Table 1**), but they suffer from similar problems when assessing desired outcomes or the fulfilment of the definition for a probiotic: only routine hematology and biochemistry parameters of questionable relevance were investigated[41] alongside fecal scores,[42–44] fecal pH, dry matter, and fermentation end products.[45–48] In some instances, experimental systems were used that are difficult to translate into clinical practice (dogs with permanent jejunal fistulas,[49] genetically modified LAB[50]). For the assessment of intestinal or fecal bacterial composition, culture-based methods have been used most frequently,[46,47,51] although they provide an inadequate representation of fecal bacterial richness, diversity and composition. In the few studies where next-generation sequencing methods like 16S rRNA gene 454-pyrosequencing were used, fecal microbiota composition changes were as expected (increase in Lactobacillaceae[44]) or absent.[52]

In healthy cats, 3 studies investigated the effect of potential probiotics on fecal characteristics like visual fecal scores, volatile compounds, pH and selected bacteria based on culture methods, as well as assessment of physical examination and routine clinicopathological data findings.[53–55] Changes in these latter parameters were generally not observed, while fecal scores either remained the same or slightly improved.[53–55] Fecal pH decreased in 1 study,[53] and volatile compounds were either not changed (with administration of a *Lactobacillus acidophilus*[53]). In another study (administration of *Bifidobacterium pseudocatenulatum*) a reduction of fecal ammonia, lactic acid, n-valeric, and isovaleric acid in combination was reported with increases in acetic acid.[55] Fecal culture results generally showed an increase in LAB[53–55] and a decrease in coliform bacteria[54,55] and *Clostridia* spp.,[53] respectively. Only 1 study assessed the effects of a synbiotic LAB mixture in both dogs and cats beyond fecal characteristics and performed a more in-depth analysis on fecal microbiota composition (see **Table 1**).[52] They also observed a significant increase in *Lactobacillus* spp. during synbiotic supplementation, although major bacterial phyla as assessed by 454-pyrosequencing were not altered. In cats, a decrease in microbiota species diversity was observed during synbiotic supplementation,[52] but, overall, the significance of any of these observed changes remains unclear.

USE OF PROBIOTICS IN SMALL ANIMAL GASTROINTESTINAL DISEASES

Peer-reviewed studies investigating the in vivo use of probiotics or synbiotics in the prevention or treatment of GI disease in dogs and cats are sparse. In a recent

Table 1
Suspected probiotics or synbiotics tested for health-promoting effects in healthy dogs and cats

Micro-Organism Used (Source)	Dose and Duration	Test Animals (n)	Control Group	Measured Outcomes	Reference
Bacillus subtilis C-3102 (no information on source, but available as commercial product)	1×10^{10} cfu/g (0.01%) purpose made feed	6 Beagle dogs (7–8 month old), purpose bread	Yes (6 Beagle dogs receiving control diet w/o *Bacillus* spp.)	Diet adaptation period of 25 d, followed by 5 d of total fecal collection in both groups *Fecal output and pH* (no difference) *Fecal score*: higher in treatment group (but "optimal" in both groups) *Fecal % dry matter*: higher in treatment group *Fecal crude protein, crude fiber, mineral matter, ether extract in acid hydrolysis (AEE), non-nitrogen extract and ME* (no difference) *Fecal ammonia content*: lower in treatment group	Felix et al,[42] 2010

(continued on next page)

Table 1
(continued)

Micro-Organism Used (Source)	Dose and Duration	Test Animals (n)	Control Group	Measured Outcomes	Reference
Bifidobacterium animals AHC7 (isolated from healthy dog)	Group 1: 1×10^9 cfu/d for 12 wk Group 2: 5×10^{10} cfu/d for 12 wk	6-month-old Beagle dogs: 10 per group → total of 20	No	Week 0, 6, 12 and 16 *Fecal scores:* firmer stools in group 2 from week 2 to 16, but "acceptable" in both groups throughout *Body weight, BCS and food intake* (no difference) *Fecal culture:* Total bacterial concentrations or percentage of total lactobacillus was not affected *Complete blood count* (no difference) *Serum biochemistry:* none outside the reference ranges *Neutrophil phagocytic activity:* improved	Kelley et al,[51] 2010

Bifidobacterium pseudocatenulatum (BP-B82) (isolated from a healthy cat) + galacto-oligosaccharides	10^{10} cfu/d for 15 d	10 client-owned healthy cats	No	*Fecal volatile compounds:* Reduced fecal ammonia concentration, higher fecal acetic acid concentration, lower fecal lactic, n-valeric and isovaleric acid concentration, no change in fecal polyamines. *Fecal cultures:* fecal bifidobacteria increased, while counts of C perfringens, coliforms and enterococci were unchanged	Biagi et al,[55] 2013
EF 10,415 SF68 (Fortiflora, Nestle Purina)	5×10^8 cfu/d from weaning to 1 y	7 purpose-bread dogs, various breeds	Yes (n = 7)	Time points: weeks 0, 10, 18, 32 and 44: *Food intake, body weight* (no difference) *Complete blood count* (no difference) *Serum biochemistry* (no difference) *Total fecal IgA:* higher in treated group *Total serum IgG and IgA* (no difference)	Benyacoub et al,[38] 2003

(continued on next page)

Table 1
(continued)

Micro-Organism Used (Source)	Dose and Duration	Test Animals (n)	Control Group	Measured Outcomes	Reference
				Canine distemper virus vaccine-specific serum IgG (no difference) and IgA: higher in treated group *Quantitative assessment of circulating lymphocyte subsets by flow cytometry (no difference)*	
E faecium 10,415 SF68	5×10^9 cfu/d	10 SPF kittens	Yes (n = 10 SPF kittens)	Randomised to treatment or placebo at 7 wk of age, duration of study 20 wk. Sampling at week 7 (before supplementation) and week 9, 15, 21 and 27 in all cats *Attitude and behavior* monitored daily (no difference) *Blood:* routine hematology and biochemistry (no difference),	Veir et al,[40] 2007

immunization-
specific antibodies
(no difference),
flow cytometry for
CD4$^+$ (higher at
week 27 in treated
group), CD8$^+$,
CD44$^+$, B220$^+$ and
CD21$^+$ lymphocytes
and MHCII (no
difference for the
rest)

*Serum total IgA and
IgG* (no difference)
*Saliva total IgA and
IgG* (no difference
in IgA, IgG not
detected)

*Fecal total IgA and
IgG* (week 9 and 27)
(no difference)

*Fecal samples
(isolation of EF):* in
7/9 treatment cats
EF was isolated at
least once, in week
28: no isolation of
EF from any of the
treated cats

Fecal pathogens: no
Salmonella spp,
Campylobacter spp,
no difference in
samples positive for

(continued on next page)

Table 1
(continued)

Micro-Organism Used (Source)	Dose and Duration	Test Animals (n)	Control Group	Measured Outcomes	Reference
				C difficile toxin A/B or *C perfringens* enterotoxin. *Fecal scoring:* 5 fecal samples from each group (communal litter box) per day (no difference)	
E faecium EE3 (isolated from a commercially available dog food)	2–3 × 10⁹ cfu/d for 1 wk	11 dogs, various breeds	No	Before and 1, 2 and 3 mo after administration: *Fecal cultures:* total concentration of LAB increased, *Pseudomonas*-like bacteria and *Staphylococcus* spp. decreased, no influence on *E coli*. *Serum biochemistry:* total lipids and total protein decreased with serum cholesterol being within the reference range in all dogs at the end of the treatment period	Marcinakova et al,[39] 2006

| LAB mixture: L fermentum LAB8, L salivarius LAB9, Weissella confuse LAB10, L rhamnosus LAB11, L mucosae LAB12 (all isolated from dog feces) | 1.4–5.9 cfu/mL of pooled cultures, stored at −20°F, then administered for 1 wk | 5 (Beagle dogs with permanent jejunal fistula) | No | *16S rRNA polymerase chain reaction followed by DGGE and sequencing of dominant bands:* reduced diversity of indigenous dominant LAB during feeding trial, not completely reestablished after supplementation ended. A dominant band was identified by sequencing as *Lactobacillus acidophilus* NCBI AY773947 *Enumeration of LAB:* reduction/ replacement of total number of jejunal LAB during supplementation | Manninen et al,[49] 2006 |

(continued on next page)

Table 1
(continued)

Micro-Organism Used (Source)	Dose and Duration	Test Animals (n)	Control Group	Measured Outcomes	Reference
LAB mixture: E faecium S salivarus ssp thermophilus B longum L acidophilus L casei ssp. rhamnosus L plantarum L delbrueckii ssp. Bulgaricus +FOS, arabinogalactans (Proviable-DC, Nutramax Laboratories, Inc.)	5 × 10⁹ cfu/d (exact proportions are proprietary) for 3 wk	12 privately owned healthy cats (mostly domestic short hair) and 12 privately owned healthy dogs (various breeds)	No	*Fecal scores:* normal with the exception of 2 cats and 2 dogs (pulpy feces for 2 d) *Complete blood count and serum biochemistry, serum cobalamin/folate, fI cTLI and fI cPL (day 0, 21 [last day of supplementation] and day 42 [3 wk after cessation of supplementation]):* decrease in lymphocytes (cats) and neutrophils (dogs) during supplementation. Other parameters unchanged. *Fecal total IgA (day 0, 21 and 42):* no change *Canine/feline fecal α1-proteinase inhibitor (day 0, 21, and 42):* no change *16S rRNA polymerase chain reaction followed by DGGE (day 0, 21, day 38 [2 wk after cessation*	Garcia-Mazcorro et al,[52] 2011

of supplementation]):
11/12 (92%) of cats
and 5/11 (45%) of
dogs specific DGGE
bands observed
during
supplementation that
were absent at
baseline or after
supplementation.
Sequencing identified
E faecium.

*16S rRNA gene clone
libraries for
Lactobacillus and
Bifidobacterium spp.*
(days 14–17 [last week
of supplementation]
and 2 wk after
cessation of
supplementation): At
least 1 LAB was
detected during
supplementation in 8/
11 (73%) of cats and
9/11 (82%) of dogs,
but were
undetectable before
or after
supplementation
*for bacterial targets of
interest:
Bifidobacterium spp.,
Enterococcus spp.,
Lactobacillus spp.,
Streptococcus spp.*

(continued on next page)

Table 1
(continued)

Micro-Organism Used (Source)	Dose and Duration	Test Animals (n)	Control Group	Measured Outcomes	Reference
				(day 1, 8, and 17 in cats, and days 3, 5, and 17 in dogs): Abundances of *Enterococcus* and *Streptococcus* spp. increased in at least 1 time point during supplementation in both cats and dogs. In cats, *Lactobacillus* spp. increased significantly on day 17 of supplementation *Massive parallel 16S rRNA 454-pyrosequencing* (day 0, 5, and 23): no changes in major bacterial phyla, no clustering on PCoA, no differences in diversity indices in dogs. Cats had higher Shannon-Weaver diversity index before supplementation when compared with during or after supplementation.	

Organism	Dose	Animals	Healthy	Findings	Reference
Lactobacillus acidophilus D2/CSL (CECT 4529) (commercial culture)	5×10^9 cfu/kg feed over 5 wk	10 adult cats (5 each in control and probiotic group)	Yes (feed alone)	Body weight and BCS (no change) Fecal characteristics: less fecal moisture and better fecal scores on probiotics Fecal culture: increase in lactobacilli and decrease in *E coli*	Fusi et al,[54] 2019
Lactobacillus acidophilus DSM13241 (commercial culture)	3×10^9 cfu/d for 4 wk	15 dogs, various breeds	No	Assessments before, after 4 wk of supplementation, and after additional 2 wk w/o supplementation: *Body weight;* assessed weekly (no change) *Fecal score;* assessed daily (no change) *Complete blood count:* increased RBC, Hct, Hb, WBC, monocytes *Total serum IgG:* increased (total serum IgE undetectable) *Serum haptoglobin* (no change) *Serum C-reactive protein* (no change) Quantitative assessment of	Baillon et al,[41] 2004

(continued on next page)

Table 1
(continued)

Micro-Organism Used (Source)	Dose and Duration	Test Animals (n)	Control Group	Measured Outcomes	Reference
				circulating lymphocyte subsets by flow cytometry (no change) *RBC osmotic fragility:* reduced after supplementation *Serum NO concentrations:* reduced after supplementation *Fecal pH* (no change) *Fecal culture or FISH:* Lactobacilli increased with supplementation. Total numbers of anaerobes, coliforms, enterococci, and clostridia: unchanged	

| Lactobacillus acidophilus DSM13241 | 2×10^8 cfu/d for 4.5 wk | 15 adult cats | No | Assessments before, after 4.5 wk of supplementation, and after additional 4 wk w/o supplementation: *No change in physical examination findings, haematology, biochemistry, food intake and body weight* *Fecal scores (no change)* *Fecal volatile compounds:* hydrogen sulphide, and ammonia (no change) *Fecal pH decreased* *Fecal culture:* clostridia reduced during probiotic feeding and increased after cessation; coliform and Enterococcus decreased during the study | Marshall-Jones et al,[53] 2006 |

(continued on next page)

Table 1
(continued)

Micro-Organism Used (Source)	Dose and Duration	Test Animals (n)	Control Group	Measured Outcomes	Reference
Lactobacillus acidophilus NCFM (commercial culture)	1×10^9 cfu/d (freeze-dried) with or without FOS, FOS alone, control	5 dogs in each of 4 treatment groups (repeated once) → total of 40 dogs	Yes (control treatment consisted of sucrose and cellulose)	Each experiment: 23-d adaptation period followed by a 5-d collection period: *Food intake and fecal weight:* reduced with LAC *Fecal % dry matter, % organic matter and pH* (no change) *Fecal culture* (no change with LAC) *Fecal fermentation end products* (ammonia, biogenic and monogenic amines, branched-chain fatty acids, indoles, lactate, phenols, SCFA) (no change with LAC) *Total macronutrient digestibilities* (no change)	Swanson et al,[45] 2002

Lactobacillus animalis LA4 (isolated from 8 healthy adult dogs)	0.5×10^9 cfu/d (freeze dried) for 10 d	9 client-owned dogs (no information on signalment)		Days 0, 11 and 15: *Fecal culture:* increased lactobacilli in all samples on day 11 and in 4/9 samples on day 15, reduced enterococci *Fecal ammonia* (no change) *Fecal SCFA* (no change)	Biagi et al,[46] 2007
Lactobacillus fermentum AD1-CCM7421 (isolated from a healthy 6-year-old Tibetan Terrier)	1×10^9 cfu/d for 1 wk	15 dogs, various breeds	No	Before and after 7 d of supplementation: *Fecal culture:* increase of lactobacilli, enterococci *Serum biochemistry:* increases of total protein, total lipids and reduction of blood glucose	Strompfova et al,[47] 2006

(continued on next page)

Table 1
(continued)

Micro-Organism Used (Source)	Dose and Duration	Test Animals (n)	Control Group	Measured Outcomes	Reference
Lactobacillus fermentum AD1-CCM7421 (same as above)	*Experiment I:* 2×10^8 cfu/d (freeze dried) for 2 wk *Experiment II:* 1×10^7 cfu/d (freeze dried) for 1 wk	*Experiment I:* 12 dogs *Experiment II:* 11 dogs	No	*Experiment I:* days 0, 7, 14, 21, 28, 49 *Experiment II:* days 0, 7, 21 *Fecal score* (no change) *Fecal pH:* decrease in both experiments at day 21 *Fecal SCFA:* increased at day 21 *Fecal culture:* increases in LAB in both experiments during treatment phase and after cessation. Decrease in *Clostridia* (experiment I only) and gram-negative bacteria (coliforms, *Aeromonas* sp., *Pseudomonas* sp.) in experiment II only	Strompfova et al,[48] 2012

Probiotic	Dose	Subjects	Placebo	Results	Reference
Recombinant *Lactobacillus casei* (no further strain designation available) producing cGM-CSF (isolated from human)	1×10^9 cfu/d for 7 wk	7-week-old Beagle puppies: 6 per treatment group → 18 dogs total	Yes (both placebo and *L casei* not producing cGM-CSF)	Assessment before and then weekly for 7 wk: *Weight gain* (no difference) *Complete blood count*: higher monocyte counts in treatment group at week 4–7 *Total serum IgA*: high in treated group at week 4 *Total serum IgG* (no difference) *Total fecal IgA and IgG* (no difference) Canine coronavirus-specific vaccination-associated IgG: higher in treated group at week 5 and 6	Chung et al,[50] 2009

Abbreviations: BCS, body condition score; c/fPL, species-specific (canine/ feline) pancreatic lipase; c/fTLI, species-specific (canine/ feline) trypsin-like immunoreactivity; cfu, colony-forming units; cGM-CSF, canine granulocyte macrophage co ony stimulating factor; DGGE, denaturing gradient gel electrophoresis; FISH, fluorescent in-situ hybridization; IgA/IgE, IgG, different classes of immunoglobulins; LAC, *Lactobacillus acidophilus*; ME, metabolizable energy; PCoA, principle component analysis; qPCR, quantitative (real-time) polymerase chain reaction; SCFA, short-chain fatty acids; SPF, specific pathogen-free.
Data from Refs.[38–42,45–55]

Table 2
Probiotics or synbiotics assessed for their effect in acute GI conditions in dogs and cats

Probiotics or Synbiotic Used (Trade Name, Manufacturer)	Dose	Target Species: Dog (D), cat (C)	Animals (n)	Disorder	Observed Outcomes	Reference
B animalis AHC7 (isolated from healthy dog)	1 × 10^10 cfu BID	D	31 (no detail on number in treatment and placebo group)	Acute idiopathic diarrhea	Significantly shorter duration to resolution of diarrhea in probiotic group (3.9 ± 2.3 d) compared with placebo group (6.6 ± 2.7 d)	Kelley et al,[61] 2009
B animalis AHC7 (isolated from healthy dog)	Either 1 × 10^7 cfu/d, 1 × 10^8 cfu/d or 1 × 10^9 cfu/d (or placebo)	D	121 (no detail on number in treatment and placebo groups)	Kennel-stress associated diarrhea	No difference between fecal scores at week 1–2 Significantly better fecal score for all probiotic groups compared with placebo at week 3 No difference in diarrhea occurrences between groups	Kelley et al,[62] 2012
E faecium DSM 10663 NCIMB 10415 4 b/ E1707 + FOS and gum Arabic (Synbiotic D-C, Protexin Ltd.)	2 × 10^9 cfu/d	D	733 (399 treated, 374 placebo)	Shelter-associated diarrhea	Significantly fewer treated dogs have diarrhea (2% vs 3% in placebo group) Number of treated dogs with >1 d of diarrhea was lower (18.8% vs 27.2% in placebo group)	Rose et al,[63] 2017

Probiotic		Dose	Condition	Results	Reference
E faecium SF68 NCIMB 10415 (Fortiflora, Nestle Purina)	D, C	2.1 × 10⁹ cfu/d	*Dogs:* 182 (102 treated with EF, 80 treated with placebo) *Cats:* 217 (130 treated with EF, 87 treated with placebo)	Shelter-associated diarrhea (some animals also positive for various parasites)	*Dogs:* No difference in number of dogs having diarrhea (9.8% with EF, 12.5% with placebo) *Cats:* No difference in prevalence or duration of diarrhea (26% with EF, 32% with placebo)	Bybee et al,[56] 2011
E faecium SF68 NCIMB 10415 (Fortiflora, Nestle Purina)	D	5 × 10⁸ cfu/d	20 (10 treatment, 10 placebo)	Giardia cyst shedding (subclinical natural infection)	No statistical difference in fecal score All dogs remained subclinical	Simpson et al,[68] 2009
E faecium SF68 NCIMB 10415 (Commercial product not specified)	C	Not disclosed	27 (13 EF, 14 placebo)	Antibiotic-induced diarrhea (potentiated amoxicillin)	No statistical difference in fecal scores between treatment groups No difference in number of observed species of the fecal microbiota between treatment groups	Torres-Henderson et al,[57] 2017
LAB mixture in sour milk: *L fermentum* VET 9A, *L rhamnosus* VET 16A, *L plantarum* VET 14A	D	4 × 10¹¹ cfu/d (either SID or BID)	44 (25 probiotic, 19 placebo)	Acute or intermittent, mild to moderate diarrhea	Statistical difference in change in mean fecal score on day 7, but not days 1–6 No difference in mean fecal score on day 28	Gomez-Gallego et al,[65] 2016

(continued on next page)

Table 2
(continued)

Probiotics or Synbiotic Used (Trade Name, Manufacturer)	Dose	Target Species: Dog (D), cat (C)	Animals (n)	Disorder	Observed Outcomes	Reference
LAB mixture: B bifidum, E faecium, E thermophilus, L acidophilus, L bulgaricus, L casei, L plantarum + FOS and arabinogalactan (Proviable-DC, Nutramax Ltd.)	1×10^{10} cfu/d	C	16 (8 treatment, 8 placebo)	Antibiotic-induced diarrhea (clindamycin)	Greater abundance of fecal Ruminococcaceae in probiotic-treated group. No difference of dysbiosis index, microbiota richness or diversity indices between treatment groups. Some complex metabolomic changes were observed, but most likely owing to antibiotics rather than probiotics	Whittemore et al,[58] 2019
LAB mixture: L acidophilus ATCC 4536, L plantarum ATCC 8014, L delbrueckii UFV H2B20	1×10^{6} cfu/d	D	20 (10 treatment, 10 placebo)	Ancylostoma egg shedding	At day 28 of treatment, eggs per gram of feces decreased by 88.8% in the probiotic group, compared with 11.8% in the placebo group. This was not sustained by day 42	Coelho et al,[69] 2013

Probiotic	Dose	Species	N	Condition	Results	Reference
LAB mixture: L acidophilus, Pediococcus acidilactici, Bacillus subtilis, Bacillus licheniformis, L farciminis (ZooLac ProPaste, Natural Instinct)		D	36 (15 probiotic treatment, 21 placebo)	Acute gastroenteritis	Treatment resulted in significantly shorter duration of diarrhea. Days to last abnormal feces: probiotic 1.3 d (0.5–2.1 d); control 2.2 d (1.3–3.1 d)	Herstad et al,[64] 2010
LAB mixture "de Simone" formulation[a]: L casei, L plantarum, L acidophilus, L delbrueckii spp. bulgaricus, B longum, B breve, B infantis, Scc salivarus spp. thermophilus (VSL#3, VSL Pharmaceuticals)	4.5×10^{10} cfu/d	D	20 (10 standard treatment alone, 10 standard treatment and probiotics)	Parvoviral enteritis	Significant improvement in clinical scores between groups on day 3 and day 5	Arslan et al,[66] 2012

(continued on next page)

Table 2
(continued)

Probiotics or Synbiotic Used (Trade Name, Manufacturer)	Dose	Target Species: Dog (D), cat (C)	Animals (n)	Disorder	Observed Outcomes	Reference
LAB mixture: L plantarum DSM 24730, Scc thermophilus DSM 24731, B breve DSM 24732, L paracasei DSM 24733, L. delbrueckii subsp. bulgaricus DSM 24734, L acidophilus DSM 24735, B longum 120 DSM 24736, B infantis DSM 24737 (Visbiome, ExeGi Pharma)	225 × 10⁹ cfu for 1– 10 kg dogs; 450 × 10⁹ cfu for 10– 20 kg dogs; 900 × 10⁹ cfu for 20– 40 kg dogs	D	25 (13 treatment, 12 control)	Acute hemorrhagic diarrhea syndrome	Significantly lower clinical severity on day 3 and 4 in probiotic group compared with placebo Increased fecal abundances of Turicibacter sp. and Faecalibacterium sp. on day 7 in probiotic group Significantly lower abundance of C perfringens on day 7 in probiotic group Significantly lower C perfringens enterotoxins on day 7 in probiotic group	Ziese et al,[67] 2018

Saccharomyces boulardii (Reflor, Biocodex)	1000 mg/d	D	24 (8 in each group): group I: AB (until diarrhea) and then placebo, group II: AB (until diarrhea) and then probiotic, Group III: AB and probiotic simultaneously	Antibiotic-induced diarrhea (lincomycin)	Duration of diarrhea significantly shorter in group II (2.9 ± 0.4 d) than group I (6.5 ± 1.2 d) Group III not compared with other groups	Aktas et al,[70] 2007

Abbreviations: BID, 2 times per day; Cfu, colony-forming units; EF, Enterococcus faecium; FOS, fructo-oligosaccharides; LAB, lactic acid bacteria; SID, 1 time per day.

[a] The "de Simone" formulation was marketed under the trade name VSL#3 until 2016. Since then, the composition of VLS#3 has changed and the "de Simone" blend is available under the trade name of Visbiome in the United States and Canada and VivoMix in Europe.

Data from Refs.[56–58,61–70]

Table 3
Probiotics or synbiotics assessed for their effect in chronic GI conditions in dogs and cats

Probiotics or Synbiotic Used (Trade Name, Manufacturer)	Dose	Target Species: Dog (D), cat (C)	Animals (n)	Disorder	Observed Outcomes	Reference
E faecium (isolated from commercial product containing E faecium SF68 NCIMB10415[a]) or E hirae (isolated from a healthy kitten) vs placebo ([a]Fortiflora, Nestle Purina)	1×10^5–10^8 cfu/cell culture well	n/a (indirectly C)	n/a (no clinical trial)	Tritrichomonas fetus infection of IECs in vitro: co-culture experiment using enterococci with T fetus infecting porcine intestinal epithelial cells (IPEC-J2)	When enterococci and TF were added simultaneously, enterococci completely inhibited TF growth When enterococci were added after TF had achieved early log-phase growth (18 h), enterococci significantly inhibited growth Viable enterococci were needed for this effect, as direct interaction and colonization of the IEC was necessary. This effect was also shown to be partially pH dependent	Dickson et al,[60] 2019
E faecium DSM 10663 NCIMB 10415 4 b/E1707 + FOS and gum Arabic, kaolin, montmorillonite, pectin, alpha-glucan butyrogenic, patented mucopolysaccharide starch (Pro-Kolin paste, Protexin Ltd.)	Dose not disclosed	C	26 (13 ronidazole 10–30 mg/kg q24 h and placebo; 13 ronidazole 10–30 mg/kg q24 h and synbiotic)	Natural T fetus infection	In both groups fecal scores and body weight improved Cats on synbiotic had significantly less relapses (2/13) compared with placebo treated cats (8/13)	Lalor et al,[61] 2012 (congress abstract)

Probiotic	Dose	Species	Population/Study	Results	Reference
E faecium DSM 10663 NCIMB 10415 4b/E1707 + FOS and gum Arabic (Synbiotic D-C, Protexin Ltd.)	1×10^9 cfu/d	D	12 (7 with synbiotic, 5 with placebo [on top of hydrolyzed protein diet]) FRE	No effect of synbiotic treatment on CCECAI after start of diet; Dog in synbiotic group had significantly lower serum folate values after 6 wk of treatment; No effect of synbiotic on endoscopic or histopathologic findings; No significant difference in duodenal or colonic gene expression of Th-lymphocyte signature cytokines	Schmitz et al,[72] 2015
E faecium DSM 10663 NCIMB 10415 4b/E1707 + FOS and gum Arabic (Synbiotic D-C, Protexin Ltd.)	1×10^9 cfu/d	D	12 (7 with synbiotic, 5 with placebo [on top of hydrolyzed protein diet]) FRE (+healthy control dogs receiving diet alone)	Small increase in fecal microbiota diversity in dogs treated with synbiotic; No significant differences in microbial community composition before and after 6 wk of treatment in either synbiotic or placebo group or healthy controls	Pilla et al,[73] 2019
E faecium DSM 10663 NCIMB 10415 4b/E1707 + FOS and gum Arabic (Synbiotic D-C, Protexin Ltd.)	1×10^7 cfu/mL culture medium	D	Ex vivo culture of duodenal biopsies from 17 dogs with CE (+11 Beagles as controls) FRE	TNF-α gene expression was suppressed by EF in both healthy and CE samples; IL-2 gene expression was suppressed by EF only in samples from healthy dogs; Expression of other investigated cytokines was not changed	Schmitz et al,[79] 2014

(continued on next page)

Table 3
(continued)

Probiotics or Synbiotic Used (Trade Name, Manufacturer)	Dose	Target Species: Dog (D), cat (C)	Animals (n)	Disorder	Observed Outcomes	Reference
L acidophilus DSM13241	6×10^6 cfu/g dry food	D (German Shorthair Pointers only)	6	Nonspecific dietary sensitivity *Control period 1:* 12 wk control diet, *Probiotic period:* 12 wk probiotic diet, *Control period 2:* 12 wk control diet	Unacceptable fecal consistency/defecation rates observed in 50% of the samples/study days during control period 1, but was reduced during the probiotic period and persisted in control period 2 Fecal dry matter was significantly higher in the probiotic period compared with both control periods Culturable bacteria concentrations (*C perfringens, E coli, Lactobacillus* spp., *Bifidobacterium* spp.) were similar in each dietary period	Pascher et al,[75] 2008

L rhamnosus GG	5×10^9 cfu BID D	14	Tylosin-responsive diarrhea *Period I:* asymptomatic on tylosin; *Period II:* tylosin discontinued: 2 wk of tylosin if relapse, stopped when asymptomatic and probiotic started; *Period III:* prednisolone upon relapse, if not responding: stop prednisolone, restart tylosin)	The second time tylosin was discontinued (in 9/14 dogs), diarrhea reappeared in all 9 dogs after a median of 7 d (range 3–26 d)	Westermarck et al,[78] 2005

(continued on next page)

Table 3
(continued)

Probiotics or Synbiotic Used (Trade Name, Manufacturer)	Dose	Target Species: Dog (D), cat (C)	Animals (n)	Disorder	Observed Outcomes	Reference
LAB mixture: *L acidophilus* NCC2628, *L acidophilus* NCC2766, *L johnsonii* NCC2767	1×10^{10} cfu/d	D	21 (10 dogs on novel protein diet and placebo; 11 dogs on novel protein diet and LAB)	FRE	Both groups had significant reduction of clinical severity (but no between-group effect) No difference in cytokines assessed in duodenal biopsies before and after treatment in both groups TNF-α mRNA levels in colonic biopsies increased during placebo-treatment (but not LAB treatment) In both groups, numbers of culturable *Enterobacteriacea* decreased, whereas *Lactobacillus* spp. and *Enterococcus* spp. remained similar, and *Bifidobacterium* spp. were present in very low counts.	Sauter et al,[74] 2006
LAB mixture: *L acidophilus* NCC2628, *L acidophilus* NCC2766, *L johnsonii* NCC2767	1×10^7 cfu/mL culture medium	D (ex vivo)	Ex vivo culture of duodenal biopsies (12 from dogs with CE, 4 from healthy controls) with LABs	Unspecified CE (+healthy controls)	LAB significantly increased mRNA and protein levels of IL-10 in samples from dogs with CE (not controls)	Sauter et al,[80] 2005

Probiotic	Dose	Grade	Population	Model	Results	Reference
Saccharomyces boulardii	1×10^{10} cfu/d	D	20 dogs included, 13 finished trial (6 treated, 7 placebo [both on top of "standard" treatment of elimination diet, tylosin or metronidazole, prednisolone ± second immunosuppressant])	IBD with or without PLE	CCECAI improved significantly more in dogs receiving *S boulardii* compared with placebo at day 45 and day 60 Stool frequency was significantly reduced in the *S boulardii* group at day 30, 45 and 60 In the subgroup of PLE dogs, serum albumin was >2 g/dL in 3/3 dogs in the treatment and 2/3 dogs in the placebo group	D'Angelo et al,[76] 2018
SLAB51 blend: *Scc thermophilus* DSM32245, *L acidophilus* DSM32241, *L plantarum* DSM32244, *L casei* DSM32243, *L helveticus, DSM32242, L brevis* DSM27961, *B lactis* DSM32246, *B lactis* DSM32247 (Sivoy/ SivoMixx, Mendes/ Omendes)	2×10^{11} cfu lyophilized bacteria per 5 kg body weight	C	10 with naturally occurring disease (10 healthy cats used as controls for tissue, but not treated with probiotic)	Chronic constipation (7/10)/idiopathic megacolon (3/10)	Clinical severity score significantly reduced at end of probiotic treatment Number of ICC increased significantly Significant increase in fecal streptococci and lactobacilli after treatment (of total of 9 analyzed taxa)	Rossi et al,[82] 2018

(continued on next page)

Table 3
(continued)

Probiotics or Synbiotic Used (Trade Name, Manufacturer)	Dose	Target Species: Dog (D), cat (C)	Animals (n)	Disorder	Observed Outcomes	Reference
LAB mixture "de Simone" formulation: *L casei, L plantarum, L acidophilus, L delbrueckii* spp. *bulgaricus, B longum, B breve, B infantis, Scc salivarus* spp. *thermophiles* (VSL#3, VSL Pharmaceuticals)	112–225 × 10⁹ cfu/10 kg BW/d	D	10 dogs probiotic treatment, 10 dogs combination treatment (metronidazole and prednisolone), 10 healthy control dogs (no treatment; as controls for microbiota analysis)	IBD	CIBDAI decreased in both treatment groups, but clinical improvement was faster in the combination drug treatment group (median, 4.8 d; range, 2.5–7 d) compared with probiotic treatment (median, 10.6 d; range, 5–15 d) TGF-β expression, in duodenal tissue increased in both groups, but at greater magnitude in the probiotic-treated group Number of CD3⁺ cells in the duodenum reduced in both groups (no difference between treatments)	Rossi et al,[77] 2014

Formulation	Dose		Condition	Subjects	Results	Reference
LAB mixture "de Simone" formulation: L casei, L plantarum, L acidophilus, L delbrueckii spp. bulgaricus, B longum, B breve, B infantis, Scc salivarus spp. thermophiles (Visbiome, ExeGi Pharma LLC)	112–225 × 10⁹ cfu/10 kg BW/d	D	IBD (all dogs treated with elimination diet and prednisolone)	17 dogs randomised to standard treatment + probiotic (14 dogs completed study); 17 dogs randomised to standard treatment + placebo (12 dogs completed the study)	FoxP3+ cells increased significantly in the duodenum of probiotic treated group (not the placebo treatment) No difference in occluding or claudin-2 protein expression in duodenal tissues between groups Plasma citrulline increased significantly in probiotic-treated dogs only Abundance of *Faecalibacterium* spp. increased significantly in the probiotic-treated group, but not in the placebo group Clinical remission: no difference Total histopathology score did not differ before or after treatment between groups Total number of mucosal bacteria assessed by FISH increased in probiotic group Increased number of intestinal mucosal and fecal *Lactobacillus* spp. in treated group, but	White et al,[81] 2017

(continued on next page)

Table 3
(continued)

Probiotics or Synbiotic Used (Trade Name, Manufacturer)	Dose	Target Species: Dog (D), cat (C)	Animals (n)	Disorder	Observed Outcomes	Reference
					decreased *Bifidobacteria* spp. (FISH) Intestinal tight junction proteins (assessed by IHC) E-cadherin, occluding and zonulin: upregulated in the treated group qPCR for specific fecal bacteria: increased bifidobacteria with probiotic treatment at week 3, otherwise no difference between groups.	

Abbreviations: BW, body weight; CCECAI, canine chronic enteropathy clinical activity index; CE, chronic enteropathy; cfu, colony-forming units; CIBDAI, canine inflammatory bowel disease activity index; *EF, Enterococcus faecium*; FISH, fluorescent in-situ hybridization; FOS, fructo-oligosaccharides; FRE, food-responsive chronic enteropathy; ICC, interstitial cells of Cajal; IEC, intestinal epithelial cells; IHC, immunohistochemistry; IL, interleukin; LAB, lactic acid bacteria; PLE, protein-losing enteropathy; qPCR, quantitative polymerase chain reaction; TF, Tritrichomonas foetus; TGF-β, transforming growth factor beta; TNFα, tumor necrosis factor alpha.

a The "de Simone" formulation was marketed under the trade name VSL#3 until 2016. Since then, the composition of VSL#3 has changed and the "de Simone" blend is available under the trade name of Visbiome in the United States and Canada and VivoMix in Europe.

Data from Refs.[60,61,72–82]

systematic review, only 17 studies carried out in dogs were identified.[56] Of these, 7 were categorized as randomized controlled trials, 7 as controlled clinical trials without randomization, 1 as low evidence trial and a pseudo-randomized controlled trial, respectively, 4 were claimed to be randomized but randomization was not described, and 2 were crossover uncontrolled trials.[56]

In cats, 5 clinical trials report the use of probiotics or synbiotics in GI diseases. One of them is an randomized controlled trials,[57] 1 is an open treatment trial with a healthy nontreated control group, 3 are experimental[58,59] or in vitro[60] studies, and 1 is a conference abstract that has so far not been published in a peer-reviewed journal.[61]

In both dogs and cats, a variety of different probiotics and synbiotics from different sources have been assessed, making a comparison of individual studies difficult (**Tables 2** and **3**).

Probiotics in Acute Gastrointestinal Conditions of Dogs and Cats

Acute GI diseases in which the merit of probiotics or synbiotic treatment has been investigated can be roughly divided in 3 categories: "proven" infectious diseases (viral, bacterial, parasitic/protozoal), "idiopathic" or otherwise ill-defined gastroenteritis (in which an infectious component might or might not be present), and antibiotic-induced diarrhea (see **Table 2**).

In dogs with acute uncomplicated diarrhea ("idiopathic" gastroenteritis not further classified or due to kenneling stress/being admitted to a shelter), the benefits of probiotics are mixed, even when similar bacterial strains (eg, *Bifidobacterium animals* AHC7[62,63] or *EF*[57,64]) are used. Overall, reported significant differences may also be of some clinical relevance (1–3 days shorter duration of diarrhea,[62,65] 1% less occurrence of diarrhea,[64] better fecal score after 1–3 weeks of treatment[63,66]). Only one of these studies also included cats, and no effect on the prevalence or duration of shelter-associated diarrhea was found.[57] It is, however, noteworthy that this latter study included animals regardless of their parasitic burden at the time of diarrhea, which might have influenced the results.

In canine parvoviral enteritis, 1 study reports a significant clinical improvement with a commercially available LAB mixture added to standard treatment compared with standard treatment alone.[67] The mortality rate was decrease by probiotic administration, with 90% of dogs in the oral probiotic group surviving compared with 70% of the nonprobiotic group. In addition, total WBC and lymphocyte counts were markedly increased in all animals after probiotic treatment, whereas these parameters remained low in dogs receiving standard treatment only.[67] However, no relationship between probiotic administration and shortening of treatment duration, improvement in disease evolution, antibody production, or fecal virus excretion was established, and the mechanism by which probiotics improved clinical outcomes remains unclear. These puppies were treated under optimal conditions and the study group was small.[67] Because strain specificity is important, the documented benefits only apply to the mixture used in the study.

In acute hemorrhagic diarrhea syndrome, a disease possibly associated with acute "overgrowth" of toxin-producing *Clostridium perfringens* strains in dogs, the "de Simone" LAB probiotic blend lowered clinical severity, and increased fecal abundances of bacterial markers of gut health (eg, *Faecalibacterium* sp.), while *C perfringens* abundance as well as enterotoxins were reduced.[68]

In parasitic disease, the probiotics or synbiotics tested so far had limited to no effects (dogs only). Giardia cyst shedding was not altered by the administration of *EF*,[69] and subclinical Ancylostoma egg shedding was significantly, but only transiently, suppressed using a LAB mixture.[70]

Antibiotic-induced intestinal dysbiosis was assessed in a total of 3 experimental studies (2 in cats[58,59] and 1 in dogs[71]). Healthy cats were either given potentiated amoxicillin[58] or clindamycin,[59] and different probiotics were used to counter their effects on the GI tract (EF[58] and a LAB mixture,[59] respectively). No statistical difference was noted in fecal scores,[58] fecal dysbiosis index,[59] or fecal microbiota characteristics.[58,59] In one of the studies, complex metabolic changes of the microbiota were described, but these were more likely associated with the administration of antibiotics than the probiotics.[59] In dogs, duration of lincomycin-induced diarrhea was significantly shortened by administration of S boulardii in comparison to placebo.[71]

Probiotics in Chronic Gastrointestinal Conditions of Dogs and Cats

In dogs, the potential benefits or mechanisms of action of probiotics or synbiotics on chronic GI conditions have been assessed using both clinical trials and ex vivo experiments (see **Table 3**). Clinical trials included 3 randomized controlled trials on food-responsive chronic enteropathy (FRE),[72–74] a treatment trial in nonspecific dietary sensitivity,[75] 2 studies on IBD,[76,77] and 1 on tylosin-responsive diarrhea.[78] In addition, 2 studies involved ex vivo stimulation of biopsies from dogs with either FRE[79] or chronic enteropathy.[80] In the latter study, dogs were diagnosed with chronic enteropathy mainly based on exclusion of infectious or extra-GI causes and the demonstration of intestinal inflammation on histopathology. In canine FRE, the probiotics used (EF[79] and a LAB mixture,[80] respectively) seemed to show promising results in ex vivo experiments (ie, shift of cytokines toward a more tolerogenic microenvironment[79,80]), but failed to produce similar responses when assessed in clinical trials.[72,74] L acidophilus DSM13241 improved fecal consistency in dogs with dietary sensitivity in a very small study.[75] In dogs with tylosin-responsive diarrhea, Lactobacillus rhamnosus GG failed to prolong the asymptomatic period once clinical remission was achieved and tylosin administration discontinued.[78] In canine IBD, defined as refractory to dietary and antibiotic treatment trials, specific probiotics seem to be a promising adjunctive or possibly even sole treatment. One study administering the de Simone LAB mixture (see comments in **Table 2**) demonstrated that it was not inferior to the standard treatment consisting of a combination of metronidazole and prednisolone in inducing clinical remission (as assessed by the Canine Inflammatory Bowel Disease Index) and reduction of inflammatory cells in duodenal biopsies.[77] In addition, this study demonstrated that only the probiotic-treated dogs showed an increase in tissue markers representative of a more tolerogenic intestinal microenvironment (ie, increase in TGF-β and FoxP3$^+$ regulatory T cells).[77] There is also evidence that probiotic mixtures modulate intestinal epithelial permeability by changing expression of tight junction proteins like E-cadherin, occludin and zonulin.[77,81] In another study, a significant improvement in clinical signs (as assessed by the Canine Chronic Enteropathy Clinical Activity Index) and defecation frequency was achieved using S boulardii in IBD dogs with and without protein-losing enteropathy.[76] This also resulted in significant improvement of serum albumin in all S boulardii-treated dogs with protein-losing enteropathy, however, the number of dogs was very small with only 3 protein-losing enteropathy dogs each treated with and without S boulardii.[76]

In cats, probiotics have been assessed in the context of chronic Tritrichomonas fetus infection[60,61] and chronic constipation[82] (see **Table. 3**). Evidence for the adjunctive use of EF in feline T fetus infections is based on a small clinical trial, where it did not accelerate time to clinical improvement compared with ronidazole alone, but significantly reduced relapses[61]; and on a recent study investigating the effects of different enterococci on *T fetus* growth and cytotoxicity in a intestinal epithelial cell culture model. The enterococci (one of them sourced from a commercial product) were able to completely inhibit *T fetus* growth both "prophylactically" (before cell infection) as well as "therapeutically" (after log-phase growth had been achieved).[60]

There is some preliminary evidence that another LAB probiotic blend might be beneficial in feline chronic constipation or idiopathic megacolon.[82] This finding is based on a small pilot study in which 10 cats were included. It has several limitations besides the relatively small number of cases, mainly involving a poorly defined clinical diagnosis and the lack of a control group. All constipated cats were reported to improve clinically. There were also some changes of fecal bacterial species of unclear significance.[82] There are no studies assessing the use of probiotics or synbiotics in IBD in cats. One open-label trial showed that a probiotic mixture given to cats with chronic diarrhea resulted in an improved fecal scores after 21 days of administration alongside other treatments.[83]

SUMMARY

Many products or strains marketed or tested as probiotics or synbiotics in small animals do not strictly fulfill the criteria required of a probiotic, especially the necessity of a proven beneficial effect on the host. Although there are only a few clinical trials in the correct target species with results clinically applicable to small animal practice, studies investigating mechanisms of action of potential probiotics in dogs or cats are even more sparse. The studies available in both acute and chronic GI conditions of small animals suffer from a number of limitations. In several clinical trials, there was no control group, animals with ill-defined diseases were included, or inappropriate and nonspecific inclusion criteria were applied: examples include using animals with diarrhea of poorly defined origin,[64-66] allowing animals with infectious diseases to be part of a study of idiopathic or stress-related diarrhea,[57] and so on. In these instances, a poorly defined disease phenotype may fail to reveal a clinical benefit of the tested probiotic in a subset of the animals. Most studies with better defined inclusion criteria had better stratification of the conditions they were investigating. However, they were conducted in small groups of animals (see **Tables 2** and **3**), with either unknown or insufficient statistical power. These inappropriate study designs would most likely lead to type II statistical errors (falsely accepting that there is no difference between treatment and control). In addition, a wide range of different potential probiotics has been used at different dosages and in various conditions. This result is problematic because there is evidence that the molecular effects of probiotics are not only specific to the genus of the bacteria used, but even species or strain specific.[29] This, together with a huge discrepancy in measured outcomes (ranging from assessment of nonspecific routine clinicopathologic parameters and purely observational assessments like fecal scores to complex fecal microbiota sequencing and metabolic profiles), makes it extremely difficult to compare studies. Especially when assessing fecal microbial diversity and function, very few studies have applied modern molecular techniques like quantitative (real-time) polymerase chain reaction or next-generation sequencing[59,68,73] that allow a more realistic assessment of the microbiota composition and diversity compared with culture-based techniques.

There is preliminary evidence that certain probiotics or synbiotic preparations could be beneficial in some acute or infectious GI conditions, namely parvovirus infection[67] and acute hemorrhagic diarrhea syndrome[68] in dogs and *T fetus* infection in cats,[60,61] whereas results in nonspecific or idiopathic acute enteritis are mixed. The effect on well-defined chronic noninfectious GI conditions has only been investigated in dogs, where little benefit was observed with adjunctive administration of probiotics to dogs with FRE[72–74] or tylosin-responsive diarrhea.[78] In immunosuppressive-responsive diarrhea or chronic enteropathy (often synonymously used with idiopathic IBD); however, there is evidence that specific probiotic strains (S boulardii[76]) or mixtures (de Simone formulation[77]) can decrease clinical severity as well as induce a more tolerogenic microenvironment in the intestinal mucosa. Probiotics might be beneficial in cats with constipation,[82] but further studies are needed into this.

Despite the need for more evidence of probiotic use in small animals, it is the author's opinion that too many acute and chronic GI conditions in dogs and cats are treated empirically—and often erroneously and unnecessarily—with antibiotics. An increased awareness of the availability and safety of probiotics or synbiotics products could (and should) lead to a decrease in antibiotic usage—especially in otherwise uncomplicated cases of diarrhea. This allows veterinarians to make a significant contribution to global health and to fight and spread awareness of increasing antimicrobial resistance around the world.

In summary, more well-designed studies evaluating the potential benefit of potential probiotics in GI diseases of small animals are needed. These studies should be designed to include animals with well-defined clinical phenotypes and have sufficient statistical power. Future research should focus on assessing functional outcomes that can further the understanding of probiotic-specific mechanisms of action and inform and drive rational and evidence-based clinical use of probiotics and synbiotics.

CLINICS CARE POINTS

- When considering treatment for acute uncomplicated diarrhoea, probiotics are likely a better choice (unlikely to cause harm, possible shortening of recovery time) than antibiotics (can cause significant and long standing gut dysbiosis).
- When considering probiotics as adjunctive treatment to infectious disease, there is so far only some evidence for the benefit of Enterococcus faecium for Tritrichomonas foetus infection in cats.
- Saccharomyces boulardii is an interesting potential probiotic, that has shown promising results in reducing antibiotic-induced diarrhoea in dogs as well as improve clinical scores in dogs with chronic enteropathy and PLE.
- Specific probiotic blends can be as efficient in treating canine chronic enteropathy than antibiotic and glucocorticoid treatment combined.
- When treating feline chronic constipation, a specific probiotic blend can be considered as adjunctive treatment.

DISCLOSURE

The author's PhD was sponsored by a BBSCR studentship with Protexin Ltd. (Somerset, UK). The author has been a consultant for Boehringer Ingelheim (Germany) and has given CPDs sponsored by Vetplus Tangerine Group (UK) and Hill's Pet Nutrition (UK). In her capacity as president of the European Society of Comparative Gastroenterology, the author has accepted sponsorship for said society from Hill's Pet Nutrition (Germany), Mendes S.A. (France) and Nestle Purina PetCare Global.

REFERENCES

1. FAO/WHO. Probiotics in food - Report of a Joint FAO/WHO Expert Consultation on Evaluation of Health and Nutritional Properties of Probiotics in Food including

Powder Milk with Live Lactic Acid Bacteria - Cordoba, Argentina, 1-4 October 2001. 2006. doi: ISBN 92-5-105513-0.

2. Hill C, Guarner F, Reid G, et al. The International Scientific Association for Probiotics and Prebiotics consensus statement on the scope and appropriate use of the term probiotic. Nat Rev Gastroenterol Hepatol 2014;11:506–14.

3. de Simone C. The Unregulated Probiotic Market. Clin Gastroenterol Hepatol 2019;17(5):809–17.

4. Metchnikoff E. Lactic acid as inhibiting intestinal putrefaction. In: Heinemann W, editor. The Prolongation of Life; Optimistic Studies. London; 1907. p. 161–83.

5. Tissier H. Traitement des infections intestinales par la methode de la flore bacterienne de l'intestin. Soc Biol 1906;60:359–61.

6. Lilly D, Stillwell R. Probiotics: Growth promoting factors produced by microorganisms. Science 1965;147:747–8.

7. Fuller R. Probiotics in man and animals. J Appl Bacteriol 1989;66:365–78.

8. Havenaar R, Huis in't Veld J. Probiotics: A general view. In: Wood B, editor. The lactic acid bacteriavol. 1. New York: Chapman & Hall; 1992. p. 209–24. The lactic acid bacteria in health and disease.

9. Guarner F, Schaafsma G. Probiotics. Int J Food Microbiol 1998;39:237–8.

10. Gibson GR, Roberfroid MB. Dietary modulation of the human colonic microbiota: introducing the concept of prebiotics. J Nutr 1995;125(6):1401–12.

11. Andersson H, Asp N-G, Bruce Å, et al. Health effects of probiotics and prebiotics: A literature review on human studies. Näringsforskning. 2001;45(1):58–75.

12. Patel RM, Denning PW. Therapeutic use of prebiotics, probiotics, and postbiotics to prevent necrotizing enterocolitis: what is the current evidence? Clin Perinatol 2013;40(1):11–25.

13. Degnan FH. The US Food and Drug Administration and probiotics: regulatory categorization. Clin Infect Dis 2008;46(s2).S133–6.

14. Food and Drug Administration FDA. Dietary supplements: new dietary ingredient notifications and related Issues: guidance for industry. 2016. Available at: https://www.fda.gov/media/99538/download.

15. Giordano-Schaefer J, Ruthsatz M, Schneider H. Distinctive regulatory barriers for the development of medical foods. Regul Focus Regul Aff Prof Soc 2017.

16. Council for Responsible Nutrition C. CRN-IPA best practices guidelines for probiotics. 2017. Available at: https://www.fda.gov/ICECI/EnforcementActions/WarningLetters/ucm367142.htm.

17. Food and Drug Administration FDA. Policy regarding quantitative labeling of dietary supplements containing live microbials: guidance for industry. draft guidance. 2018. Available at: https://www.crnusa.org/sites/default/files/pdfs/CRN-IPA-Best-Practices-Guidelines-for-Probiotics.pdf.

18. Weese JS, Arroyo L. Bacteriological evaluation of dog and cat diets that claim to contain probiotics. Can Vet J 2003;44(3):212–6.

19. Weese J, Martin H. Assessment of commercial probiotic bacterial contents and label accuracy. Can Vet J 2011;52(1):43–6.

20. Sanders ME, Akkermans LMA, Haller D, et al. Safety assessment of probiotics for human use. Gut Microbes 2010;1(3):164–85.

21. Didari T, Solki S, Mozaffari S, et al. A systematic review of the safety of probiotics. Expert Opin Drug Saf 2014;13(2):227–39.

22. Sanders ME, Merenstein DJ, Ouwehand AC, et al. Probiotic use in at-risk populations. J Am Pharm Assoc 2016;56(6):680–6.

23. Vallabhaneni S, Walker TA, Lockhart SR, et al. Notes from the field: Fatal gastrointestinal mucormycosis in a premature infant associated with a contaminated

dietary supplement–Connecticut, 2014. MMWR Morb Mortal Wkly Rep 2015; 64(6):155–6.

24. Besselink MG, van Santvoort HC, Buskens E, et al. Probiotic prophylaxis in predicted severe acute pancreatitis: a randomised, double-blind, placebo-controlled trial. Lancet 2008;371(9613):651–9.

25. Lee Y-K, Puong K-Y, Ouwehand AC, et al. Displacement of bacterial pathogens from mucus and Caco-2 cell surface by lactobacilli. J Med Microbiol 2003; 52(Pt 10):925–30.

26. Collado MC, Grześkowiak Ł, Salminen S. Probiotic strains and their combination inhibit in vitro adhesion of pathogens to pig intestinal mucosa. Curr Microbiol 2007;55(3):260–5.

27. Saarela M, Mogensen G, Fondén R, et al. Probiotic bacteria: safety, functional and technological properties. J Biotechnol 2000;84(3):197–215.

28. Oelschlaeger TA. Mechanisms of probiotic actions - A review. Int J Med Microbiol 2010;300(1):57–62.

29. Thomas CM, Versalovic J. Probiotics-host communication: Modulation of signaling pathways in the intestine. Gut Microbes 2010;1(3):148–63.

30. Allaart JG, van Asten AJAM, Vernooij JCM, et al. Effect of Lactobacillus fermentum on beta2 toxin production by Clostridium perfringens. Appl Environ Microbiol 2011;77(13):4406–11.

31. Jones SE, Versalovic J. Probiotic Lactobacillus reuteri biofilms produce antimicrobial and anti-inflammatory factors. BMC Microbiol 2009;9:35.

32. Pagnini C, Saeed R, Bamias G, et al. Probiotics promote gut health through stimulation of epithelial innate immunity. Proc Natl Acad Sci U S A 2010;107(1):454–9.

33. Soo I, Madsen KL, Tejpar Q, et al. VSL#3 probiotic upregulates intestinal mucosal alkaline sphingomyelinase and reduces inflammation. Can J Gastroenterol 2008; 22(3):237–42.

34. Lin PW, Myers LES, Ray L, et al. Lactobacillus rhamnosus blocks inflammatory signaling in vivo via reactive oxygen species generation. Free Radic Biol Med 2009;47(8):1205–11.

35. Vitetta L, Briskey D, Alford H, et al. Probiotics, prebiotics and the gastrointestinal tract in health and disease. Inflammopharmacology 2014;22(3):135–54.

36. Fijan S. Microorganisms with claimed probiotic properties: An overview of recent literature. Int J Environ Res Public Health 2014;11(5):4745–67.

37. Schmitz S, Suchodolski J. Understanding the canine intestinal microbiota and its modification by pro-, pre- and synbiotics - what is the evidence? Vet Med Sci 2016;2(2):71–94.

38. Benyacoub J, Czarnecki-Maulden GL, Cavadini C, et al. Supplementation of food with Enterococcus faecium (SF68) stimulates immune functions in young dogs. J Nutr 2003;133(4):1158–62.

39. Marciňáková M, Simonová M, Strompfová V, et al. Oral application of Enterococcus faecium strain EE3 in healthy dogs. Folia Microbiol (Praha) 2006;51(3): 239–42.

40. Veir JK, Knorr R, Cavadini C, et al. Effect of supplementation with Enterococcus faecium (SF68) on immune functions in cats. Vet Ther 2007;8(4):229–38.

41. Baillon ML a, Marshall-Jones ZV, Butterwick RF. Effects of probiotic Lactobacillus acidophilus strain DSM13241 in healthy adult dogs. Am J Vet Res 2004;65(3): 338–43.

42. Félix AP, Netto MVT, Murakami FY, et al. Digestibility and fecal characteristics of dogs fed with Bacillus subtilis in diet. Ciência Rural 2010;40(10):2169–73.

43. Biourge V, Vallet C, Levesque a, et al. The use of probiotics in the diet of dogs. J Nutr 1998;128(12 Suppl):2730S–2S.

44. Gagné JW, Wakshlag JJ, Simpson KW, et al. Effects of a synbiotic on fecal quality, short-chain fatty acid concentrations, and the microbiome of healthy sled dogs. BMC Vet Res 2013;9:246.

45. Swanson KS, Grieshop CM, Flickinger E a, et al. Fructooligosaccharides and Lactobacillus acidophilus modify gut microbial populations, total tract nutrient digestibilities and fecal protein catabolite concentrations in healthy adult dogs. J Nutr 2002;132(12):3721–31.

46. Biagi G, Cipollini I, Pompei A, et al. Effect of a Lactobacillus animalis strain on composition and metabolism of the intestinal microflora in adult dogs. Vet Microbiol 2007;124(1–2):160–5.

47. Strompfová V, Marciňáková M, Simonová M, et al. Application of potential probiotic Lactobacillus fermentum AD1 strain in healthy dogs. Anaerobe 2006; 12(2):75–9.

48. Strompfová V, Lauková a, Gancarčíková S. Effectivity of freeze-dried form of Lactobacillus fermentum AD1-CCM7421 in dogs. Folia Microbiol (Praha) 2012; 57(4):347–50.

49. Manninen TJK, Rinkinen ML, Beasley SS, et al. Alteration of the canine small-intestinal lactic acid bacterium microbiota by feeding of potential probiotics. Appl Environ Microbiol 2006;72(10):6539–43.

50. Chung JY, Sung EJ, Cho CG, et al. Effect of recombinant Lactobacillus expressing canine GM-CSF on immune function in dogs. J Microbiol Biotechnol 2009; 19(11):1401–7.

51. Kelley R, Soon Park J, O'Mahony L, et al. Safety and Tolerance of Dietary Supplementation With a Canine-Derived Probiotic (Bifidobacterium animalis Strain AHC7) Fed to Growing Dogs. Vet Ther 2010;11(3):E1–14.

52. Garcla-Mazcorro JF, Lanerie DJ, Dowd SE, et al. Effect of a multi-species synbiotic formulation on fecal bacterial microbiota of healthy cats and dogs as evaluated by pyrosequencing. FEMS Microbiol Ecol 2011;78(3):542–54.

53. Marshall-Jones ZV, Baillon M-LA, Croft JM, et al. Effects of Lactobacillus acidophilus DSM13241 as a probiotic in healthy adult cats. Am J Vet Res 2006;67(6): 1005–12.

54. Fusi E, Rizzi R, Polli M, et al. Effects of Lactobacillus acidophilus D2/CSL (CECT 4529) supplementation on healthy cat performance Companion or pet animals. Vet Rec 2019;6(1):e000363.

55. Biagi G, Cipollini I, Bonaldo A, et al. Effect of feeding a selected combination of galacto-oligosaccharides and a strain of Bifidobacterium pseudocatenulatum on the intestinal microbiota in cats. Am J Vet Res 2013;74(1):90–5.

56. Jensen AP, Bjørnvad CR. Clinical effect of probiotics in prevention or treatment of gastrointestinal disease in dogs: A systematic review. J Vet Intern Med 2019; 33(5):1849–64.

57. Bybee SN, Scorza aV, Lappin MR. Effect of the probiotic Enterococcus faecium SF68 on presence of diarrhea in cats and dogs housed in an animal shelter. J Vet Intern Med 2011;25(4):856–60.

58. Torres-Henderson C, Summers S, Suchodolski J, et al. Effect of Enterococcus Faecium Strain SF68 on gastrointestinal signs and fecal microbiome in cats administered amoxicillin-clavulanate. Top Companion Anim Med 2017;32(3): 104–8.

59. Whittemore JC, Stokes JE, Price JM, et al. Effects of a synbiotic on the fecal microbiome and metabolomic profiles of healthy research cats administered clindamycin: a randomized, controlled trial. Gut Microbes 2019;10(4):521–39.

60. Dickson R, Vose J, Bemis D, et al. The effect of enterococci on feline Tritrichomonas foetus infection in vitro. Vet Parasitol 2019;273:90–6.

61. Lalor S, Gunn-Moore D. Effects of concurrent ronidazole and probiotic therapy in cats with Tritrichomonas foetus-associated diarrhoea. J Feline Med Surg 2012; 14(9):650–8.

62. Kelley RL, Minikhiem D, Kiely B, et al. Clinical benefits of probiotic canine-derived Bifidobacterium animalis strain AHC7 in dogs with acute idiopathic diarrhea. Vet Ther 2009;10(3):121–30.

63. Kelley R, Levy K, Mundell P, et al. Effects of varying doses of a probiotic supplement fed to healthy dogs undergoing kenneling stress. Int J Appl Res Vet Med 2012;10(3):205–16.

64. Rose L, Rose J, Gosling S, et al. Efficacy of a probiotic-prebiotic supplement on incidence of diarrhea in a dog shelter: a randomized, double-blind, placebo-controlled trial. J Vet Intern Med 2017;31(2):377–82.

65. Herstad HK, Nesheim BB, L'Abée-Lund T, et al. Effects of a probiotic intervention in acute canine gastroenteritis - A controlled clinical trial. J Small Anim Pract 2010;51(1):34–8.

66. Gómez-Gallego C, Junnila J, Männikkö S, et al. A canine-specific probiotic product in treating acute or intermittent diarrhea in dogs: A double-blind placebo-controlled efficacy study. Vet Microbiol 2016;197:122–8.

67. Arslan HH, Aksu DS, Terzi G, et al. Therapeutic effects of probiotic bacteria in parvoviral enteritis in dogs. Rev Vet Med 2012;163(2):55–9.

68. Ziese AL, Suchodolski JS, Hartmann K, et al. Effect of probiotic treatment on the clinical course, intestinal microbiome, and toxigenic Clostridium perfringens in dogs with acute hemorrhagic diarrhea. PLoS One 2018;13(9):e0204691.

69. Simpson KW, Rishniw M, Bellosa M, et al. Influence of Enterococcus faecium SF68 probiotic on giardiasis in dogs. J Vet Intern Med 2009;23(3):476–81.

70. Coêlho MDG, Coêlho FADS, Mancilha IM De. Probiotic therapy: A promising strategy for the control of canine hookworm. J Parasitol Res 2013;2013. https://doi.org/10.1155/2013/430413.

71. Aktas MS, Borku MK, Ozkanlar Y. Efficacy of Saccharomyces Boulardii As a Probiotic in Dogs With Lincomycin Induced Diarrhoea. 2007;(2004):365–9.

72. Schmitz S, Glanemann B, Garden OA, et al. A prospective, randomized, blinded, placebo-controlled pilot study on the effect of enterococcus faecium on clinical activity and intestinal gene expression in canine food-responsive chronic enteropathy. J Vet Intern Med 2015. https://doi.org/10.1111/jvim.12563.

73. Pilla R, Guard BC, Steiner JM, et al. Administration of a synbiotic containing enterococcus faecium does not significantly alter fecal microbiota richness or diversity in dogs with and without food-responsive chronic enteropathy. Front Vet Sci 2019;6. https://doi.org/10.3389/fvets.2019.00277.

74. Sauter SN, Benyacoub J, Allenspach K, et al. Effects of probiotic bacteria in dogs with food responsive diarrhoea treated with an elimination diet. J Anim Physiol Anim Nutr (Berl) 2006;90(7–8):269–77.

75. Pascher M, Hellweg P, Khol-Parisini A, et al. Effects of a probiotic Lactobacillus acidophilus strain on feed tolerance in dogs with non-specific dietary sensitivity. Arch Anim Nutr 2008;62(2):107–16.

76. D'Angelo S, Fracassi F, Bresciani F, et al. Effect of Saccharomyces boulardii in dogs with chronic enteropathies: double-blinded, placebo-controlled study. Vet Rec 2018;182(9):258.

77. Rossi G, Pengo G, Caldin M, et al. Comparison of microbiological, histological, and immunomodulatory parameters in response to treatment with either combination therapy with prednisone and metronidazole or probiotic VSL#3 strains in dogs with idiopathic inflammatory bowel disease. PLoS One 2014;9(4). https://doi.org/10.1371/journal.pone.0094699.

78. Westermarck E, Skrzypczak T, Harmoinen J, et al. Tylosin-responsive chronic diarrhea in dogs. J Vet Intern Med 2005;19(2):177–86.

79. Schmitz S, Henrich M, Neiger R, et al. Stimulation of duodenal biopsies and whole blood from dogs with food-responsive chronic enteropathy and healthy dogs with toll-like receptor ligands and probiotic enterococcus faecium. Scand J Immunol 2014;80(2):85–94.

80. Sauter SN, Allenspach K, Gaschen F, et al. Cytokine expression in an ex vivo culture system of duodenal samples from dogs with chronic enteropathies: Modulation by probiotic bacteria. Domest Anim Endocrinol 2005;29(4):605–22.

81. White R, Atherly T, Guard B, et al. Randomized, controlled trial evaluating the effect of multi-strain probiotic on the mucosal microbiota in canine idiopathic inflammatory bowel disease. Gut Microbes 2017;8(5):451–66.

82. Rossi G, Jergens A, Cerquetella M, et al. Effects of a probiotic (SLAB51™) on clinical and histologic variables and microbiota of cats with chronic constipation/megacolon: A pilot study. Benef Microbes 2018;9(1):101–10.

83. Hart ML, Suchodolski JS, Steiner JM, et al. Open-label trial of a multi-strain synbiotic in cats with chronic diarrhea. J Feline Med Surg 2012;14(4):240–5.

Fecal Microbiota Transplantation in Dogs

Jennifer Chaitman, VMD[a], Frédéric Gaschen, Dr med vet, Dr habil[b],*

KEYWORDS

- Fecal microbiota transplantation • Intestinal microbiome • Intestinal metabolome
- Dog • Acute enteritis • Chronic enteropathy

KEY POINTS

- Fecal microbiota transplantation (FMT) is used with success in the treatment of recurrent *Clostridioides difficile* infections in people, and its benefits in other diseases of the digestive tract and additional organ systems are currently being investigated in human medicine.
- In canine medicine, FMT administered via enema seems to be beneficial in acute gastrointestinal disorders. Repeat FMT treatments shortened duration to return of formed feces and hospital stay in puppies with parvovirus infections. In addition, a single FMT was superior to metronidazole in the treatment of acute enteritis.
- The effects of FMT in chronic gastrointestinal disorders are much less well documented, although the existing data consisting of case reports and small case series seem to document that the technique may be beneficial in some instances. However, more data are needed to define which canine patients could be helped by FMT.

INTRODUCTION

Fecal microbiota transplantation (FMT) describes the transfer of feces from a healthy donor into the gut of a diseased recipient with the goal of modulating the recipient's intestinal microbiome.[1] The procedure can be done via enema, colonoscopy, duodenoscopy, nasogastric/nasojejunal tube, or by ingesting oral capsules.[2,3]

FMT is not a new medical technique. It has been used in various forms to treat patients in China since the fourth century of our era.[3] More recently, the first report describing the use of FMT in North American patients with pseudomembranous colitis was published in 1958,[4] and the technique has gained great popularity and approval for use in patients with *Clostridiodes difficile* infections (CDI) in the last years.[1,5] At this

---

Conflict of Interest Declaration: The authors declare no conflict of interest.
[a] Veterinary Internal Medicine and Allergy Specialists, 207 East 84th Street, New York, NY 10028, USA; [b] Department of Veterinary Clinical Sciences, Louisiana State University School of Veterinary Medicine, Skip Bertman Drive, Baton Rouge, LA 70803, USA
* Corresponding author.
E-mail address: fgaschen@lsu.edu

Vet Clin Small Anim 51 (2021) 219–233
https://doi.org/10.1016/j.cvsm.2020.09.012
0195-5616/21/© 2020 Elsevier Inc. All rights reserved.
vetsmall.theclinics.com

time, the value of FMT continues to be explored in the treatment of other gastrointestinal (GI) and non-GI disorders.[5,6]

In veterinary medicine transfer of GI microbiota is not new either. First, several mammalian species are coprophagic. Coprophagy is of nutritional significance in rodents and lagomorphs, allowing the animal to absorb nutrients produced by their large intestinal microbiota.[7] Conspecific coprophagy occurs in 16% of privately owned dogs and seems to be a positive behavioral trait already present in the ancestors of the domestic dog aiming at limiting the risk of parasite infestation in the den.[8]

Therapeutic transfer of rumen content (transfaunation) has been documented in Europe as early as in the seventeenth century.[9,10] More recently, following the successful use of FMT in people with CDI, the technique has gained notoriety in small animal gastroenterology as well. FMT products are available commercially in the United States and elsewhere. However, to date there are only few peer-reviewed scientific publications that establish the value of FMT in the treatment of canine and feline GI diseases.[11]

MECHANISMS OF ACTION OF FECAL MICROBIOTA TRANSPLANTATION

Humans, cats, and dogs host trillions of microorganisms in their gastrointestinal tracts, including bacteria, archaea, fungi, and protozoa. The gut microbiota contributes to the health of the host through several functions: development and support of the immune system, production of metabolites with nutritional value or signaling function, maintenance of homeostasis (eg, maintenance of the intestinal barrier), and resistance to colonization with pathogenic bacteria, and these important functions ultimately exert an essential and positive influence the host's general health.[12,13]

The intestinal microbiome is severely affected by acute and chronic GI inflammatory diseases[13-15] or by administration of antibiotics.[16-18] Although it is not known if the intestinal microbiota exerts a triggering role or is a mere innocent bystander in the pathogenesis of chronic enteropathies such as inflammatory bowel disease (IBD), the resulting dysbiosis has measurable repercussions on the metabolome that may negatively affect the host's health. For more details, the reader is referred to the review by Anna-Lena Ziese and Jan. S. Suchodolski's article, "Impact of Changes in GI Microbiota in Canine and Feline Digestive Diseases," in this issue.

The beneficial effects of FMT on the intestinal microbiota and the host have not been clearly identified yet. They likely occur in response to multiple events associated with fecal transfer. An increase in richness in the microbiome and a shift of recipient microbial profiles toward those of the healthy donor are recognized as essential benefits of FMT in people with CDI and typical extreme dysbiosis.[19,20] In addition, these microbial changes also create less favorable conditions for the growth of *C difficile*, for instance by providing bacteriocins and reestablishing the prominence of secondary bile acids over primary bile acids in the feces.[19,20] Concentrations of secondary bile acids are also decreased in the feces of dogs with chronic intestinal diseases, and *Clostridium hiranonis*, a bacteria with the capacity to transform primary into secondary bile acids, is present in only diminished concentration.[21] Transplanted fecal microbiota may also contribute to restoring the integrity of the intestinal barrier through secretions of mucin to support the mucous layer separating the epithelial cells from the gut lumen.[20] Furthermore, a significant shift toward butyrate-producing species of bacteria following FMT may induce regulatory T cells and promote interleukin-10 production, ultimately resulting in favorable modulation of the mucosal immune response and decreased inflammation.[20,22] Finally, it is possible that bacteriophages present in the donor's feces contribute to the beneficial effects as well.[23]

USE OF FECAL MICROBIOTA TRANSPLANTATION IN PEOPLE

The therapeutic value of FMT was demonstrated during several outbreaks of severe recurring CDI in Europe and North America early in the twenty-first century.[5] Fecal microbiota transplantation is now recognized as the treatment of choice for recurrent CDI.[2,5] The technique has also been applied with more limited success to patients with other intestinal diseases such as Crohn's disease, ulcerative colitis, IBD, and colorectal cancer with promising perspectives in some instances.[5,19] Interestingly, there is also preliminary evidence about the effect of FMT as an added modality on outcomes of diseases that affect organs located outside the GI tract and are associated with intestinal dysbiosis. Examples include hepatic encephalopathy, psoriasis, some neurologic disorders, metabolic syndrome, and cancer.[6] For instance, FMT improved gastrointestinal and behavioral symptoms of patients with autism spectrum disorders,[24] and studies described increased insulin sensitivity after FMT in people with metabolic syndrome.[25] These preliminary results need to be confirmed, and the mechanisms through which the alteration in intestinal microbiota exerts a beneficial effect on the disease processes need to be elucidated. However, these studies offer a perspective on the very broad potential of FMT as an adjunctive treatment in human medicine.

Complications of FMT in human patients seem to be generally limited to abdominal discomfort, bloating, cramping, diarrhea/constipation, nausea/vomiting, and low-grade fever.[1,26] However, rarely more serious infectious complications have been reported such as high-grade fever and bacteremia with multidrug resistant (MDR) bacteria, and death was described recently in 2 patients.[27] This underscores the essential importance of diligent donor screening including fecal MDR bacteria in human medicine.

EXPERIENCE WITH FECAL MICROBIOTA TRANSPLANTATION IN DOGS

There are only few studies describing the use of FMT in dogs. Data obtained from studies and case reports published in peer-reviewed journals (**Table 1**) and published conference abstracts and university thesis (**Table 2**) include results from 5 clinical trials, a few case series, and several case reports.

Daily FMT administered orally to puppies for 5 days before weaning using feces from their dam was not helpful in preventing postweaning diarrhea.[28] In puppies with parvovirus infection, FMT did not significantly improve survival but increased the percentage of survivors who had resolution of diarrhea within 48 hours (61.5% with FMT plus standard treatment vs 4.5% with standard treatment alone) and shortened hospitalization time from a median of 6 days (range 2–15) to 3 days (range 1–6).[29] However, puppies treated with FMT were significantly older than those not receiving FMT (4-month-old vs 3-month-old, respectively), which may represent a confounding factor, as better survival might be expected in older puppies.[29]

One of the authors (JC) performed a study comparing the outcome of treatment with a single FMT administered by enema or with a 7-day course of oral metronidazole at 15 mg/kg q12 hours in adult dogs with noninfectious acute diarrhea of less than 14 days duration and no or only mild systemic signs.[30] Although fecal consistency was equally improved after 7 days of treatment in both groups, by day 28 the dogs receiving FMT had firmer feces than those treated with antibiotics. The fecal dysbiosis index (FDI) is a value computed based on qPCR result of 8 bacterial taxa in the feces, which provides a reliable indication of changes in fecal microbiota composition.[31] FDI normalized at day 7 and remained within the reference range at day 28 in most dogs treated with FMT, whereas it did not normalize in most dogs receiving metronidazole.

Table 1
Cases of fecal microbiota transplantation in dogs reported in the literature (in chronologic order)

Author, Year	Indication	Format	Number of Animals, Frequency of FMT	Route	Clinical Effect	Effect of Fecal Microbiome	Comments
Burton et al,[28] 2016	Puppies at weaning age, postweaning diarrhea.	RCT	11 puppies received FMT daily for 5 d, 12 received sham treatment.	O	No difference in fecal consistency between FMT and sham-treated puppies.	Wide variability of microbiome in puppies, no clustering with donor microbiome observed.	10 mL fecal suspension (100 g pooled dam feces mixed with 200 mL 2% fat cow's milk after filtration).
Bottero et al,[32] 2017	IBD refractory to conventional treatment.	CS	16 adult dogs with severe, refractory IBD of >1 y duration. Oral treatment group received FMT q48–72h	Endo + O (9). O (7)	Overall, mean CCECAI seemed to decrease in most dogs following FMT. Heterogenous clinical presentation and concurrent treatments complicate evaluation.	Not done.	60–80 g feces for dogs <20 kg BW, 100–150 g for dogs >20 kg BW. 1/1 dilution with 0.9% saline, filtered and mixed with low-fat yoghurt as enrichment solution.
Pereira et al,[29] 2018	Parvovirus infection.	CT	33 received standard treatment, 33 received FMT in addition. FMT administered within 6–12 h of admission and q48 h thereafter.	E	No difference in mortality rate, quicker resolution of diarrhea, and shorter hospital stay in dogs receiving FMT.	Not done	10 g feces administered per puppy. 1/1 dilution with saline. Possible confounding factor: treatment group was statistically older than control group.

Study	Indication	Design	Route	Population/Treatment	Outcome	Microbiota	FMT protocol
Niina et al,[34] 2019	IBD refractory to antibiotic and immune-suppressive treatment over time.	CR	E	One 10-year-old toy poodle.	Improved CIBDAI and fecal scores throughout treatment period.	Increase in Fusobacteria, Firmicutes and Bacteroidetes, decrease in Proteobacteria. Clustered phylogenetically with donor.	1 vol. feces diluted with 3 vol. Ringer lactate. Dog received approx. 3 g feces/kg body weight. Nine treatments within 6 mo
Sugita et al,[35] 2019	Intermittent large bowel diarrhea, 4 mo duration, feces positive for Clostridioides difficile (PCR and toxins A & B).	CR	O	One 8-month-old French bulldog.	Normalization of fecal consistency and defecation frequency within 2–3 d, no recurrence of C difficile or diarrhea over 190 d.		30 mL fecal suspension (60 g feces diluted in 50 mL tap water after filtration) given orally. Equivalent to approx. 2.5–3 g feces/kg BW
Chaitman et al,[30] 2020	Uncomplicated acute diarrhea of < 14 d duration.	CT	E	11 dogs received a single FMT, 7 dogs received MTZ 15 mg/kg q12 h for 7 d, 14 healthy control dogs	Lower (better) fecal score at days 7 and 28 for both treatments, FMT fecal score lower than MTZ at day 28.	Fecal dysbiosis index better with FMT than MTZ at days 7 and 28. FMT dogs tended to cluster with healthy dogs at day 28 unlike MTZ dogs.	See **Table 3**

None of the comparative studies was blinded.

Abbreviations: CCECAI, canine chronic enteropathy clinical activity index; *C. difficile, Clostridioides difficile*; CIBDAI, canine IBD activity index; CR, case report; CS, case series; CT, non-randomized clinical trial; E, enema; Endo, delivery in the duodenum through endoscope; FMT, fecal microbiota transplantation; IBD, inflammatory bowel disease; MTZ, metronidazole; O, oral; RCT, randomized clinical trial.

Data from Refs.[28–30,32,34,35]

Table 2
Cases of fecal microbiota transplantation in dogs reported in congress proceedings and theses (in chronologic order)

Author, Year	Indication	Format	Number of Animals, Frequency of FMT	Route	Clinical Effect	Effect of Fecal Microbiome	Comments
Weese et al,[41] 2013	Eosinophilic IBD, 2 y duration, insufficiently controlled with conventional treatment.	CR	One 3-year-old dog received a single FMT.	E	Fecal consistency normalized within 24 h, dog clinically normal for 3 mo except one bout of diarrhea responsive to antibiotics.	Increased species richness, clustered phylogenetically with donor 24h after FMT.	10 mL/kg BW fecal suspension (unknown concentration) after warm water enema, 45 min retention time.
Murphy et al,[42] 2014	C. perfringens infections unresponsive to MTZ and amoxicillin and clavulanate	CS	8 dogs receiving between 1 and 3 FMT.	E	Immediate resolution of diarrhea after FMT in all dogs.	6/8 dogs had negative fecal PCR for C. perfringens toxin after FMT.	See Table 3.
Gerbec, 2016,[45]	Various chronic GI diseases associated with diarrhea and vomiting	CS	3 dogs receiving 1 single FMT	Endo	Owners reported clinical improvement for 1–2 mo followed by relapse in 2 dogs, no change in 1 dog.	Improvement of the fecal dysbiosis index in 2of 3 dogs.	10 mL/kg BW fecal solution, equivalent to 1.45 g feces/10 kg BW.
Chaitman et al,[33] 2017	Chronic diarrhea refractory to diet and antibiotic treatment, or refractory Giardia infection.	CS	8 dogs <8-month-old with treatment-refractory Giardia infections and 8 dogs with chronic enteropathy and no response to a novel protein diet or antibiotics.	E	No data available.	Fecal dysbiosis index normalized 7 d after FMT, improved concentrations of C. hiranonis and Faecalibacterium, improved fecal concentration of primary bile acids.	5 g feces per kg BW. See Table 3.

Burchell et al,[43] 2019	Acute hemorrhagic diarrhea syndrome.	RCT	4 dogs received a single FMT and 4 dogs received saline.	E	No difference in clinical score between FMT and saline.	Diversity index improved in FMT dogs at discharge but not 30 d later.	No further details available.
Dwyer et al,[44] 2019	Heathy dogs receiving tylosin.	RCT	6 dogs received a single FMT via enema, 6 dogs received FMT orally for 14 d.	E/O	No difference in fecal score between control dogs and dogs treated with either form of FMT.	Normalization of qPCR for *C. hiranonis* and *Faecalibacterium* delayed in controls but not in FMT dogs.	See **Table 3**.

Abbreviations: CCECAI, canine chronic enteropathy clinical activity index; CIBDAI, canine IBD activity index; CR, case report; CS, case series; CT, nonrandomized clinical trial; E, enema; Endo, delivery in the duodenum through endoscope; O, oral; PCR, polymerase chain reaction; RCT, randomized clinical trial.
Data from Refs.[33,41–44]

Similarly, there was an increase in fecal bacterial diversity and concentration of desirable bacterial taxa such as *C. hiranonis* and *Faecalibacterium* and a decrease of *Escherichia coli* only in dogs receiving FMT at both times. Finally, the increased percentage of primary bile acids (when compared with total fecal bile acids) documented at presentation normalized after FMT only, and generally the fecal metabolome of dogs treated with FMT was closer to that of healthy controls at days 7 and 28 than was the case for metronidazole-treated dogs. The superiority of FMT over metronidazole treatment is not surprising in light of the changes in fecal microbiota and metabolome reported in healthy dogs treated with metronidazole.[18]

Unfortunately, the available evidence is less compelling in dogs with chronic enteropathies. In a case series of 16 adult dogs with treatment-refractory chronic IBD of greater than 12 months duration, FMT was delivered endoscopically in the duodenum, followed by oral FMT (n = 9) or only orally (n = 7).[32] In the latter group, oral FMT was administered every 48 hours for 1 month, then every 72 hours for another 2 months. The chronic canine enteropathy clinical activity index was calculated for these dogs before and 1 and 3 months after initial FMT and seemed to improve in many dogs. However, the confounding effects of the different clinical presentations and the other treatments given to these dogs make the interpretation of the impact of FMT on their clinical outcome impossible. In another study performed by one of the authors (JC) and presented as an abstract, 16 dogs with chronic diarrhea were enrolled, 8 were younger than 8 months and had treatment-refractory *Giardia* infections, whereas the other 8 were of undisclosed age and had a chronic enteropathy that had not responded to a novel protein diet or to antibiotics.[33] All dogs received one single FMT treatment administered via enema. Their mean FDI normalized 1 week after FMT, and there was an increase in the fecal concentration of desirable taxa such as *C. hiranonis* and *Faecalibacterium*. In addition, the initially increased proportion of primary fecal bile acids compared with total fecal bile acids normalized 1 week after FMT. Fecal bile acid metabolism is abnormal in dogs with chronic enteropathy[21] and other chronic diseases. This seems to be associated with subnormal fecal concentrations of *C. hiranonis*.[21]

The remaining data on the effect of FMT on dogs with chronic intestinal diseases consists of case reports. A 10-year-old toy poodle with treatment refractory IBD received 9 FMT via enema over 6 months, which improved the dog's Clinical IBD Activity Index and fecal consistency during the treatment period, and caused the recipient's fecal microbiome to cluster with that of the donor.[34] An 8-month-old French bulldog with chronic colitis and a positive *C difficile* fecal culture showed improved defecation frequency and fecal appearance and consistency within 2 to 3 days of receiving a single oral FMT. No recurrence was observed for at least 6 months.[35] Further case reports and case series presented at conferences are listed in **Table 2**.

Based on the available data, dogs with acute diarrhea often respond well to a single FMT,[30] and the technique is commonly used in clinical patients by one of the authors (JC). A single FMT should be considered instead of antibiotic therapy in order to prevent the effects of antibiotics on the intestinal microbiome and to decrease overall antibiotic use in the treatment of these conditions. FMT also shows promise as a therapeutic modality for dogs with chronic intestinal diseases and associated dysbiosis including various chronic enteropathies and exocrine pancreatic insufficiency. However, dogs with chronic diarrhea may improve for a few days to a week after FMT, but generally relapse thereafter. Therefore, multiple FMTs may be needed in most situations (Chaitman and Gaschen, unpublished observations, 2020). In one author's experience (JC), FMT is helpful in patients with *Giardia* infections who are not responding to conventional therapy. In many instances, the infection seems to subside a few weeks after FMT. If it does not, it generally responds to an additional treatment with fenbendazole and metronidazole (Chaitman, unpublished observations).

CURRENT RECOMMENDATIONS FOR USE OF FECAL MICROBIOTA TRANSPLANTATION IN DOGS
Patient (Recipient) Selection

Although FMT may help in any patient with diarrhea, a proper diagnostic workup to identify the cause of the problem is recommended, as diarrhea is likely to recur if underlying causes are not addressed. Therefore, parasitic infections, atypical hypo-adrenocorticism, diet-responsive enteropathy, antibiotic-associated diarrhea, and other causes of diarrhea should be identified and appropriately treated before considering FMT. It is not generally recommended to give FMT to patients who are simultaneously receiving antibiotics because it is likely that antibiotics will negatively affect the microbiome and limit the beneficial effects of FMT as was shown in people with CDI.[36] However, based on existing case reports and the authors' experience, FMT can be safely given to dogs with uncontrolled IBD treated with immunosuppressive steroids, chlorambucil and/or cyclosporine. Nevertheless, immune-suppressed patient should receive FMT from carefully screened donors and be monitored carefully after FMT to ensure they do not develop infectious complications.

Donor Dog Selection

In human medicine, fecal donors are subjected to very strict screening procedures aimed at preventing transmission of infections or other diseases and ensuring transplantation of a desirable fecal microbiome and metabolome. Potential donors are screened for dietary habits, recent use of antibiotics, immune-suppressants, chemotherapy drugs, proton pump inhibitors, and for history of chronic diseases including GI diseases, diabetes, obesity, and psychiatric disorders. Candidates with risk behaviors for infections including travel, drug use, etc. are generally unacceptable. A complete blood count, chemistry panel, and protein C concentration are obtained as well as titers for common infectious diseases such as hepatitis viruses and human immunodeficiency virus. Parasitic diseases need to be ruled out as well as the presence of enteric pathogens and MDR bacteria in the feces.[1,37] More details on fecal donor selection can be found in recent medical literature.[1,37]

In canine medicine, screening protocols vary among published studies. The authors propose general screening criteria that donor dogs should meet before to be used (**Box 1**). The goal of these criteria is to ensure that the feces used for FMT will not infect the recipient with known parasites or enteropathogens and that the transplanted microbiome and metabolome are of optimal quality. A comparable but less stringent approach is used by a commercial canine fecal bank that states that they collect feces from "healthy dogs that regularly go outdoors for walks, have not had antibiotic treatment in the prior 6 months, have diverse and species-rich microbiomes, are not over-weight, and have no behavioral issues"; in addition, feces are screened for pathogens and toxins including C difficile toxin B, Cryptosporidium spp, Salmonella spp, Giardia spp, and canine parvovirus 2 (https://www.animalbiome.com/fecal-microbiota-transplant-capsules-aka-poo-pills, last accessed September 2, 2020). Ultimately, the desired depth of screening depends on the personal preference of the veterinarian in charge and could also include intestinal function tests (serum cobalamin and folate concentrations), pancreatic enzymatic immunoassays (pancreatic lipase

> **Box 1**
> **Recommended selection criteria for canine fecal donors**
>
> History and physical examination
> • Preferably between the ages of 1 and 10 years
> • Preferably no travel history outside the local area
> • No health issues in the last 6 or 12 months
> • No history of chronic GI diseases, allergies, and immune-mediated diseases
> • Has not received any antibiotics in the last 12 months
> • Regularly vaccinated according to existing guidelines
> • Fed a balanced diet
> • Not overweight or underweight (9-point body condition score between 4 and 6)
> • Normal fecal consistency
> • Deemed healthy on physical examination
>
> Laboratory screening
> • Normal CBC and serum biochemistry
> • Consider evaluation of basal cortisol, thyroxine
> • Negative for parasite ovas on fecal floatation, consider empirical deworming with a broad-spectrum anthelmintic drug
> • Negative for Giardia oocysts on fecal floatation and ELISA fecal test, see above for empirical deworming
> • Consider testing for fecal pathogens such as *Salmonella* spp., *Campylobacter* spp., etc.
>
> Fecal microbiome evaluation
> • Fecal dysbiosis index[31] less than 0
>
> *Abbreviations:* CBC, complete blood count, ELISA, enzyme-linked immunosorbent assay.

immunoreactivity and trypsin-like immunoreactivity) and endocrine tests (serum cortisol, thyroxine, and thyroid-stimulating hormone concentrations) to more definitely rule out abnormal intestinal function, pancreatitis, exocrine pancreatic insufficiency, hypothyroidism, and atypical hypoadrenocorticism. One of the authors (JC) prefers to feed canine donors a hydrolyzed or limited ingredient diet for several weeks before and during collection.

Preparation and administration of the fecal solution

In human medicine, it is recommended that fresh feces be used within 6 hours after defecation (storage at room temperature is adequate during that time). Storage and preparation should be as brief as possible in order to protect anaerobic bacteria. Fecal material is suspended in saline using a blender or manual effort and sieved in order to avoid the clogging of infusion syringes and tubes. Staff should wear gloves and facial masks while processing feces. If the fecal solution is frozen, glycerol should be added up to a final concentration of 10%. The fecal solution should be stored at −80°C, warmed in a water bath at body temperature, and used within 6 hours of thawing.[1]

A very similar protocol is generally used to prepare fecal solution from canine feces. The methods used by both authors are described in **Table 3**. The quantity of donor feces transplanted into the recipient is derived from human medicine where 20 to 100 g of donor feces are typically used for each FMT procedure.[1,2] Recently, the viability of fecal bacteria was shown to be maintained in homogenized fecal samples for 1 week in a refrigerator (4°C). This suggests that canine feces could be kept refrigerated for more than 6 to 12 hours after defecation and maintain their efficacy for use in FMT. However, after 3 months adequate bacterial viability was maintained only in

Table 3
Authors' protocols for preparation of fecal solution and administration of fecal micrrobiota transplantation to dogs

Author	Fecal Amount	Preparation	Administration	Sedation of Recipient	Post-FMT Care
Chaitman (from Chaitman et al,[30] 2020)	2.5–5 g feces per kg BW recipient	Mix fresh feces with 60 mL 0.9% NaCl in blender. Blend on high until the stool is liquefied and no large pieces are seen. For very large dogs a larger volume of saline may be needed to obtain sufficiently liquefied fecal solution	Rectally via 12–14 French red rubber catheter pushed all the way into the colon	Not necessary in most dogs	Do not feed, restrict activity for 4–6 h post-FMT to decrease risk of defecation
Gaschen (adapted from Kao et al,[2] 2018, unpublished observations)	1–2 g feces per kg BW recipient	Use feces within 6–12 h of defecation. Mix 1 volume feces with 4 volumes of 0.9% NaCl (20% solution) and filter solid material using gauze or other method. If freezing, add glycerol (10 mL per 100 mL final solution) and store at −80C	Rectally via large bore red rubber catheter (5–10 mL solution per kg BW recipient)	Mild sedation is beneficial to keep the recipient calm during and 30 min after the procedure	Same as above

Data from Kao D, Roach B, Silva M, et al. Effect of oral capsule- vs colonoscopy-delivered fecal microbiota transplantation on recurrent clostridium difficile infection: a randomized clinical trial. JAMA. 2017;318(20):1985-1993 and Chaitman J, Ziese AL, Pilla R, et al. Fecal microbial and metabolic profiles in dogs with acute diarrhea receiving either fecal microbiota transplantation or oral metronidazole. Front Vet Sci 2020;7:192.

frozen samples (−20°C and −80°C) with added glycerol (10% of total volume) and after 6 months only in samples stored at −80°C with 10% glycerol.[38]

In human medicine, a recent systematic review identified FMT via colonoscopy and oral capsules as superior to FMT via nasogastric tube and enema for the treatment of CDI.[39] In another study, poor bowel preparation and administration of antibiotics after FMT were associated with poorer outcomes in patients with CDI.[36] However, a randomized clinical trial showed high efficacy of FMT administered as enema without colonic lavage.[40] The same study also demonstrated that both fresh and frozen fecal solution were equally effective.[40] So there is still some debate on the optimal preparation and delivery of FMT in human medicine. There are no corresponding studies for FMT in dogs. The situation could be different because FMT is used in the treatment of canine diseases affecting both small and large intestine. Moreover, enema is a procedure that can easily be applied in veterinary clinical settings and is often preferred because it does not require general anesthesia. Human FMT recipients are requested to remain on their back for approximately 30 minutes after completion of the procedure in order to limit the urge to defecate.[1] For the same reason, one of the authors (FG) prefers to keep canine recipients sedated for approximately 30 minutes after FMT is completed.

OUTLOOK

In human medicine, ongoing investigations are exploring the therapeutic potential of FMT in the treatment of digestive diseases and other conditions associated with intestinal dysbiosis.[5,6,24,25] It is likely that in the near future microbe-based therapies will replace transplantation of the whole fecal microbiome. They may consist of specific combinations of microbes or microbe-derived products.[6]

In canine medicine, there is a need for well-designed studies further investigating the benefits of FMT in dogs with intestinal dysbiosis due to acute and chronic GI diseases and disorders of other organ systems. Ease of administration of fecal products will likely improve in coming years so that repeated treatments will not be as fastidious to plan. The efficacy of lyophilized fecal preparations, some of them already available commercially through animal fecal banks, will need to be investigated. Moreover, it is likely that advancement of knowledge about the value of FMT in human medicine will guide further research in canine medicine as well.

REFERENCES

1. Cammarota G, Ianiro G, Tilg H, et al. European consensus conference on faecal microbiota transplantation in clinical practice. Gut 2017;66(4):569–80.
2. Kao D, Roach B, Silva M, et al. Effect of oral capsule- vs colonoscopy-delivered fecal microbiota transplantation on recurrent Clostridium difficile infection: a randomized clinical trial. JAMA 2017;318(20):1985–93.
3. Zhang F, Cui B, He X, et al. Microbiota transplantation: concept, methodology and strategy for its modernization. Protein Cell 2018;9(5):462–73.
4. Eiseman B, Silen W, Bascom GS, et al. Fecal enema as an adjunct in the treatment of pseudomembranous enterocolitis. Surgery 1958;44(5):854–9.
5. Borody TJ, Eslick GD, Clancy RL. Fecal microbiota transplantation as a new therapy: from Clostridioides difficile infection to inflammatory bowel disease, irritable bowel syndrome, and colon cancer. Curr Opin Pharmacol 2019;49:43–51.
6. D'Haens GR, Jobin C. Fecal microbial transplantation for diseases beyond recurrent Clostridium difficile infection. Gastroenterology 2019;157(3):624–36.

7. Soave O, Brand CD. Coprophagy in animals: a review. Cornell Vet 1991;81(4): 357–64.

8. Hart BL, Hart LA, Thigpen AP, et al. The paradox of canine conspecific coprophagy. Vet Med Sci 2018;4(2):106–14.

9. DePeters EJ GL. Rumen transfaunation. Immunol Letters 2014;G Model IMLET-5525. Immunology Letters 2014;162:69–76.

10. Klein W, Müller R. Das Eiweißminimum, die zymogene Symbiose und die Erzeugung von Mikrobeneiweiß im Pansen aus Stickstoff-verbindungen nicht eiweißartiger Natur. Zeitschrift für Tierzüchtung und Züchtungsbiologie 1941;48(3): 255–76.

11. Chaitman J, Jergens A, Gaschen FP, et al. Commentary on key aspects of fecal microbiota transplantation in small animal practice. Vet Med Res Rep 2016; 7:71–4.

12. Redfern A, Suchodolski J, Jergens A. Role of the gastrointestinal microbiota in small animal health and disease. Vet Rec 2017;181(14):370.

13. Pilla R, Suchodolski JS. The role of the canine gut microbiome and metabolome in health and gastrointestinal disease. Front Vet Sci 2019;6:498.

14. Honneffer JB, Minamoto Y, Suchodolski JS. Microbiota alterations in acute and chronic gastrointestinal inflammation of cats and dogs. World J Gastroenterol 2014;20(44):16489–97.

15. Suchodolski JS, Markel ME, Garcia-Mazcorro JF, et al. The fecal microbiome in dogs with acute diarrhea and idiopathic inflammatory bowel disease. PLoS One 2012;7(12):e51907.

16. Gronvold AM, L'Abee-Lund TM, Sorum H, et al. Changes in fecal microbiota of healthy dogs administered amoxicillin. Fems Microbiol Ecol 2010;71(2):313–26.

17. Manchester AC, Webb CB, Blake AB, et al. Long-term impact of tylosin on fecal microbiota and fecal bile acids of healthy dogs. J Vet Intern Med 2019;33(6): 2605–17.

18. Pilla R, Gaschen FP, Barr JW, et al. Effects of metronidazole on the fecal microbiome and metabolome in healthy dogs. J Vet Intern Med 2020;34:1853–66.

19. Kelly CR, Kahn S, Kashyap P, et al. Update on fecal microbiota transplantation 2015: indications, methodologies, mechanisms, and outlook. Gastroenterology 2015;149(1):223–37.

20. Khoruts A, Sadowsky MJ. Understanding the mechanisms of faecal microbiota transplantation. Nat Rev Gastroenterol Hepatol 2016;13(9):508–16.

21. Guard BC, Honneffer JB, Jergens AE, et al. Longitudinal assessment of microbial dysbiosis, fecal unconjugated bile acid concentrations, and disease activity in dogs with steroid-responsive chronic inflammatory enteropathy. J Vet Intern Med 2019;33(3):1295–305.

22. Quraishi MN, Shaheen W, Oo YH, et al. Immunological mechanisms underpinning faecal microbiota transplantation for the treatment of inflammatory bowel disease. Clin Exp Immunol 2020;199(1):24–38.

23. Zuo T, Wong SH, Lam K, et al. Bacteriophage transfer during faecal microbiota transplantation in Clostridium difficile infection is associated with treatment outcome. Gut 2018;67(4):634–43.

24. Vendrik KEW, Ooijevaar RE, de Jong PRC, et al. Fecal microbiota transplantation in neurological disorders. Front Cell Infect Microbiol 2020;10:98.

25. Zhang Z, Mocanu V, Cai C, et al. Impact of fecal microbiota transplantation on obesity and metabolic syndrome-a systematic review. Nutrients 2019;11(10).

26. Dailey FE, Turse EP, Daglilar E, et al. The dirty aspects of fecal microbiota transplantation: a review of its adverse effects and complications. Curr Opin Pharmacol 2019;49:29–33.

27. DeFilipp Z, Bloom PP, Torres Soto M, et al. Drug-resistant E. coli bacteremia transmitted by fecal microbiota transplant. N Engl J Med 2019;381(21):2043–50.

28. Burton EN, O'Connor E, Ericsson AC, et al. Evaluation of fecal microbiota transfer as treatment for postweaning diarrhea in research-colony puppies. J Am Assoc Lab Anim Sci 2016;55(5):582–7.

29. Pereira GQ, Gomes LA, Santos IS, et al. Fecal microbiota transplantation in puppies with canine parvovirus infection. J Vet Intern Med 2018;32(2):707–11.

30. Chaitman J, Ziese AL, Pilla R, et al. Fecal microbial and metabolic profiles in dogs with acute diarrhea receiving either fecal microbiota transplantation or oral metronidazole. Front Vet Sci 2020;7:192.

31. AlShawaqfeh MK, Wajid B, Minamoto Y, et al. A dysbiosis index to assess microbial changes in fecal samples of dogs with chronic inflammatory enteropathy. Fems Microbiol Ecol 2017;93(11).

32. Bottero E, Benvenuti E, Ruggiero P. Fecal microbiota transplantation (FMT) in 16 dogs with idiopatic IBD. Veterinaria 2017;31(1):31–45.

33. Chaitman J, Guard B, Sarwar F, et al. Fecal microbial transplantation decreases the dysbiosis index in dogs presenting with chronic diarrhea [abstract]. J Vet Intern Med 2017;31(4):1287.

34. Niina A, Kibe R, Suzuki R, et al. Improvement in clinical symptoms and fecal microbiome after fecal microbiota transplantation in a dog with inflammatory bowel disease. Vet Med (Auckl) 2019;10:197–201.

35. Sugita K, Yanuma N, Ohno H, et al. Oral faecal microbiota transplantation for the treatment of Clostridium difficile-associated diarrhoea in a dog: a case report. BMC Vet Res 2019;15(1):11.

36. Tariq R, Saha S, Solanky D, et al. Predictors and management of failed fecal microbiota transplantation for recurrent Clostridioides difficile Infection. J Clin Gastroenterol 2020. https://doi.org/10.1097/MCG.0000000000001398. Published ahead of print.

37. Bibbo S, Settanni CR, Porcari S, et al. Fecal microbiota transplantation: screening and selection to choose the optimal donor. J Clin Med 2020;9(6).

38. Rodriguez E, Khattab MR, Lidbury JA, et al. Bacteria viability in stored canine feces for use in fecal microbiota transplantation. ACVIM Forum 2020.

39. Ramai D, Zakhia K, Fields PJ, et al. Fecal Microbiota Transplantation (FMT) with colonoscopy is superior to enema and nasogastric tube while comparable to capsule for the treatment of recurrent Clostridioides difficile infection: a systematic review and meta-analysis. Dig Dis Sci 2020. https://doi.org/10.1007/s10620-020-06185-7. Published ahead of print.

40. Lee CH, Steiner T, Petrof EO, et al. Frozen vs fresh fecal microbiota transplantation and clinical resolution of diarrhea in patients with recurrent Clostridium difficile Infection: a randomized clinical trial. JAMA 2016;315(2):142–9.

41. Weese JS, Costa MC, Webb JA. Preliminary clinical and microbiome assessment of stool transplantation in the dog and the cat [abstract]. J Vet Intern Med 2013;27(3):604.

42. Murphy T, Chaitman J, Han E. Use of fecal transplant in eight dogs with refractory Clostridium perfringens associated diarrhea [abstract]. J Vet Intern Med 2014;28:976.

43. Burchell RK, Pazzi P, Biggs PJ, et al. Faecal microbial transplantation in a canine model of haemorrhagic diarrhoea syndrome [abstract]. J Vet Intern Med 2019;33: 1026–7.
44. Dwyer EL, Marclay M, Suchodolski J, et al. Effect of fecal microbiota transplantation on the fecal microbiome of healthy dogs treated with antibiotics [abstract]. J Vet Intern Med 2019;33:2467.
45. Gerbec Z. Evaluation of therapeutic potential of restoring gastrointestinal homeostasis by fecal microbiota transplant in dogs. Thesis. Faculty of Pharmacy, University of Ljubljana 2016.

Printed and bound by CPI Group (UK) Ltd, Croydon, CR0 4YY

03/10/2024

01040477-0003